Medical Sociology on the Move

William C. Cockerham
Editor

Medical Sociology on the Move

Revised Edition including New Directions in Theory

Second Edition

Springer

Editor
William C. Cockerham
University of Alabama at Birmingham
Birmingham, AL, USA

ISBN 978-3-031-92455-2 ISBN 978-3-031-92456-9 (eBook)
https://doi.org/10.1007/978-3-031-92456-9

This Springer imprint is published by the registered company Springer Nature Switzerland AG
The registered company address is: Gewerbestrasse 11, 6330 Cham, Switzerland

This book is dedicated to the memory of Kathy Charmaz (1939–2020) and Peter Conrad (1945–2024), both friends and colleagues, who authored chapters published in the first edition of this book. Charmaz was a major figure in symbolic interaction theory in medical sociology, and Conrad formulated the often-cited concept of medicalization, which still influences the work of numerous scholars. In their honor, their chapters in the first edition of this book are reprinted here so the quality of their significant theoretical perspectives can be displayed to new readers.

Contents

Notes on Contributors

Ellen Annandale is Professor of Sociology at the University of York, UK. She has a longstanding interest in feminist and gender theory and the sociology of health. Her book publications include *The Sociology of Health and Medicine* (Polity, 2014) and *Women's Health and Social Change* (Routledge, 2009). Between 2004 and 2012, she was Editor-in-Chief of *Social Science & Medicine*. She is currently Chair of Trustees for the Foundation for the Sociology of Health and Illness.

Linda Liska Belgrave is retired from the Department of Sociology and Criminology at the University of Miami, USA. Her scholarly interests included medical sociology, grounded theory, social psychology, and social justice. She pursued research on the daily lives of African American caregivers of family members living with Alzheimer's disease, the conceptualization of successful aging, academic freedom, and the value of the work of George Herbert Mead for understanding meanings and selves in illness. She also explored the social meanings of infectious disease. She is honored to have worked with Kathy Charmaz.

Claudine Burton-Jeangros is professor at the University of Geneva's Department of Sociology, Switzerland, and is affiliated with the Institute of Sociological Research and the LIVES Swiss Center of Expertise for Life Course Research. She earned her PhD in sociology from the University of Geneva in 2001 and a Master of Sciences in Health Promotion and Health Education from the University of Cardiff in 1994. She is conducting research on health inequalities in a life course perspective and co-edited the book *A Life Course Perspective on Health Trajectories and Transitions* (Springer, 2015). Her research also examines the co-existence of contrasted understandings of public health risks in a range of domains including the prevention of infectious diseases (HIV/AIDS, H1N1, COVID-19) and different forms of screening (prenatal, cancer, genetic), discussed in her book *Experiences of Health Risks: Prevention, Power Dynamics and Inequalities* (Palgrave Macmillan, 2025).

Kathy Charmaz (1939–2020) was Professor of Sociology Emerita and former Director of the Faculty Writing Program at Sonoma State University, USA. She was a leading figure in symbolic interaction theory in medical sociology. Originally trained as an occupational therapist, she was in the first cohort of doctoral students in the Ph.D. program in sociology at the University of California, San Francisco, working with Anselm Strauss and Barney Glaser. She authored 14 books and numerous other publications, which included *Good Days, Bad Days: The Self in Chronic Illness* (Rutgers University Press, 1991) that received the Charles Horton Cooley Award from the Society from the Study of Symbolic Interaction, followed by the Feminist Mentors Award and the George Herbert Mead Award for Lifetime Achievement. She also authored *Constructing Grounded Theory: A Practical Guide Through Qualitative Analysis* (Sage, 2006) that received an award from the American Educational Studies Association. Additionally, she served as President of the Pacific Sociological Association (1990–2000) and the Society for the Study of Symbolic Interaction (2009–2010), as well as Editor of *Symbolic Interaction* (1999–2003).

William C. Cockerham is Distinguished Professor of Sociology and Chair Emeritus at the University of Alabama at Birmingham (UAB) and Research Professor of Sociology at the University of Maryland, College Park, USA. He earned his doctorate from the University of California, Berkeley, and specializes in medical sociology and sociological theory. He is past President (2006–2010) of the Research Committee on Health Sociology of the International Sociological Association and author or editor of 23 books, including Editor-in-Chief of the *Wiley Blackwell Encyclopedia of Health, Illness, Behavior, & Society*, 2nd edition (2025). His most recent books Social Causes of Health and Illness, 4th edition (Polity, 2026); include *Medical Sociology*, 16th edition (Routledge, 2025); *Sociology of Mental Disorder*, 12th edition (Routledge, 2024); *The COVID-19 Reader: The Science and What It Says About the Social* (with Geoffrey Cockerham, Routledge, 2021); and *Sociological Theories of Health and Illness* (Routledge, 2021).

Peter Conrad (1945–2024) was Harry Coplan Professor of Social Sciences at Brandeis University, USA. He received his Ph.D. in sociology from Boston College in 1975 and was on the sociology faculty at Brandeis from 1979 until his death. He was the author of over 120 articles and book chapters and nine books, including the award-winning, *Deviance and Medicalization: From Badness to Sickness* (with Joseph Schneider, Mosby, 1980) and *The Medicalization of Society: On the Transformation of Human Conditions into Treatable Disorders* (Johns Hopkins University Press, 2007). He was President of the Society for the Study of Social Problems (1995–1996). Honors include the Charles Horton Cooley Award (1981) from the Society for the Study of Symbolic Interaction and the Reeder Award (2004) from the American Sociological Association for distinguished contributions to medical sociology.

Brian Hinote serves as Professor of Sociology and Vice Provost for Faculty & Strategic Initiatives at Middle Tennessee State University, USA. Hinote's past research agenda stretches globally from South America to the former Soviet Union to the United States. In addition to clinical and research experience in areas as diverse as pediatrics, neurology, and cell biology, his interdisciplinary work appears in multiple books and peer-reviewed journals in social science, nursing, and medicine. He is co-author of *Social and Behavioral Science for Health Professionals* (Rowman & Littlefield, 2020, with Jason Wasserman) and *Amazon Town TV: An Audience Ethnography in Gurupá, Brazil* (University of Texas Press, 2013). A practitioner of multiple research methods, he serves as affiliated research faculty in the Free Speech Center at MTSU and as a reviewer for more than a dozen academic journals.

Bruce G. Link is Distinguished Professor of Public Policy and Sociology at the University of California, Riverside and Professor Emeritus of Epidemiology and Sociomedical Sciences at Columbia University, USA. Dr. Link received his Ph.D. in Sociology (1980) from Columbia University. He received career awards from the American Sociological Association's Mental Health Section (Pearlin Award 2002) and Medical Sociology (Reeder Award 2007) and the Rema Lapouse Award from the Mental Health Section of the American Public Health Association. He was elected to the US National Academy of Medicine in 2002. His interests are centered on topics in psychiatric and social epidemiology as they bear on policy issues. With Jo Phelan, he has advanced the theory of social conditions as fundamental causes of disease and produced a widely used definition and conceptualization of stigma. His current work focuses on the contribution of relatively more privileged groups to social inequalities in health.

Sigrún Ólafsdóttir is a Professor of Sociology at the University of Iceland. Dr. Ólafsdóttir received her Ph.D. in Sociology (2007) from Indiana University. Her research has appeared in the *American Journal of Sociology*, the *Journal of Health and Social Behavior*, *Social Science & Medicine*, and other journals. Her work has been funded by various agencies, including the US National Institutes of Health, the Icelandic Centre for Research, and Nordforsk. She served as the Editor of *Acta Sociologica* (2018–2022) and leads Iceland's participation in several international surveys, including the International Social Survey Program (ISSP). Her research lies at the intersection of medical, political, and cultural sociology. In her work, she examines the impact of broader institutional factors, such as the welfare state and/or the health care system on individual outcomes. For example, she has focused on health inequalities in a cross-national perspective, stigma toward mental health, and social attitudes toward health systems.

Bernice Pescosolido is Distinguished Professor of Sociology at Indiana University and Founding Director of both the Indiana Consortium for Mental Health Services Research and the Irsay Institute for Sociomedical Sciences, USA. She is an elected member of the National Academy of Medicine and the National Academy of

Sciences. Trained as a medical sociologist at Yale University, her research focuses on connectedness and suicide, the stigma of mental illness and addiction, international issues in health and health care, and social networked pathways to treatment. She co-edited the volumes *Personal Networks: Classic Readings and New Directions in Egocentric Analysis* (Cambridge University Press, 2021) and *The Sociology of Health, Illness, and Healing: Blueprint for the 21st Century* (Springer, 2011).

Jo Phelan is Emerita Professor of Sociomedical Sciences at Columbia University's Mailman School of Public Health, USA. She received the Best Publication Award (with Carol Aneshensel) and the Leonard I. Pearlin Award for Distinguished Contributions to the Sociological Study of Mental Health from the American Sociological Association's Section on the Sociology of Mental Health and the James R. Greenley Award for Distinguished Contributions to the Sociology of Mental Health from the Society for the Study of Social Problems Division of Mental Health. Dr. Phelan is perhaps best known for her collaboration with Bruce Link in developing "fundamental cause" theory, which attempts to explain the persistent connection between social conditions such as socioeconomic status and favorable health outcomes. She has also studied stigma and discrimination associated with mental illness, obesity, homelessness, socioeconomic status, and race. She has also been concerned with the role of the genomic revolution in stigma and discrimination.

Graham Scambler is Emeritus Professor of Sociology at University College London and a Fellow of the Academy of Social Sciences, UK. He has been a visiting professor at Emory University in the USA and an honorary professor at Surrey University, UK. He is the author of many books, chapters, and articles, principally on social theory, health, and sport. He was editor of the pioneering textbook for British medical students, *Sociology as Applied to Medicine*, which went into seven editions. He co-founded the international journal *Social Theory & Health* in 2003. His book *Sociology, Health and the Fractured Society* (Routledge, 2018) won the 2018 Cheryl Frank Memorial Prize for the best book on critical realism. His latest book is *Healthy Societies*, published by Policy Press in 2024. He continues to be active in academia in retirement.

Sasha Scambler is Professor of Medical Sociology and Dean for People and Culture in the Faculty of Dentistry, Oral and Craniofacial Sciences at King's College London, UK. Sasha is a member of the International Association for Disability and Oral Health Scientific Advisory Group and a contributing editor of the British Sociological Association (BSA) affiliated "Cost of Living Blog." She was previously Editor of the *Sociology of Health & Illness* and Chair of the British Sociological Association Medical Sociology Group. Her research focuses on the experiences of people living with long-term conditions and disability, inequality and the application of social theory to empirical research and she has published widely in these areas.

Jason Adam Wasserman is Dean's Distinguished Professor of Foundational Medical Studies and Pediatrics at Oakland University William Beaumont School of Medicine, USA, the Founding Director of the Center for Moral Values in Health and Medicine, and he leads the Holocaust and Medicine program. He co-authored the book *Social and Behavioral Science for Health Professionals* with Brian Hinote (Rowman and Littlefield, 2020) and has published numerous articles in journals including *Social Science and Medicine*, *Pediatrics, JAMA-Pediatrics, American Journal of Bioethics, Hastings Center Report, Mayo Clinic Proceedings*, and *The New England Journal of Medicine.*

Chapter 1
The Rise of Theory in Medical Sociology

William C. Cockerham

The purpose of this book is to provide readers with a single source reviewing and updating developments in theories commonly used today in medical or health sociology. The first edition originated in papers and discussions in a session on new developments in theory in medical sociology at the International Sociological Association's 2010 World Congress of Sociology held in Gothenburg, Sweden. The session was scheduled because theoretical work had increasingly become a major feature of medical sociology. Much of the work was atheoretical when the field first appeared as a new sociological specialty in the mid-twentieth century. Over time, this situation changed dramatically, and this book's task was to not only discuss the major theoretical approaches that had emerged but also to identify new directions in theory in medical sociology. This second edition continues this theme.

Three of the chapters are contributed by the original theorists—Bruce Link and Jo Phelan on fundamental cause theory, the late Peter Conrad on medicalization, and William Cockerham on health lifestyle theory—and the other chapters are all written by selected senior scholars (the late Kathy Charmaz, Linda Liska Belgrave, Bryan Turner, Graham Scambler, Ellen Annandale, and Bernice Pescosolido) and the next generation of medical sociologists (Sigrun Olafsdottir, Sasha Scambler, Brian Hinote, Jason Wasserman, and Claudine Burton-Jeangros) with special expertise in theory.

Theory is critically important to every academic discipline because it conceptualizes how sets of phenomena or particular phenomena work in the empirical world. As Karl Popper pointed out several decades ago in *The Logic of Scientific Discovery* (1934/1992, p. 59), theories are "nets" that allow us to catch what we call the world in order to understand and explain it, and we endeavor to make the net's mesh ever

W. C. Cockerham (✉)
University of Alabama at Birmingham, Birmingham, AL, USA

University of Maryland, College Park, MD, USA
e-mail: wcocker@uab.edu

W. C. Cockerham (ed.), *Medical Sociology on the Move*,
https://doi.org/10.1007/978-3-031-92456-9_1

finer and finer. Theories in sociology provide definitions and sets of propositions explaining some facet or facets of social reality. Usually, these propositions are testable, so the validity of the theory can be either confirmed, modified, or rejected. Over time, theories are discarded as social conditions change or better theories emerge; consequently, theoretical work is continually ongoing and evolving. Many techniques developed by sociologists have been adopted by other disciplines, including both quantitative and qualitative research methodologies, such as social surveys and participant observation. However, sociological theory remains *the* most important pillar of medical sociology's uniqueness in studies of health and disease.

It is the sociological perspective, as exemplified by its theoretical gaze, which gives medical sociology its distinctiveness in comparison to research in public health, health psychology, medical anthropology, health services research, and behavioral medicine. Therefore, one of the most important developments in medical sociology since the 1950s is the increased use of sociological theory to provide explanatory models of the social processes affecting health and disease. In fact, medical sociology now has a robust theoretical literature of its own, and the use of theory is now a significant strength of the field, as demonstrated by the chapters in this book.

In the beginning, as noted, medical sociology was largely atheoretical. This is understandable, given that its origins in the early twentieth century were in medicine, not sociology (see Cockerham, 2021). The field did not emerge more fully until after World War II when Western governments sought to improve the lives of the populations in their respective countries. One strategy was to address the social conditions associated with poor health through sociological research that could be applied to health-related policies and improving medical care (Bloom, 2002; Cockerham & Scambler, 2021). This meant funding, research opportunities, and jobs for sociologists on topics that paired work in their specialty with research in public health and medicine. At this time, some people working in medical sociology had little or no formal sociological training and switched to the new specialty because of the employment opportunities (Claus, 1983). The questions they researched tended to be more relevant for medical practice than sociology, and the new specialty began to develop largely outside of mainstream sociology until several practitioners petitioned the American Sociological Society for section sponsorship in 1959 (Bloom, 2002).

While contributing to medical practice and health policy is an essential role of medical sociology, a lack of theoretical insight undermined the capability of medical sociologists to make systematic analyses and conclusions. A theoretical base was needed for medical sociology to fully establish itself as a scientific subdiscipline. Karl Marx, Emile Durkheim, and Max Weber—the three most noted classical theorists in sociology—did incorporate notions of health and disease into some of their writings that are still cited in medical sociology (Collyer, 2010). However, they "did not formulate sociological theories of health and medicine, nor recognize medical sociology as a potential field of sociological inquiry, deliberately promote it, organize it, give it a name, or provide evidence they were even aware of it" (Cockerham, 2021, pp. 36–37). A theoretical grounding for medical sociology was missing at the mid-point of the twentieth century. An exception was a 1935 paper published in the *New England Journal of Medicine* by Lawrence Henderson, a physician teaching sociology at Harvard College. Henderson's paper, "Physician and Patient as a Social System," advanced a theory that social relationships constituted systems of mutual dependence in which all parties were interconnected. His example was the doctor-patient relationship. Talcott Parsons (1951, p. 428) was one of his students and referred to Henderson's paper for a general comparison with his concept of the sick role.

Parsons' Sick Role

The catalyst for the development of theory in medical sociology was the publication of Talcott Parsons' *The Social System* in 1951. Within its pages (pp. 428–479) was his concept of the sick role, the first theoretical statement directly applicable to medical sociology. The propositions he listed about the roles and norms associated with being sick still have some relevance in certain types of doctor-patient interaction (i.e., doctors' offices), along with Parsons' notion of a social imperative existing for patients to *try* to get well. Parsons was a world figure in sociology, and anything he published at the time attracted considerable attention from the global sociological community. His book *The Social System* had a wide readership because he intended to provide the ultimate theory about how large social systems worked based upon the then-popular structural-functionalist perspective.

As we know now, Parsons was unsuccessful in providing the definitive theory of society, and structural-functionalism is no longer an active theory. In fact, one of Parsons' most lasting contributions may have been to call attention to medical sociology as a fertile theoretical field. At the time, during the 1950s and 1960s, when medical sociology was established as an academic specialty in the United States, the structural-functionalist perspective advocated by Emile Durkheim and Parsons was the dominant theory in all of sociology. Parsons demonstrated that the topic of sickness could be embraced by mainstream sociology. More than any other sociologist of his generation, Parsons made medical sociology academically attractive by providing its inaugural theoretical orientation and calling attention to its potential for developing sociological theory (Cockerham, 2021).

As for structural-functionalism, no one today refers to themselves as a structural-functionalist, and the perspective joins another major twentieth-century theory, conflict theory, in the category of what George Ritzer and William Yagatich (2012, p. 105) describe as "zombie theories." Zombie theories are theories that may seem alive to some supporters, but they are actually either dead or "at least in the process of dying while moving toward a zombie-like state" (Ritzer & Yagatich, 2012, p. 105). Conflict, of course, is ongoing in the social world and the topic remains important, yet finding conflict in social situations does not make one a conflict theorist in their view. The theory sparked opposition because, like structural-functionalism, it accorded the individual little opportunity for creativity. Additionally, it was never fully developed and was severely criticized for ignoring social order and stability, just as it had earlier attacked structural-functionalism's failure to account for conflict and change (Ritzer & Stepnisky, 2021). Once structural-functionalism largely disappeared, conflict theory's value as an alternative faltered, leading Ritzer and Yagatich (2012) to rank it in the zombie category. Moreover, conflict theory never evolved as a leading theory in medical sociology. It gained even less of a foothold than structural-functionalism, which could at least point to the significance of Parsons' (1951) concept of the sick role.

Among the once so-called "big three" sociological theories—structural-functionalism, conflict theory, and symbolic interaction—that dominated all of sociology, including medical sociology in the 1960s, symbolic interaction has survived the best, although Ritzer and Yagatich suggest it might be on life support. Oddly, they note that these three theories are still featured in many introductory sociology textbooks today, even though they are no longer prominent.

Agency Theories: Symbolic Interaction and Social Construction

Symbolic Interaction

Symbolic interaction emerged in the 1960s as the leading agency-oriented theoretical paradigm. Agency is a term referring to the capacity of the individual to select their behavior freely. The primacy of agency is embedded in the core of the symbolic interactionist perspective whose popularity signaled the beginning of the end of the dominance of structural-functionalism in sociological theorizing.

Symbolic interaction was expressly concerned with understanding the individual's stream of consciousness, internal self-conversations, the development of the individual's self-concept in relation to social experiences with other people, self-definitions of social situations, and the merging of individual behavior into collective expressions of joint or group activities (Blumer, 1969; Mead, 1934). While it stressed the distinctly social character of everyday group life, the initial focus was deeply lodged in the socialization of individuals and how they came to recognize and adopt as their own the social perspectives of their significant others, groups, communities, and societies (Mead, 1934). Thus, the starting point for symbolic interactionist theorizing invariably begins with how self-awareness and agency emerge in the individual through social experience.

Symbolic interaction flourished in 1963–1970 and brought with it a corresponding increase in the influence of agency in sociology generally. By the 1980s, however, symbolic interaction entered a period of decline that extended to its use in medical sociology. Labeling theory, a major variant of symbolic interaction, likewise came under criticism. Despite its merits in accounting for the powerful and often lasting effects of social "labels" (e.g., HIV-infected, ex-mental patient, ex-convict) placed by others on individuals and affecting the way they are treated, labeling theory could not explain the causes of deviance (other than the reactions of other people), nor whether deviants themselves shared common characteristics like poverty, stress, or social backgrounds relevant to their deviance. Moreover, as pointed out by Norman Denzin (1992), a major figure in symbolic interaction at the time, the larger body of theory represented by symbolic interaction generally seemed to have reached its limits and taken on the image of a "fixed doctrine." The theory seemed to have gone as far as it could, and no new developments were forthcoming. Furthermore, symbolic interaction suffered from a methodological handicap in that studies using the perspective employed qualitative methodologies (e.g., participant observation, focus groups), and most research in American sociology was generally quantitative and based on statistical analyses of survey data.

Even though less influential than in the past, symbolic interaction continued in the late twentieth century, with some interactionists moving into postmodern theory and others into the study of emotions and social constructionism. Postmodern theory, despite its early promise of explaining contemporary social change, was unable to account for the social conditions and structures following the transition from modernity to postmodernity and never gained a foothold in medical sociology (Cockerham, 2007). In contrast, research on the sociology of emotions has increased as interactionism fills an analytic gap between biological approaches and nonbiological social theories like social constructionism.

To investigate whether symbolic interaction is indeed headed toward "zombie" status in health or medical sociology, Chap. 2, reprinted from the first edition, examines modern symbolic interaction theory and its application to health. Written by Kathy Charmaz and Linda Liska Belgrave, the chapter begins with a brief review of the central tenets of symbolic interaction, followed by a discussion of how the theory is used to account for the lived experience of illness and aging, before examining ways in which it can be applied beyond the micro or small group level that could give the perspective a longer life. Charmaz and Belgrave observe that contrary to some of its critics, there are new developments in symbolic interaction theory.

Social Construction

An important legacy of symbolic interaction is its influence on social construction theory, often called social constructionism. As Bryan Turner (2004) noted, the classic text of social constructionism is Peter Berger and Thomas Luckmann's *Social Construction of Reality* (1967), which is solidly grounded in the symbolic interactionist perspective. Other works are also important, such as Eliot Freidson's (1970a, b) analysis of medical knowledge in his study of the American medical profession and the views of the French theorist Michel Foucault (1979) depicting the social control of the body as a product or outcome of power and knowledge utilized by dominant groups such as the state, church, and medical profession.

Social constructionism is a dominant theoretical perspective in the UK, although its use has been much slower to expand in the US. It does not have a uniform doctrine and is divided into branches. One major branch, reflecting its symbolic interaction roots, is influenced by Berger and Luckmann (1967) and strongly emphasizes agency. Another branch virtually ignores agency and is influenced by the work of Foucault (1979) emphasizing the tight relationship between knowledge and power. These different types of constructionism present differing versions of agency and thus have different implications for understanding the relationship between health and disease (Turner, 2004, p. 43). Nevertheless, social constructionism as a whole does have some unity in that its various practitioners agree that scientific knowledge and biological discourses about the body, health, and illness are produced by subjective, historically determined human interests and are therefore subject to change and reinterpretation (Gabe et al., 2004, p. 130). A diagnosis, for example, represents the transformation of physiological symptoms into socially appropriate behavior for the person who has been diagnosed and carries a changed social status with it.

While doctrinal uniformity is lacking, there are other difficulties, such as sometimes failing to acknowledge the biological realities of specific illness scenarios, rejecting the possibility that knowledge can be discovered (by insisting that knowledge can only be socially constructed), and adopting a relativist position that no one form of knowledge is more valid than another which calls the validity of all theories into question, including social construction (Gabe et al., 2004; Turner, 2004). Nevertheless, social constructionism remains popular in studies of the body, the use of genetic information and other medical knowledge, women's health, patient-physician interaction, physical disability, aging, and other topics.

Chapter 3 in this book, by Sigrún Ólafsdóttir, provides a update on social constructionism and its merits for medical sociology. Following the Berger and Luckmann path, she employs a cross-national perspective to determine its value. Ólafsdóttir concludes that it is an important perspective for understanding cultural influences on the meanings of illness, distinctions between normal and abnormal, ways in which illness responses are embedded in the community, and how social factors impact medical knowledge. She then discusses the strengths and weaknesses of this approach. She considers future directions, noting how health and illness are simultaneously impacted by biological realities, cultural traditions, historical patterns, and institutional arrangements.

Fundamental Cause, Gender, Health Lifestyle, and Life Course Theories

There is increasing evidence of the capability of social factors to cause health and disease, with theories in medical sociology emerging that explain the social processes and conditions involved. The basic thesis is that such factors are not just background or secondary variables when it comes to causation but have *direct* causal effects on physical health and longevity. This relatively recent development requires a paradigm shift from an emphasis on studying individual attitudes and behaviors regarding health to a more balanced conceptual approach that includes a renewed focus on structural effects. Variables beyond the level of individuals and small groups in determining health outcomes are required because people can find their health and longevity directly influenced—either positively or negatively—by social structures. Therefore, a comprehensive understanding of health and disease is impossible without considering the role of macro-level social structures.

Fundamental Cause Theory

The seminal work on the role of social factors in disease causation in medical sociology is that of Bruce Link and Jo Phelan who are co-authors of Chap. 4. Link and Phelan (1995) maintain that social conditions are *fundamental* causes of disease when social variables (1) influence multiple diseases, (2) affect these diseases through multiple pathways of risk, (3) are reproduced over time, and (4) involve access to resources that can be used to avoid the disease or minimize the consequences if it occurs. In addition to stratification variables such as class, race, and gender, stressful life events and stress-process variables like social support qualify as social factors in their view. Also included is a sense of control over one's life because people with such control typically feel good about themselves, cope with stress better, and have the capability and living situations to adopt healthy lifestyles. This situation applies especially to people in powerful social positions than persons at the bottom of society who are less able to control their lives, have fewer resources to cope with stress, live in more unhealthy circumstances, confront powerful constraints in adopting a healthy way of life, and die earlier. In this chapter, Link and Phelan refine and update their influential fundamental cause theory. Noteworthy is the addition of racism as a fundamental cause of poor health.

Gender Theories

Chapter 5, on gender theories and health by Ellen Annandale, reviews the feminist origins of research on gender and health, the theoretical approaches currently employed, subsequent critical transformations, and a critique of the current state of gender theory. She then considers the development of new directions in research on gender and health as gender binary and cisgendered approaches have emerged and researchers have investigated the increasingly complex realities of gender on various health issues. The final part of the chapter observes the growing utilization of intersectionality theory in health-related gender studies. Intersectionality theory focuses on the intersection of race, gender, sexuality, and class, and the ways in which these variables simultaneously interact to disadvantage marginalized groups.

Health Lifestyle Theory

William Cockerham provides an updated version of his health lifestyle theory in Chap. 6. Drawing initially on the early twentieth-century work of Max Weber, the theory adopts Pierre Bourdieu's (1984) emphasis on class distinctions, and his concept of habitus is accorded a major role. The decisive role of social structures in determining health lifestyles is stressed. This is because lifestyles tend to cluster in particular patterns reflecting distinct differences by class, age, gender, and other structural variables. The argument here is that health lifestyles are shaped from the top down by structural influences that influence people to adopt them as their own. In this scenario, structure channels health and other lifestyle practices down particular pathways. People still have the option to choose and exercise agency, but generally do so along class lines and in accordance with other structural influences that might be situationally relevant. Consequently, lifestyles are not the random behaviors of socially disconnected individuals. Instead, they have an aggregate form characteristic of particular groups and social classes in which individuals hold membership. This chapter updates health lifestyle theory by adding health-protective lifestyle practices for infectious diseases seen in epidemics and pandemics, along with connectivities (electronic networks) as a structural computational authority influencing health lifestyles through health apps and other digital resources.

Life Course Theory

In Chap. 7, Claudine Burton-Jeangros discusses how life course theory, which joins fundamental cause theory as one of the two most popular theories currently in medical sociology, contributes to studies of health and medical sociology. She summarizes the perspective by noting its emphasis on the lifelong development of individuals that maintains early life circumstances are significant, as well as later conditions, throughout the life course. The timing of transitions in one's life, whether expected or unexpected, and the context within they occur are also important. Since individuals co-exist within social networks and do not go through their lives alone or detached from others, their life trajectories can be importantly affected by the persons with whom they live, as seen the notion of "linked lives." As for the core sociological question of the relative influence of structure and agency, attention is given to agency and the capacities of individuals to shape their own trajectories amidst social structural constraints.

After introducing the life course perspective, Burton-Jeangros examines (1) mechanisms related to changes in social positions throughout the life course; (2) interactions across life domains, including the relationships between work, family and health trajectories; (3) the importance for health of social locations and social identities from an intersectionality perspective; (4) the integration of a life course perspective from the institutional perspective on health inequalities; and (5) the importance of social meanings attached to health and illness as a measure of agency.

The Medical Profession and Medicalization

Another area of study in medical sociology is the evolution of the medical profession from a position of extraordinary professional dominance and control over their work at the mid-twentieth century to a profession whose status and power have somewhat eroded at this time in history. In Chap. 8, Bernice Pescosolido examines the rise and fall of the medical profession and the theories that explain its upward and downward movement. She discusses the mechanisms causing the change and poses key questions about the future.

This chapter is followed by Chap. 9, in which Peter Conrad reviewed and updated his concept of medicalization for the first edition of this book. In it, Conrad wrote about the factors he considered in formulating his thoughts about medicalization and explained why his concept turned out the way it did. Medicalization occurs when problems previously considered to be non-medical, such as hyperactivity, obesity, male baldness, and short stature, are defined, assimilated, and treated by the medical profession as medical problems. As trends toward medicalization continue in society and medicine expands its jurisdiction over the mind and body, Conrad's medicalization perspective remains important in medical sociology.

A New Look at Marx and Critical Realism

Chapter 10 by Graham and Sasha Scambler is based largely on the work of Marx, but in a novel approach, they combine Marx with critical realism. In doing so, they suggest a provisional post-Marxist perspective of health inequalities grounded on critical realism. The critical realism perspective in sociology has been advanced by Margaret Archer (1995) and is based on the work of British social philosopher Roy Bhaskar (1998) who trained as a sociologist. Critical realism highlights the openness of social systems to process and change. People are depicted as agents with the critical capacity, reflexivity, and creativity to shape social structures, yet, in turn, are shaped by structure. But the key feature for the critical realist is the capability of the individual to transform these structures and produce variable outcomes. That is, individuals are able to withstand or strategically circumvent structure, thereby minimizing its effects. Structure, for its part, is relatively enduring, although it can be modified, and deep structures have generative mechanisms going beyond the superficially observable that influence behavior. In this theoretical context, Scambler and Scambler use Marxist views on the contradictions of capitalism and the need for policy reform to theorize ways to reduce health disparities with a focus on the UK.

Reflexive Modernity

This book also includes Chap. 11 by Jason Wasserman and Brian Hinote utilizing the work of German sociologist Ulrich Beck on reflexive modernity to examine the social transformation of medicine. They suggest that discussions of the challenges facing contemporary medicine reflect an idiosyncratic vision of how the field is changing. Beck's conceptualization of reflexive modernization is used to organize and analyze critical developments in contemporary medicine in ways that allow them to connect changes in medicine in a more comprehensive fashion. These changes, in their view, appear to signal the end of modern medicine and the beginning of a new medical era defined by unprecedented complexity and, in some instances, uncertainty. For its part, medical sociology must effectively articulate and theorize the changing nature of health, illness, and health care delivery in which sociological variables play an increasingly important role.

Conclusion

Theory binds medical sociology to the larger discipline of sociology more extensively than any other aspect of sociological work. Theory is also what usually distinguishes research in medical sociology from socially-oriented studies in allied fields, like public health and health services research and allows it to remain unique among the health-related social and behavioral sciences. This could be considered a somewhat surprising statement because medical sociology has often been described in the past as atheoretical. It is true that much of the work in the field historically has been applied to practical problems rather than theoretical questions, but this situation has changed dramatically. The use of sociological theory is now widespread. There has been a general evolution of work in medical sociology that combines both applied and theoretical perspectives, with the utilization of theory an increasingly common framework for explaining or predicting health-related social behavior. This book represents an effort to capture some of the best current theoretical thinking in medical sociology.

References

Archer, M. (1995). *Realist social theory: The morphogenetic approach*. Cambridge University Press.
Berger, P. L., & Luckmann, T. (1967). *The social construction of reality*. Anchor.
Bhaskar, R. (1998). *The possibility of naturalism: A philosophical critique of the contemporary human sciences*. Routledge.
Bloom, S. W. (2002). *The word as scalpel: A history of medical sociology*. Oxford University Press.
Blumer, H. (1969). *Symbolic interaction*. Prentice-Hall.

Bourdieu, P. (1984). *Distinction: A social critique of the judgement of taste*. Harvard University Press.

Claus, L. (1983). *The growth of a sociological discipline: The development of medical sociology in Europe* (Vol. II). Katholieke Universiteit.

Cockerham, W. C. (2007). A note on the fate of postmodern theory and its failure to meet the basic requirements for success in medical sociology. *Social Theory and Health, 8*, 285–296.

Cockerham, W. C. (2021). *Sociological theories of health and illness*. Routledge.

Cockerham, W. C., & Scambler, G. (2021). Medical sociology and sociological theory. In W. Cockerham (Ed.), *The new Blackwell companion to medical sociology* (pp. 22–42). Wiley Blackwell.

Collyer, F. (2010). Origins and canons: Medicine and the history of sociology. *History of the Human Sciences, 23*, 86–108.

Denzin, N. K. (1992). *Symbolic interactionism and cultural studies*. Blackwell.

Foucault, M. (1979). *History of sexuality*. Allen Lane.

Freidson, E. (1970a). *Professional medicine: A study of the sociology of applied knowledge*. Dodd, Mead.

Freidson, E. (1970b). *Professional dominance*. Aldine.

Gabe, J., Bury, M., & Elston, M. A. (2004). *Key concepts in medical sociology*. Sage.

Henderson, L. J. (1935). Physician and patient as a social system. *New England Journal of Medicine, 212*, 819–823.

Link, B. G., & Phelan, C. J. (1995). Social conditions as fundamental causes of disease. *Journal of Health and Social Behavior* (extra issue), 80–94.

Mead, G. H. (1934). *Mind, self, and society*. University of Chicago Press.

Parsons, T. (1951). *The social system*. Free Press.

Popper, K. (1934/1992). *The logic of scientific discovery*. Routledge.

Ritzer, G., & Stepnisky, J. (2021). *Sociological theory* (11th ed.). Sage.

Ritzer, G., & Yagatich, W. (2012). Contemporary sociological theory. In G. Ritzer (Ed.), *The Wiley-Blackwell companion to medical sociology* (pp. 98–118). Wiley-Blackwell.

Turner, B. S. (2004). *The new medical sociology: Social forms of health and illness*. Norton.

Chapter 2
Modern Symbolic Interaction Theory and Health

Kathy Charmaz and Linda Liska Belgrave

As sociologists we know that people are connected both to and through society. Individuals share much in the way of values and understandings of the world and their actions generally appear to be coordinated—yet human actors are more than well-socialized cogs in a machine. The symbolic interactionist perspective helps us understand relationships between the individual and the larger society as dynamic. This theoretical perspective views concepts of self, social situations, and society as accomplished through people's actions and interactions. Through its concepts and guiding assumptions, symbolic interactionism fosters theoretically driven research with implications for medical sociology, which we address here.

In this chapter, we show how symbolic interactionism has informed theorizing in medical sociology—and beyond.[1] Symbolic interactionism is one of the least understood and most misrepresented theoretical perspectives. Hence, we include a short statement of the perspective before addressing the manner in which it informs conceptualizing the experience of illness, an area in which symbolic interactionism has

EDITOR'S NOTE: This chapter is reprinted from the first edition in honor of the late Kathy Charmaz to whom this book is co-dedicated.

[1] We have selected several main ideas to discuss how the symbolic interactionist perspective influences theorizing in medical sociology but have not detailed its significance in areas such as stigma and social constructionism as other chapters in this volume cover these topics. We realize that the influence of symbolic interactionism in medical sociology extends far beyond the boundaries of this chapter and the borders of North America and Northern Europe although many of the ideas we discuss emanate from these regions.

K. Charmaz
Sonoma State University, Rohnert Park, CA, USA

L. L. Belgrave (✉)
University of Miami, Coral Gables, FL, USA

W. C. Cockerham (ed.), *Medical Sociology on the Move*,
https://doi.org/10.1007/978-3-031-92456-9_2

played a significant role. Medical sociologists working from a micro-symbolic interactionist perspective have created inductive concepts: including biographical disruption, loss of self, and the moral status of suffering. Such concepts illustrate the form, content, and direction of theorizing the illness experience and provide fertile ground for other researchers to develop and refine. Symbolic interactionism offers a way of looking at experience which our discussion of embodiment illustrates. We also show how medical sociologists have taken up micro approaches to study health and illness in the field of aging. Micro symbolic interactionist research can produce knowledge of meso level phenomena, particularly at the organizational level, as evident in past knowledge and present conceptions of the negotiated order and social worlds. Because many symbolic interactionists have relied on grounded theory[2] methods to guide inquiry, we conclude with a brief discussion of symbolic interaction and grounded theory as a theory-methods package (Clarke, 2005; Clarke & Fujimura, 1992; Clarke & Star, 2008).

Symbolic interactionist theorizing in health and illness occurs within and beyond medical sociology. As our reference list attests, many relevant symbolic interactionist contributions appear in other places than medical sociology journals. Boundaries blur between symbolic interactionist research in medical sociology and general qualitative inductive research. Thus, symbolic interactionists in medical sociology have developed concepts that have informed other subfields, disciplines, and professions and, in some cases, have been further developed in them. Establishing distinct lines of theoretical development in medical sociology also poses problems. Medical sociology draws on and speaks to multiple, related theoretical perspectives, including symbolic interactionism (e.g. Crossley, 2004; Haworth-Hoeppner & Maines, 2005), phenomenology (e.g. Brown et al., 2011; Haddow, 2005), social constructionism/medicalization (e.g. Carter, 2010; Faircloth et al. 2004a; Nettleton et al., 2008), and feminist theory (e.g. Parry, 2006) and researchers frequently draw on more than one tradition. Depending on the publication outlet and the author's orientation, the theoretical framework of a particular work might not be mentioned, much less discussed. For that matter, an author's background in medical sociology may not be apparent since medical sociologists work in varied settings and scholars from other fields have adopted symbolic interactionism to study health and illness. Multiple, overlapping, theoretical and disciplinary perspectives are mutually enriching and, frankly, sometimes inseparable. Medical sociologists use such perspectives to examine empirical problems ranging from health behavior (whether or not conceived of as such) to the experience of illness and the practice of health care services. Thus, we take an inclusive but not exhaustive approach here.

[2]Grounded theory methods consist of a set of systematic strategies for conducting qualitative research. These methods begin with inductive data that the researcher codes, analyzes, and checks to construct an abstract theoretical analysis. Grounded theory methods were designed to construct middle-range theories of empirical problems. Relatively few researchers use all grounded theory strategies and perhaps fewer have constructed theories. These methods can, however, be used to sharpen qualitative analyses and have been widely adopted. For explication of the logic and practice of using grounded theory methods see Charmaz (2006, 2008a).

Those symbolic interactionists whose studies distinctly reside within medical sociology typically direct their studies toward sociological rather than medical questions. Yet William Cockerham (2012) has rightly pointed out that the lines between a sociology *of* medicine and sociology *in* medicine overlap. Symbolic interactionists have, however, had a long history of starting research from the standpoint of sociology of medicine, although their analyses increasingly inform health professionals and patients, clients, and caregivers.

Medical sociologists from the symbolic interactionist tradition have continued, joined, and sometimes led lines of analysis in a variety of other areas within and beyond the discipline such as aging, emotions, organizations, social movements, inequality, and social studies of science, as well as having been major contributors to the development of qualitative inquiry. These medical sociologists have done more than apply a theoretical perspective originating in other disciplines or subfields. Rather, their concepts travel to other fields, although their theoretical roots in symbolic interactionism may not always be recognized.

The Symbolic Interactionist Perspective

Symbolic interactionism offers an abstract theoretical framework for viewing social realities rather than a definitive explanatory theory that specifies variables and predicts outcomes. This perspective assumes that society and collective life precede the individual and form contexts for action and interpretation. Most social scientists learn about the symbolic interactionist perspective through Blumer (1969). All that many scholars know about symbolic interactionism is Blumer's analysis of interpretation, which early critics often mistook as having an astructural bias. Symbolic interactionists do not deny the existence of social structures but argue that people construct and reproduce them. Social interaction is crucial. As Blumer (1969, p. 8) stresses, social interaction *forms* human conduct instead of being merely a means of expressing or releasing it. Interaction relies on spoken and unspoken shared language, symbols, and meanings. Hence, interaction occurs within social, cultural, and historical contexts that shape but do not determine it.

Symbolic interactionism assumes a reciprocal relationship between interpretation and action—each informs the other. In Mead's (1934) view, subjective meanings emerge from grappling with experienced interactions, are given form through language, and change when subjective or collective experience prompts reassessment. Thus, social interaction is dynamic and somewhat open-ended. Symbolic interactionists start from the assumption that human life consists of *process* and *change* rather than stability and continuity. Yet structure and process intrinsically implicate each other in a dynamic process.

Mead (1934) theorized that language is pivotal for the development of self and the conduct of social life. For Mead, self and mind develop simultaneously and depend on learning the language and symbolic meanings of one's community. Thus, consciousness is inextricably linked to possessing a self which allows us to converse with ourselves. As a result, we can act toward ourselves as we act toward others.

Symbolic interactionists distinguish between several seemingly similar concepts, such as self, self-image, self-concept, and identity. Self-images rely on our use of language to understand, categorize, and deal with experience, whether or not someone else is physically present. Self–images include fleeting reflections given in experience as noted and interpreted by the individual. Symbolic interactionists view self as an unfolding process in contrast to the self-concept. As Turner (1976) outlines, the self-concept consists of relatively stable, organized attributes, values, and judgments through which a person defines him or herself. If so, a self-concept has boundaries, content, and limits—and evaluations. Self-concepts are not neutral (Charmaz, 1991). Symbolic interactionists devote much theoretical energy to these concepts because they so strongly influence action. Selves experience, suffer, and create meaning and they act.

Medical sociologists, particularly those following Erving Goffman (1959, 1961, 1963), have studied individuals' social identities and thus have attended to such concerns as creditable and discreditable identities, stigma potential, and the courtesy stigmas awarded to those closest to a stigmatized individual. Other people confer social identities on individuals and groups based on their social locations, cultural meanings, and group affiliations (Hewitt, 2000). Typically social identities have profound implications for claims to a personal identity, which means the way the individual defines "a sense of location, differentiation, continuity, and direction by and in relation to the self" (Charmaz, 1991, p. 269).

Symbolic interactionism views people as enacting meanings and making them real through interaction. Despite assuming that people's intended and taken-for-granted interactions construct society, situations, and selves, symbolic interactionists recognize that they seldom do so under conditions entirely of their own choosing. While acknowledging human agency, symbolic interactionists understand that society and its institutions and traditions precede and constrain individuals although how they respond to external constraints can vary. Structure exists and persists but some individuals may resist, circumvent, or ignore these constraints.

According to Blumer (1969, p. 3), the symbolic interactionist position rests upon three premises:

1. Human beings act toward things on the basis of the meanings that things have for them.
2. The meaning of such things is derived from, or arises out of, the social interaction that one has with one's fellows.
3. These meanings are handled in, and modified through, an interpretative process used by the person in dealing with the things he encounters.

   We can add two more premises (Charmaz, 1980):

4. Meanings are interpreted through shared language and communication.
5. The mediation of meaning in social interaction is distinguished by a continually emerging processual nature (Mead, 1934).

Blumer (1969) clarifies how symbolic interactionist views of meaning differ from common ways of attributing meaning. Rather than assume that the meaning of an object—such as an illness—emanates from this object itself, as if meaning is intrinsic to it, symbolic interactionists assume that people form meanings from what they *do* with the object. Blumer's first premise implies that meanings precede action, which over-simplifies a fundamental assumption of symbolic interactionism. People establish meanings—or *reconfirm* past meanings—through acting. Blumer also implies that social actors constantly make indications to themselves as they grapple with their situations. However, much of social life is routine. People are unlikely to change either their practices or meanings unless their situations have become problematic and their habitual responses no longer work or unanticipated situations arise (Charmaz, 1980; Snow, 2002). If others question a person's meanings or actions, such as by suggesting that this individual feigns symptoms, then this person may change these meanings and actions.

We understand situations through defining and naming them. As Strauss (1959) pointed out, naming constitutes a way of knowing, categorizing, locating, evaluating, and dealing with an object, event, individual, or group. Naming intrinsically involves boundary-setting and outlines one's relationship to what is named. Names are seldom neutral. Naming a phenomenon evokes or ensures evaluating it while renaming involves changing one's relationship to this phenomenon. Renaming clumsiness to lack of proprioception after being diagnosed with multiple sclerosis recasts its meaning, revises actions, predicts social identity, and casts shadows on the future.

Blumer's emphasis on interpretation relies heavily on communication processes. An alternative lies in the dramaturgical approach, which looks at *action* first, and then infers meaning from action. By invoking the metaphor of the drama, we see aspects of reality that might otherwise not be brought into view. Dramaturgy also draws attention to the temporal and spatial dimensions of the scene as well as the social staging of action. Scenes, actors, roles, performances, and audiences all contribute to dramaturgical analysis and concepts of self-presentation and impression management indicate how actors play their roles and what kind of performance they give. To the extent that we integrate dramaturgical analysis with more interpretive approaches, we can construct theory that is both fluid and reflective of the studied experience.

Studying the Illness Experience

The symbolic interactionist perspective leads to studying self-construction, interaction, actions, and meanings in the empirical world. To the extent possible, symbolic interactionists start inquiry from the experiencing person or collectivity's standpoints and understandings. Early symbolic interactionist studies of the experience of illness made in medical sociology purported to bring an "insider's view" into purview because their authors emphasized concrete realities rather than borrowed abstract concepts (Conrad, 1987, p. 2). Today, researchers would not claim that their analyses speak for or fully represent research participants' experience or views. We try to get close to the illness experience, and some of us may share aspects of it, but the research frame limits as well as extends our views—and therefore the form and content of our theorizing. Most researchers use single in-depth interviews to conduct their studies of the illness experience. Thus they gain insights from their research participants' stories and reflections but seldom witness their actions or silences. Taken collectively, however, symbolic interactionist studies make significant statements about experience and offer directions for theorizing.

Establishing Lines of Inquiry

Symbolic interactionists have attempted to portray what people with chronic illnesses experience, how they experience it, which actions they take toward their situations, how they understand their experiences, and when their understandings shift or change. The symbolic interactionist perspective also alerts researchers to study varied—and sometimes conflicting—definitions of the situation among actors and groups within a setting or social world, an approach that began in the early days of medical sociology and still continues (see, for example, Freidson, 1961; Roth, 1963; Nack, 2008; Shriver & Waskul, 2006). Many symbolic interactionist studies have used grounded theory methods to explore, describe, and theorize life with chronic illness.

Lines of inquiry have generated new conceptual directions, as have areas of focus. What began as descriptions of the illness experience became theoretical conceptions of experience. Making the ill person's experience the central focus moved symbolic interactionists out of hospitals and into homes, away from patients' roles and into people's problematic lives. Early concepts about stigma (Goffman, 1963), awareness, and uncertainty (Glaser & Strauss, 1965, 1968) formed the backdrop of initial and contemporary studies of experiencing chronic illness (Charmaz, 2008b; Charmaz & Rosenfeld, 2010; Foote-Ardah, 2003; Nack, 2008; Strauss & Glaser, 1975), but the early analyses remained descriptive. These studies described how people lived with chronic illness and thus addressed regimen management, dealing with uncertainty, and, following Goffman (1959, 1961, 1963), their efforts to control how others viewed them and avoided stigma. Strauss and Glaser (1975) and their colleagues depicted the kinds of work and considerable time involved in managing chronic illness at home, which numerous authors still explore and in the study of how chronically ill people engage in restructuring their lives, emphasis has increasingly turned toward analyzing biographies (see, for example, Charmaz, 1991; Corbin & Strauss, 1984, 1987, 1988; Faircloth et al., 2004a; Hubbard, Kidd & Kearney, 2010).

Each of these developments brought questions about self and identity into view— and simultaneously altered views of people with chronic illness. Managing illness and care commonly poses knotty concrete problems as Strauss and Glaser's volume documents. Dealing with these problems developed two lines of analysis: (1) substantive analyses of the work that ill people and their caregivers perform and (2) subsequent theoretical statements about the reconstruction of self, as Bury (1982), Charmaz (1983, 1987, 1991, 2011), and Galvin (2005) 'among many other' show. Concepts derived from a symbolic interactionist perspective, particularly those developed through grounded theory methods invite development and refinement.

Theorizing the Illness Experience

Bury's (1982) concept of biographical disruption constituted a direct attempt to theorize how chronic illness affected people's lives. This disruption involves undermining or decimating the person's taken-for-granted assumptions about their concept of self, their health, and the conduct of their life; it entails reevaluating the person's biography and self-image, and marshaling resources to deal with changes stemming from the illness. Bury's (1982, pp. 169–170) concept takes into account age, time, uncertainty, and issues of legitimacy.

Scholars (e.g., Lawton, 2003; Pierret, 2003) often link Bury's concept of biographical disruption with Charmaz's (1983) early concept of loss of self, which she ties explicitly to suffering. Charmaz defines loss of self as experiencing one's "former self-images crumbling away without the simultaneous development of equally valued new ones [self-images]" (Charmaz, 1983, p. 168). Ghaziani (2004, p. 282) interviewed a man who said, "One of the down sides of having your job be really important to you is that when it's gone, you also lose a big piece of yourself. And it's a long process to sort out who you are. I think it's one of the biggest disability issues-'Who am I without a job?'" Over time, such losses erode the person's self-concept as well as narrowing the sources of identity construction. Taken together, the concepts of biographical disruption and loss of self provide an analytic handle on crucial aspects of experiencing illness. Both concepts bring self, identity, and time into the conceptual foreground and have given numerous researchers sources of comparison and debate as well as of application (see, for example, Pierret, 2003; Sandstrom, 1990, 1998).

The concept of loss of self captured numerous researchers' attention (Pierret, 2003) although analyses of discoveries and transformation of self did not (Charmaz, 1991, 1994a, b). Some researchers who endeavor to study self and identity in chronic illness make explicit use of Mead's (1934) framework to sensitize themselves to look for the effects of illness. For example, Adams et al. (1997) adopted Mead's analysis of the self. They agree about the potential of loss of self but contend that it "will only occur in our respondents if an individual cannot reconcile the social identity of 'asthmatic' (this particular 'me') with their other social identities which, in turn, are irrevocably inter-connected with their personal identities or sense of self" (Adams et al. 1997, p. 198).

Analytic questions about awareness, timing, and action flow from a symbolic interactionist perspective. As Bury (1982) contends, a diagnosis may initiate or confirm biographical disruption. Charmaz (1991) refines the concept because she documents that people may also define a diagnosis or medical crisis as temporarily interrupting life, perhaps requiring a time-out, rather than marking a permanent change. She also shows that people experience chronic illness as intrusive or find themselves immersed in it as well as disrupted. Charmaz demonstrates temporality in multiple ways, as some people learn that they have an illness long before they receive a diagnosis and others long after. Diseases may be contested while illnesses may be present—and discounted for lengthy periods of time. Having no diagnosis at all 'or a questionable one' undermines a person's credibility to self as well as others, as this woman describes:

> Most people out there don't believe that it [chronic fatigue syndrome/environmental illness] exists, you don't look sick so no one is going to believe that I'm sick, and so it became surreal.... It became this kind of battle trying to remind myself that, Yeah, I really am sick, and then, but also [I'm] trying to meet other people's expectations. They expected me to be healthy and so I would push to do things that I didn't feel up to doing, and so in consequence I basically made myself sicker and sicker and sicker. (Charmaz, 2008b, p. 8)

People whose self-concepts are predicated on being healthy and active often insist on defining their conditions as temporary until long after health professionals dismiss their views and actions as unrealistic, or even as impairing their health. Learning about ill people's past biographies and current situations from *their* standpoints can explain their present actions. Both definitions of illness as temporary or chronic result in reconstructing the past in light of present events. In keeping with Mead's (1932) analysis of the past, Charmaz (1991) shows that the reconstructed past is a past of a particular present and Lombardo (2004, p. 539) argues that his "worried well" informants "symbolically reconstructed their pasts in order to make sense of their present beliefs in being HIV-positive".

Bury recognizes that biographical timing of illness influences the extent of its defined disruptiveness and like others finds defining loss varies with age (see, for example, Sanders et al., 2002). Moreover, using self, identity, and time as sensitizing concepts, fosters attending to the aftermath of biographical disruption, which is seldom a single event for chronically ill people. People form implicit or explicit identity goals that congeal into an identity hierarchy (Charmaz, 1987, 1995). Where they locate themselves on this hierarchy depends on their age, situations, and experience with illness. The levels of the identity hierarchy include the supernormal social identity, the restored self, a contingent personal identity, and a salvaged self, all of which allowed people claims to avoid being what they saw as invalid. A successful surgery or new medication allowed some people to move up identity levels, but over years many people plummeted down the hierarchy, as further crises accrued and with these events, their preferred identities crumbled.

Concrete empirical study in multiple settings refines the concept of biographical disruption. Heather McKenzie and Mira Crouch (2004) agree that the diagnosis of cancer constitutes a critical situation consistent with Bury's concept. But they point out that unlike people with chronic illnesses, many people who have had cancer do not feel sick. Instead, they feel enormous uncertainty and fear of illness and death, but suffer from others disallowing expression of these feelings. Thus, these authors identify lasting uncertainty without experienced illness as a condition under which biographical disruption arises. As we explore below in greater detail, experiencing disturbing bodily cues induces action. Cynthia Mathieson and Henderikus Stam's (1995) narrative analysis pinpointed tacit forewarnings among cancer patients of biographical disruption and identity changes: bodily cues and troubled interactions with medical workers. These signs prompted changed narratives of self and elicited a renegotiation of identity.

Earlier marginalization, crises, and problematic lives affect the extent to which illness is a disruption. Illness may frame a way of life but it occurs within a life. What happened before illness counts. Desirée Ciambrone (2001, p. 517) finds that women with HIV/AIDS experienced an initial disruption but in hindsight saw it as causing them less disruption than violence, separation from children, and drug use. Daniéle Carricaburu and Janine Pierret (1995) find serious chronic illness may mean "biographical reinforcement" rather than a disruption among marginalized people. Pierret (2007) further refines the concept of biographical disruption. She found that people who had chaotic lives became passive, withdrawn, and unable to cope when they were diagnosed with HIV or AIDS. These people's identities changed when they gained the respectable label of "patients" due to French social policy. They gained stability because as patients, they could receive sufficient welfare benefits to live. Subsequently, their meanings of illness, self, and disruption changed. Pierret not only shows how people receive biographical reinforcement while ill but also makes important connections between meanings of subjective experience and structural conditions.

Symbolic interactionists scrutinize their studied empirical worlds and the assumptions on which their concepts rest. Under certain conditions, acknowledging disruption may be disallowed. Sinding and Wiernikowski (2008, p. 289) find that "broad cultural and moral discourses, patterns of social interaction and structures of power combine to foreclose older women's accounts of disruption". Studies of biographical disruption assume "good" health until illness occurs. Lowton and Gabe (2003) turn from disruption and illness to the converse: continuity of illness and health as they explore what *health* means to people who have been diagnosed as chronically *ill* since early infancy. Their study nicely brings continuity in the life of the chronically ill individual into focus and provides a strong counterpoint to the concept of disruption. Nonetheless, the concept of biographical disruption has applications beyond the sick person. Karner and Bobbit-Zeher (2005) show that it can be usefully applied to caregivers as well as sufferers.

Disruption, intrusive illness, and immersion in illness all lead to marginalization, and loss of self contributes to it. But what is marginalization? Everyone knows what marginalization is, but few researchers define it. Symbolic interactionists would look at how marginalizing processes are enacted and given meaning and grounded theorists would define an extant concept by its empirical indicators and identify its properties, if the concept earned its way into the analysis. Thus, Charmaz (2008b), p. 9) compared accounts in her data and arrived at this definition: "Marginalization means boundaries or barriers, distance or separation, and division or difference. Disconnection, devaluation, discrimination, and deprivation exemplify experiences of marginalization". Marginalization is both psychological and social; it assumes structure. Beyond the obvious observation that marginalized people and groups hold problematic statuses in society, Charmaz contends that marginalization assumes the following: (1) some identifiable social entity constitutes a core, a center; (2) implicit or explicit measures locate certain people as part of this core; (3) these measures separate or distance other people from the core; and (4) marginalizing processes are inherently comparative.

The stories of people with visible disabilities tell tales of experiencing marginalization. Anthropologist Murphy (1987) and sociologist Robillard (1999) each became paralyzed and used wheelchairs. Each man discovered that his colleagues avoided or ignored him, which resulted in his growing isolation and uneasy feelings. One of Galvin's (2005, p. 397) interviewees who used a wheelchair said:

> … being rejected is the biggest part. I don't like that feeling. I mean, no one would like the feeling of being rejected, but having a disability, that rejection seems to be… it's all of you. They are not just rejecting something you might have said or done. It's because they're rejecting you… it always comes back to you being different because you have a disability.

Social acts of marginalization not only result in psychological suffering but also confer a moral status on the individual *for* suffering. This status takes relative health into account yet spreads beyond it. When suffering is deemed legitimate, others grant an ill person moral rights and entitlements that, in turn, allow this individual to make moral claims. Here, moral judgments view the person as deserving, dependent, and in need. Definitions of legitimacy can elevate an individual's moral standing and even confer a sacred moral status—for a while. Through comparing numerous accounts, Charmaz (1999, p. 368) discerned an "implicit hierarchy of moral status in suffering". Over time, the ill person's moral claims and moral status become contested, particularly when people define this person's claims and physical and/or mental condition as troublesome. Subsequently, the person tumbles down the hierarchy of moral status in suffering.

Understanding Embodied Selves in Health and Illness

By offering a general frame for looking at empirical realities, symbolic interactionism leads researchers to ask certain kinds of questions and to forge certain kinds of questions. In the studies of the illness experience questions arise about the effects of having an altered body on chronically ill people. Hence, connections between embodiment, self, and identity not only follow but also bring researchers to wider issues concerning health as well as illness. We focus on embodiment to portray how symbolic interactionists have conceptualized it and to recognize its crucial place in qualitative studies of illness—and health.

Recent growth in explicit medical sociological attention to embodiment leads one to scratch one's head and ask, why wasn't the body always a focus of our field? (e.g. Walsh, 2010; Waskul & Vannini, 2006; Williams, 2003). Bodies have been present in our work, of course, but too often relegated to the background. Williams (2003, p. 1) argues that medical sociology includes a "secret history of the body". Today, however, embodiment is an explicit focus among those using symbolic interactionist and related interpretive perspectives.

In their review, Waskul and Vannini (2006) identify five bodies of symbolic interactionism: the looking-glass body, the dramaturgical body, the phenomenological body, the socio-semiotic body, and the narrative body, all of which deal with meaning and/or reflexivity. Although symbolic interactionists use these various bodies to examine quite divergent health/illness issues, the bulk, though not all, of the sociology of the body deals in one way or another with self and identity, with issues concerning *control* and *visibility* as pivotal parts of the mix. Given space limitations, we focus on only a few substantive areas with clear relevance for medical sociology and beyond, but encourage the reader to explore further. Numerous examples below have clear implications for practice, suggesting that grounded theory research would be valuable in further pursuing those topics because it generates relevant findings for practice as well as for theory.

Authors often use embodiment to examine *self and/or identity*, topics fundamental to symbolic interactionist theory, explicitly and directly. For instance, Charmaz (1995) examines the adaptation to repeated changes in body-self unity in chronic illness. She explores substantive questions including: How do people with chronic illnesses respond to bodily changes? What meanings do they attribute to such changes? How do their meanings and actions change over time? She suggests that people adapt to their altered bodies, albeit this adaptation may be forced by the physical constraints they now have. The process of adapting to illness begins with the experience of an altered body, even a sense of bodily betrayal. Chronically ill people objectify their bodies (or the now problematic part) until they come to work *with* it, rather than *against* it. Bodily changes can lead to changes in their identity goals, a theoretical direction that Hubbard et al. (2010) continue. Adaptation to one's altered body involves tradeoffs, whereby ill people sacrifice some identity goals in order to hang on to others. Finally, surrendering to the sick body, giving up the quest for *control,* is an active process, one that brings a new unity of body and self. Symbolic interactionism guides the understanding of the process of adaptation, the interaction between self and body, explicated in this work.

Using the looking-glass self approach, Charmaz and Rosenfeld (2006) examine the intrusion of chronic illness in both mundane and ritual occasions, pointing out that people with disabilities are even more self-conscious than Goffman's ordinary strategic actors. Consider this woman's statement about other people's response to her difficulty in walking:

> I just feel real self-conscious when I'm downtown and people look at me, you know, like women or something, or they notice the way I'm not walking correctly or whatever. And it really bothers me. It's almost like it brings me up short or something....I don't know what

> they're thinking or anything, but I can see that they perceive something different about me because they're looking, and I get annoyed. (Charmaz & Rosenfeld, 2006, p. 35)

The *control* of visibility turns out to be a double-edged sword in identity management. Although visible health problems might threaten claims to competent identities, invisible problems call into question the legitimacy of requests for help.

Haworth-Hoeppner and Maines (2005) examine persistent invalidated anorexic identities and take a new look at a classic mismatch between self-identity and identity as seen by others. These researchers discover a divergence contrary to the successful reflexivity that symbolic interactionists often find. As anticipated, diet and exercise take center stage of sufferers' lives and growing ever thinner does increase their sense of self-worth. Yet traditional identity theory does not explain the persistence of invalidated identities. Sufferers cling to identity-claims of size (as huge, big, etc.), although other people typically counter these claims. Symbolic interaction theory points us to examining such seeming mismatches between theory and reality. Work like this helps advance theory, by specifying *conditions* that modify reflexivity.

Size is embodied not only by those with anorexia, of course, but also by those who are large, those living obesity. In their efforts to get at the embodiment and experience of largeness, Warin et al. (2008) quickly learned that to talk food and bodies within families is to talk motherhood and femininity. Identity, motherhood, and body are all connected. For the poor, who have experienced food insecurity, food symbolizes nurturing and is central to identity. For more affluent women, paid employment might be central to identity, but putting the family before one's self is still key, so that cooking comes before exercise. Essentially, women's embodied histories and practices of motherhood set the context for their relationships to food; medicalizing obesity and messaging for healthy lifestyles miss this boat (Warin et al., 2008).

Some (potential) disruptions come from *practices of the body*, as in the case of injury that strikes at the core of identity. The first example examines the "set up" for loss of self, while the second illustrates the process. Turner and Wainwright (2003) use the case of the injured ballet dancer to integrate embodiment and the construction of the body as a cultural object. Injuries are an expected part of the ballet career. Pain, like anorexia, comes with dance, but injury, real injury, destroys a dancer's embodiment. Because "(p)rofessional ballet is not just something you *do*—it is something you *are*… being a ballet dancer is an embodiment of identity" (Turner & Wainwright, 2003, pp. 284–285).

Injury and pain also constitute sport. In a case study of an amateur rugby player, Smith and Sparkes (2008) examine aftermath of spinal cord injury (SCI). Parallel to the dancers discussed above, for Jamie, "my life was sport" (Smith & Sparkes, 2008, p. 221). Initially following SCI the dominant narrative of restitution has Jamie telling, and seeing, his disability as temporary. Jamie looks forward to being once again able-bodied even though he can feel nothing below the neck. Jamie is a case example of what Charmaz (1991) has theorized as having a selfconcept that lags behind experience. With no improvement, Jamie moves into a state of chaos, in which he has no narrative order and only a desolate future. Finally, as he faces social-structural barriers and internalizes others' definitions of who he now is, he sees his story as being over. Jamie is overwhelmed by pain and impairment, the raw materials of his embodied disability. Thus, examining injury through the lens of embodiment helps us to integrate the social and physical sides of impairment, to better understand the meaningful interaction of self and body.

Studies of situations in which "embodied experience is front and center" (Faircloth et al., 2004b, p. 83) yield insights into dualism. Faircloth et al. (2004b) looked at the practical mechanisms used by stroke survivors to manage their newly limited bodies. Some see the body as a whole, rather than focusing on parts that don't work. Others see the body as a foreign object that just will not listen to what their mind tells it to do or, alternatively, an active body that pushes the mind. Thus, while disrupted biography is part of the story, the stroke experience centers more on dualism.

In childbearing, the central issue is that of *control* (Carter, 2010), with dualism vital to the story. This unique situation challenges symbolic interactionist theory's focus on self and the agency of the human actor, herself. Childbearing bodies are only rarely controlled and once in labor, the loss of control can extend to the self. Some bodies are autonomous, active, while others are accommodating to the needs of the self. Still other body/self relationships involve collaboration between bodies and selves that are both active agents. This point extends symbolic interactionism to recognizing that in some circumstances corporal bodies supersede the agency of symbolic selves.

Embodied knowledge has been examined at both the lay and professional levels. As more and more pregnant women are pushed into prenatal screening, with those deemed "high risk" encouraged to undergo amniocentesis, the relative power and authority of medical/scientific knowledge versus womens' experiential/embodied knowledge becomes a key issue. Markens et al. (2010) examined agency and decision-making among Mexican-origin women, finding that those who distrust medical/scientific knowledge or, at least, do not have blind faith in medicine, rely on their embodied knowledge of how their babies are doing. Those who trust medicine, find the arguments in favor of amniocentesis logical, and who express less certainty in their embodied knowledge are more likely to accept the test. The agency of these women, as they weighed various knowledge sources to make their own decisions is noteworthy, given their relative vulnerability. Work such as this demands the extension of symbolic interactionist work beyond the micro level, to deal with issues of differing status and power in the larger social system, as Nettleton et al.'s (2008) narrative analysis also confirms. Using embodiment perspectives can help symbolic interactionists understand how larger social structural actions play out at a level that is both more micro and far-reaching.

Taking an embodiment approach is not without risk. When examining the arena of childbirth with an eye toward *integration of perspectives*, Walsh (2010) notes that various approaches to embodiment, including phenomenology, feminist thought, the socially-constructed body, and more, lead to different foci and takes on childbirth and carry different shortcomings. For instance, a focus on discourse, a la

Foucault, can lose the carnal nature of the body, whereas attention to the "natural body" can lead to essentialism. One result of this diversity has been dichotomized thinking regarding natural and medical childbirth, bringing distress for laboring women caught between the two sides.

Embodied analyses call into question some of our cherished approaches. Researchers need not discard these, but need to acknowledge their limitations, in order to elaborate them and expand their usefulness. For instance, Williams (2003) warns that when we become too caught up in the social construction of disease, we leave bodies behind. He contends that we do not so much overcome reductionism as invert it, ignoring the successes of medicine. Symbolic interactionism, in concert with related, interpretive theoretical approaches, might be particularly suited to address how bodies are "lived, experienced, and expressed in sickness and in health" and the role of emotions in linking "biology and society, structure and agency, the public and the private" (Williams, 2003, p. 1). Certainly symbolic interactionist theory points us toward interrogating the relationship between body and self, a key relationship for understanding health actions. In combination with a grounded theory approach to research, symbolic interactionism can be key for designing useful interventions.

Glimpsing Selves in a Medicalized Old Age

Some might find it odd to see a section on aging included in a discussion of using theory in medical sociology. After all, aging and old age are neither diseases nor health states. Others will find it "natural" to see such a section, since growing old is "clearly" associated with increasing health problems. Symbolic interactionism is valuable for examining questions of aging and health ranging from the meaning of health and illness in old age to matters especially associated with old age, such as experiences of dementia or caregiving. This perspective can sensitize us to the downside of medicalization, the consequences of redefining phenomena of everyday life in medical terms, while acknowledging attendant benefits.

Criticisms of medicalization include Irving Zola's (1972) classic concern over medicine as a form of social control and later attention to the potential over-reach of the medical model (Irving Zola, 1991). More recently, Gabe (2005) has attended to potential benefits of medicalization and expressed concern that the drawbacks have been overstated. Certainly clinical reductionism has yielded treatments that relieve very real suffering. Symbolically, we have long recognized that labels for troubling bodily signs that evade diagnosis can bring reassurance and help organize experience, even when the labels are quite serious, such as those related to multiple sclerosis or lupus erthymatosus (e.g. Davis, 1973; Stockl, 2007). Work in a symbolic interactionist perspective continues this tradition of interest in the consequences—both positive and negative—of having the meanings of elders' lives interpreted through medical lens.

Holstein and Gubrium (2007) distinguish what they see as two distinct social constructionist perspectives, one grounded in symbolic interactionism and the other more influenced by ethnomethodology. They state that those using symbolic interactionism seek to understand the construction of the meaning of experiences. They see those pursuing the "more radical" ethnomethodological approach as bracketing the meaning of the experience to focus on the construction and use of the tacit understandings and structures that underlie that experience. Thus, Holstein and Gubrium believe that a symbolic interactionist would be interested in the construction of meanings of experiences of health and illness, but leave out the symbolic interactionist emphasis on action, which addresses how actions reveal and construct tacit understandings and structures. These approaches are inherently connected and both are relevant to symbolic interactionist work on aging, health, and illness.

Medicalization of/in Old Age: Constraint and Resource

Epidemiologically speaking, indeed, age and illness are associated, primarily due to chronic illness. However, defining old age in terms of health/illness, with an inability to separate the two, symbolizes the strong medicalization of aging, no doubt largely influenced by the dominance of the "successful aging" framework in social gerontology (Belgrave & Bisma, 2013). This framework pushes aside critical perspectives based on class, race, and gender power structures (Estes et al., 2003; Holstein & Minkler, 2003). Medicalization of old age is so strong that even critiques of equating old age with any particular health status contain implicit assumptions about the relationship. For instance, Jones and Higgs (2010) analyze natural, normal, and normative assumptions about aging, in the context of contemporary consumer society. They argue that we should attend to the lived experience of those who accept or reject these contested domains or are unable to do so, yet still refer to aging as an "important field of health" (p. 1513). The fact that we do not refer to youth or even infancy as a field of health alerts us to taken-for-granted acceptance of the medicalization of old age. Symbolic interaction theory can push us to let go of such unintended assumptions in order to focus on the meaning of health in old age for those living it. In fact, with this approach we see that meanings in old age are varied, that they can liberate or constrain.

The medicalized view of aging, the tendency to see old age in health/illness terms is hardly limited to gerontological researchers and practitioners. Life is increasingly "the business of bureaucracies and agencies" that become "primary sources of meaning for most aspects of our lives" (Holstein & Gubrium, 2007, p. 348). Subsequently, medicalized definitions of aging become common resources for constructing meanings of and in later life. Multiple findings of expectations of bodily deterioration with aging reflects reliance on medicalized definitions. People can draw on such expectations to construct continuity in the face of illness-related disruption (Hinojosa et al., 2008). However, the growing influence of the "successful aging" framework brings with it demands that we assume personal responsibility for aging in good health, no matter our ability to do so. Holstein and Minkler (2003) remind us that cultural norms matter, influencing selves even when they are resisted. The potential damage done by this framework to aging selves has to be recognized and challenged. Symbolic interactionism provides the intellectual tools to confront this unintended consequence of "successful aging" and weigh it with the positive value of encouraging elders' agency in holding on to their health.

Moreover, "although well-constructed scientific experiments can provide much needed information about what we must do (if we are able) to have a relatively healthy old age, it cannot tell us what makes that life a good one" (Holstein & Minkler, 2003, p. 790). Yet positive identities and continuous selves can be accomplished in the face of health problems (Phoenix & Sparkes, 2009). Actors' abilities to draw on their creativity to do so cutsacross ailments such as pain (Encandela, 1997), stroke (Hinojosa et al., 2008), and other conditions. However, they exercise this creativity within larger interpretive contexts, which can either encourage alternatives to defining oneself as limited or constrain such creative definitions. Encandela (1997) found that elders living with chronic pain in continuing care retirement communities that encouraged active lives found ways to remain on the go and conceal their pain. Those who failed to live up to these expectations became the source of gossip. However, in these same facilities, the meaning of needing skilled nursing care constrained patients who required it more than collective definitions of pain. Elders can invoke cultural beliefs about aging to normalize bodily changes and thus maintain a sense of continuity of self in the face of loss of function following stroke (Hinojosa et al., 2008). In effect, elders use both disruption and continuity as sources of self-construction, so that even when experiencing despair over new limitations, one could maintain "that on the whole, in the realms of self-perception, the meaning of life, and future outlook, one continues to be the same person" (p. 211). This ability might explain, at least in part, the acceptance of bodily limitations following stroke or other serious health problem (Faircloth et al., 2004b).

Regardless of one's maintenance of a positive, continuous self/identity, serious illness does present problems that must be managed. For instance, the health care system often must be navigated in some fashion. Styles of negotiating treatment and care vary by hospital patients' adaptation—or resistance to being subordinated to health care providers (Löfmark & Hammarström, 2005). Stroke survivors might use and listen to their bodies to understand what has happened to them and what it means (Faircloth et al., 2004b). Studies of pain in old age highlight the importance of the meaning of bodily conditions, an approach typical of symbolic interactionist theory. For instance, Miles et al. (2005) found that pain itself is less important for coping efforts than the bodily, activity, and identity constraints caused by that pain.

Learning from Dementia

Issues of meaning, continuity, and maintaining a positive image of self become more poignant when we turn to the experience of dementia. Alzheimer's disease/dementia provides a surprisingly valuable laboratory for examination of core principles of symbolic interaction theory while the theory guides us to a much more sensitive understanding of experiences and lives of sufferers and their caregivers.

Health professionals, social scientists, and ordinary people see dementia/Alzheimer's as qualitatively different from other ailments. This condition challenges our sociological understandings not only of the experience of illness but, moreover, of relationships and selves as well. As such, studies of dementia are especially well-poised to contribute to interactionist theory in medical sociology and beyond. At the most obvious level, dementia/Alzheimer's is distinct in that it combines "fear of losing one's mind" with medicalized notions of inevitable, irreversible decline in a condition that is unique to old age. Although early-onset dementias occur, they are left out of the cultural picture of the condition. Dementia/Alzhiemer's conditions are also distinct in that care also might be given in the home or in a long-term care institution.

Dementia disrupts two lives—the sufferer and the informal caregiver. Symbolic interactionism alerts us to the possibilities that this disruption changes relationships within this dyad, with the potential for altered selves. Disruptions directly impact caregivers because they have the responsibility of dealing with the changed circumstances and making whatever pragmatic adjustments are needed (Belgrave et al., 2004; Karner & Bobbitt-Zeher, 2005). When the relationship is spousal, the potential impact for intimacy is enormous and gendered in nature (Hayes et al., 2009). Emotional intimacy hinges on communication, which can be lost, so that physical intimacy is challenged, especially for women caregivers. Moreover, if the wife's role becomes one of "mothering," the conflict with sexual intimacy is profound. Changed relationships, as one person becomes a caregiver, imply changed selves for both parties (Karner & Bobbitt-Zeher, 2005), at least potentially. Relationships remain paramount, at least early on, as dementia/Alzheimer's sufferers rely on supportive others to help maintain their sense of leading meaningful lives (MacRae, 2010). With such confirmation available, sufferers can define their essential selves as unchanged and continuous, despite their condition. Whether or not these supportive others are fully open with the sufferer (Blum, 1994), they play key roles in defining day-today situations. In effect, the extreme example of dementia/Alzheimer's dramatically highlights the place of social interaction in constructing meaning.

Symbolic interaction theory, with its focus on interaction, subjective meaning, and self, points us to examine loss of self within the specific context under study, rather than to assume universality. The potential loss of self with dementia/Alzheimer's is less straightforward, perhaps, than with other conditions. Contrary to expectation, dementia/Alzheimer's sufferers do not necessarily experience or fear a loss of self (MacRae, 2010), although the caregiver might (Karner and

Bobbitt-Zeher 2005), particularly when he or she is the sufferer's spouse (Hayes et al., 2009). Caregivers find that they have lost their "old" loved one and, hence, the familiar relationship they once had. Some sufferers, even in the face of their ailment, use their agency to construct valued selves, disputing caregivers' definitions and normalizing their conditions (Belgrave et al., 2004; MacRae, 2010). Others are silenced while caregivers construct new meanings of their selves (Karner & Bobbitt-Zeher, 2005). The divergence between sufferer and caregiver in definitions of the sufferer's self could be connected to their disparities in responsibilities and standpoints and/or the relative advancement of the condition in different studies.

Despite medicalization of dementia/Alzheimer's, neither caregivers nor sufferers, even those in long-term care facilities, define this condition in medical terms. In the home setting, sufferers and caregivers alike may experience dementia/Alzheimer's as medicalized, but not necessarily an illness at all (Belgrave et al., 2004). Though caregivers and sufferers might differ on constructions of sufferers' selves and in their use of medicalized explanations, both draw on common, cultural stocks of knowledge as well as their joint lived experiences to define these selves (Belgrave et al., 2004; Karner & Bobbitt-Zeher, 2005; MacRae, 2010).

Elders negotiate selves, conditions, and even models of dementia/Alzheimer's in long-term care settings, where one would expect the medical model to dominate. Residents of such facilities actively define their own and others' behavior and situation, despite limited awareness of the severity of their losses. However, their definitions might not match those of staff or researchers (Clare et al., 2008). Staff, primarily CNAs, when given the freedom to do so, draw on their deep respect for the selves of residents, the residents' own contributions to the meaning of the unit, and their experience of the residents' own world(s) to construct a decidedly non-medical model (Vittoria, 1999). This model modifies, even rejects, basics of, the medical stage model. These staff change "the referent, from the disease or biological symptoms to the person of the resident" and the context, from the medical model to the "lived context" of the unit (Vittoria, 1999, p. 369). And they do much of this through non-symbolic interaction with residents, whose language abilities are so limited.

We see that medicalization *in* old age is a complex phenomenon, carrying the potential for either benefit or harm. For instance, medicalization can provide a way to normalize experiences that might otherwise diminish the self. However, there appears to be no upside to medicalization *of* old age. Medicalizing elders, as a social category, individualizes responsibility for health, cuts off critical discourse, and potentially influences the selves and experiences of elders, even as they struggle to maintain a holistic, full self.

Moving Symbolic Interactionism Beyond Microsociology

Symbolic interactionism need not remain solely a micro perspective; it can inform studies of health care policies and organizations. What begins as inductive micro explorations can end with moving beyond microsociology. The symbolic interactionist perspective has long contained the elements for developing dynamic inductive meso and macro analyses that often start with micro research, such as Horowitz's (2011) study of medical licensing boards, but lead to general principles and useful concepts. Taking action as the unit of analysis and of theoretical development leads symbolic interactionists into organizational, social movement, and other forms of collective analysis.

Many of symbolic interactionist conceptual contributions build on researchers' prior interests and lines of research, although these contributions may take on a life of their own. Strauss's (1984, 1993; Strauss et al., 1963, 1985) dual concern with the theoretical study of action and the substantive study of work is a case in point. The sociology of work animated many of Anselm Strauss's (Star, 1991; Strauss, 1984; Strauss et al., 1963, 1985) organizational analyses but these studies consistently addressed the actions that constituted the work. Like his empirical analysis of segmentation, over time Strauss's concepts segmented into separate lines of inquiry and spread across fields as other scholars engaged and developed them (see, for example, Casper, 1998a, b; Clarke, 1998; Clarke & Star, 2008; Star, 1989; Star & Griesemer, 1989; Wiener, 1991, 2000).

Conceptualizing a Negotiated Order

Strauss et al.'s (1963) portrayal of the hospital as a "negotiated order" is one prominent example of a concept that moves symbolic interactionism beyond microsociology. This concept assumes that people construct and reconstruct the division of labor in organizations and accomplish organizational work through interaction processes. It addresses how order and change occur simultaneously— and depends on an analysis of action. Nadai and Maeder (2007) contend that the negotiated order approach offers a useful theoretical tool for "connecting different levels of analysis and linking interactions to organizations and overarching societal structures".

The concept of negotiated order takes into account informal sentiments, actions, and alignments as well as formal hierarchies, communications, and the content and distribution of work. The concept answers the question: How are these aspects of organizational life played out in action and interaction? These interaction processes are dialectical in that Strauss et al. (1963) argue that informal aspects of organizational life can influence formal structure in addition to the converse. Strauss rightly contended that scholars had reified structure to the exclusion of addressing process. In his later book, Strauss (1978a) explicitly states that negotiations occur within situations that have their own structural properties. He argues here that researchers must recognize which structural conditions impinge on the studied negotiations and specify how they do so. Certainly some groups seek to exercise their power to ensure that other groups have no power to negotiate their definitions of the situation, much less to obtain more symbolic and material resources.

Strauss (1987, 1993) brought temporality, flexibility, and mutability into purview in his concept of negotiated order—all within a focus on action. It focuses on movement—shifting commitments, changing organizational environments, fluctuating organizational relationships and continued fluid discussions, compromises, concessions, and resolutions. This concept also leads to looking at processes that otherwise may remain invisible, such as the requisite background work needed to accomplish over organizational goals and activities. When do explicit negotiations arise? Disagreements, ambiguity, uncertainty, and changed conditions encourage negotiations to arise (Maines & Charlton, 1985) and often permit previously silenced voices to speak. For Strauss et al. (1963) the concept of the negotiated order corrected organizational theory and studies that assumed and over-emphasized organizational stability, rather than process and change. They based their concept on what they found in empirical settings rather than what organizational theory had prescribed. As Day and Day (1977, p. 126) note, the concept "calls into question the more static structural-functional and rational-bureaucratic explanations of complex organizations".

For over a decade after its publication, the concept of negotiated order received accolades. Its promise for developing lines of research has not, however, been fully realized, as both Davies (2003) and Griffiths (2003) point out. Davies observes that the relative absence of a sociology of organizations in medical sociology has been a source of question and consternation. However, symbolic interactionist concepts beginning with the negotiated order and its sequelae may give such studies a fresh start.

The concept of negotiated order generated a spate of studies in the 1970s and several important studies in the 1990s. Svensson (1996) calls for adopting the concept of negotiated order to understand changes in the doctor-nurse relationship which resulted in nurses taking an active role in defining patients' medical status and in interpreting hospital rules. He argues that researchers must take into account both micro processes at the hospital ward level and macro processes at the societal level and that the concept of negotiated order facilitates this type of analysis. Svensson states that the field of doctor-nurse negotiations had widened. The increased incidence of chronic illnesses meant devising strategies for managing life. Nurses had gained increased control of medical work and direct nurse-doctor communications routinely occurred in "sitting rounds" during which doctors and nurses discussed patient care. Such changes gave nurses many more opportunities to negotiate for patients and to negotiate expanding their tasks.

The studies above demonstrate how concepts born in medical sociology can serve other areas of study and disciplines and, thus, extend the reach of medical sociology. Perhaps the concept of negotiated order itself stands as boundary object between fields and disciplines, although its foundations in symbolic interactionism sometimes get lost.

Developing Social Worlds and Arenas Analysis

Like the earlier concept of negotiated order, Anselm Strauss's (1978a, b, 1982) notion of social worlds brings process into the foreground and aims to capture fluid social relationships and forms of structure. Theorizing in social worlds and social arenas analysis stands at the borders between medical sociology and social studies of science. Some scholars who have developed these lines of inquiry, such as Clarke (1998) and Star (1989), possess and build on their expertise in medical sociology; others do not have this expertise. In social worlds and arena analyses, researchers have found that actors do engage in boundary-establishment and maintenance as well as efforts to legitimize their purposes and practices. Strauss's analysis focuses on fluid actions that construct and reconstruct social worlds while Clarke and Star (2008) sharpen how discursive practices shape these actions.

A symbolic interactionist perspective combined with grounded theory methods has generated robust analyses. Clarke and Star (2008, p. 115) show how social worlds analysis has led to new concepts such as "infrastructures," which they define as "frozen discourses that form avenues between social worlds and into arenas and larger structures". There are also "implicated actors" which include both physically present individuals who powerful social world leaders silence, ignore, or render invisible and actors who are *not* physically present but are made discursively present through other participants' conceptions, representations, and intentions (Clarke & Montini, 1993, p. 119). Social worlds analysis fosters making "invisible infrastructures" (Star, 1991) visible, particularly when silences within relevant situations are explicated (Clarke, 2005).

Star's (1993) widely invoked concept of "cooperation without consensus" puts to rest the notion that symbolic interactionism is wholly anchored to a narrow consensus model. Monica Casper's (1998a, b) study of the controversial area of fetal surgery reveals that different players in the emergent specialty of fetal surgery may cooperate without consensus. Casper (1998a) herself became a player as she rejected a prevailing view of the mother as only a container for the "real" patient, the fetus. Subsequently, she advocated for the mother's health as well as that of the unborn child. The concepts of social worlds and social arenas provide particularly useful tools for understanding fast-changing relationships, policies, and practices in emergent specialties before they become hardened into stable structures that control the conditions of action and involvement.

Conclusion

Researchers can join symbolic interactionism with grounded theory to form a useful theory-methods package. True, symbolic interactionist studies may be quantitative or qualitative and grounded theory methods can be used in conjunction with varied theoretical approaches. However, the symbolic interactionist perspective and grounded theory method fit and complement each other. Symbolic interactionist emphases on meaning and action fit the inductive approach of grounded theory. Both this theoretical perspective and the method emphasize studying actions. Symbolic interactionism takes process as fundamental and thus sensitizes researchers to look for processes—and how processes constitute structures. Grounded theory is uniquely and explicitly a method for analysing processes. Symbolic interactionism follows the pragmatist call to study experiences and practices; grounded theory offers a way to reveal these experiences and practices. Both perspective and method emphasize emergent phenomena in obdurate but multiple realities. Symbolic interactionism leads researchers to study the specific, situated, and constructed nature of multiple realities and diverse definitions of a situation that grounded theory is well-positioned to examine and analyze. All these attributes of perspective and method can serve research in medical sociology.

As our analysis attests, symbolic interactionists in medical sociology have adopted qualitative, interpretive methodologies, which are not explicitly designed for applied research. However, studies from a symbolic interactionist perspective often serve applied goals. These studies address topics of relevance to participants and emphasize participants' meanings, and thus likely yield results suited for translation to practice.

Qualitative research invokes its own canon that differs from quantitative research. Qualitative findings are more explicitly interpretive than are their quantitative counterparts. As such, qualitative researchers openly debate and contest the means for evaluating the validity of their findings. Replicability, in contrast, holds less significance in qualitative than quantitative studies but qualitative researchers do seek resonance with participants and/or practitioners.

When researchers use grounded theory methods, they test and retest their developing theory against new data in keeping with the iterative process of the method. A key strategy of the method, theoretical sampling, leads researchers to gather new data to make their theoretical categories more complete and robust. From its beginnings to the present, grounded theory studies aim to contribute to theory construction. Yet researchers can and have used grounded theory methods for a variety of purposes. When they conduct studies with application in mind, the test of the robustness of the grounded theory resides in its successful, meaningful use in practice (Fig. 2.1).

Ultimately the value of a perspective lies in its products. Why do symbolic interactionist studies of health and illness matter? Interpretive medical sociology contributes to theory, of course, and produces translatable findings that can help professionals relieve suffering. Our work has offered fresh views of how health and illness affects people's lives but we can also help to move understandings of health and illness beyond the level of the individual. In the process, our theorizing can help meet Link's (2003) call to counter-balance the "blame-the-victim" approach so prevalent in North America, generally, and in practice fields pertaining to health, illness, and healing, in particular. Much of what we do as symbolic interactionists articulates the experiences of those who suffer. Symbolic interactionism and related interpretive approaches offer ideal tools for "look(ing) at things from the 'other

HIERARCHY of MORAL STATUS in SUFFERING

HIGH MORAL STATUS--VALIDATED MORAL CLAIMS

MEDICAL EMERGENCY

INVOLUNTARY ONSET

BLAMELESSNESS FOR CONDITION

"APPROPRIATE" APPEARANCE AND DEMEANOR

SUSTAINED MORAL STATUS—ACCEPTED MORAL CLAIMS

CHRONIC ILLNESS

NEGOTIATED DEMANDS

PRESENT OR PAST POWER & RECIPROCITIES

DIMINISHED MORAL STATUS—QUESTIONABLE MORAL CLAIMS

CHRONIC TROUBLE

BLAME FOR CONDITION AND COMPLICATIONS

"INAPPROPRIATE / REPUGNANT" APPEARANCE AND/OR DEMEANOR

PERSONAL VALUE

worth less

worth less

Worth Less

WORTHLESS

Institutional Traditions **Structural Conditions**

Difference—class, race, gender, age, sexual preference, resources, capabilities

Fig. 2.1 As adapted in Charmaz (2005, p. 523). (The original version of this figure has been published in K. Charmaz, "Stories of Suffering: subjective Tales and Research Narratives" in Qualitative Health Research, Volume 9 Issue 3, May 1999 p. 369 by SAGE Publications, Inc., All rights reserved. © SAGE Publications)

side'" (Link, 2003, p. 462). Let us use these tools and work together with colleagues of various theoretical orientations to produce knowledge that can challenge the dominance of the powerful.

References

Adams, S., Pill, R., & Jones, A. (1997). Medication, chronic illness and identity: The perspective of people with asthma. *Social Science and Medicine, 45*, 189–201.

Belgrave, L. L., & Bisma, A. S. (2013). Successful/productive aging, responsibility, and reflection. In J. W. Murphy & S. L. Arxer (Eds.), *The symbolism of globalization, development, and aging*. Springer.

Belgrave, L. L., Allen-Kelsey, G. J., Smith, K. J., & Flores, M. C. (2004). Living with dementia: Lay definitions of Alzheimer's disease among African American caregivers and sufferers. *Symbolic Interaction, 27*, 199–222.

Blum, N. S. (1994). Deceptive practices in managing a family member with Alzheimer's disease. *Symbolic Interaction, 17*, 21–36.

Blumer, H. (1969). *Symbolic interactionism: Perspective and method*. Prentice-Hall.

Brown, P. R., Alaszewski, A., Swift, T., & Nordin, A. (2011). Actions speak louder than words: The embodiment of trust by heatlhcare professionals in gynae-oncology. *Sociology of Health & Illness, 33*, 280–295.

Bury, M. (1982). Chronic illness as biographical disruption. *Sociology of Health & Illness, 4*, 167–182.

Carricaburu, D., & Pierret, J. (1995). From biographical disruption to biographical reinforcement: The case of HIV-positive men. *Sociology of Health & Illness, 17*, 65–88.

Carter, S. K. (2010). Beyond control: Body and self in women's childbearing narratives. *Sociology of Health & Illness, 32*, 993–1009.

Casper, M. J. (1998a). *The making of the unborn patient: A social anatomy of fetal surgery*. Rutgers University Press.

Casper, M. J. (1998b). Negotiations, work objects, and the unborn patient: The interactional scaffolding of fetal surgery. *Symbolic Interaction, 21*, 379–400.

Charmaz, K. (1980). *The social reality of death*. Addison-Wesley.

Charmaz, K. (1983). Loss of self: A fundamental form of suffering in the chronically ill. *Sociology of Health & Illness, 5*, 168–195.

Charmaz, K. (1987). Struggling for a self: Identity levels of the chronically ill. In P. Conrad & J. A. Roth (Eds.), *Research in the sociology of health care: The experience and management of chronic illness* (pp. 283–321). JAI Press.

Charmaz, K. (1991). *Good days, bad days: The self in chronic illness and time*. Rutgers University Press.

Charmaz, K. (1994a). Discoveries of self in illness. In M. L. Dietz, R. Prus, & W. Shaffir (Eds.), *Doing everyday life: Ethnography as human lived experience* (pp. 226–242). Copp Clark, Longman.

Charmaz, K. (1994b). Identity dilemmas of chronically ill men. *Sociological Quarterly, 35*, 269–288.

Charmaz, K. (1995). The body, identity, and self: Adapting to impairment. *Sociological Quarterly, 36*, 657–680.

Charmaz, K. (1999). Stories of suffering: Subjects' tales and research narratives. *Qualitative Health Research, 9*(3), 369–382.

Charmaz, K. (2005). Grounded theory in the 21st century: Applications for advancing social justice studies. In N. K. Denzin & Y. E. Lincoln (Eds.), *Handbook of qualitative research* (3rd ed., pp. 507–535). Sage.

Charmaz, K. (2006). *Constructing grounded theory: A practical guide through qualitative analysis*. Sage.
Charmaz, K. (2008a). Constructionism and the grounded theory method. In J. A. Holstein & J. F. Gubrium (Eds.), *Handbook of constructionist research* (pp. 397–412). Guilford.
Charmaz, K. (2008b). Views from the margins: Voices, silences, and suffering. *Qualitative Research in Psychology, 5*, 7–18.
Charmaz, K. (2011). A constructivist grounded theory analysis of losing and regaining a valued self. In F. J. Wertz, K. Charmaz, L. J. McMullen, R. Josselson, R. Anderson, & E. McSpadden (Eds.), *Five ways of doing qualitative analysis: Phenomenological psychology, grounded theory, discourse analysis, narrative research, and intuitive inquiry* (pp. 165–204). Guilford.
Charmaz, K., & Rosenfeld, D. (2006). Reflections of the body, images of self: Visibility and invisibility in chronic illness and disability. In D. D. Waskul & P. Vannini (Eds.), *Body/embodiment: Symbolic interaction and the sociology of the body* (pp. 35–50). Ashgate.
Charmaz, K., & Rosenfeld, D. (2010). Chronic illness. In W. C. Cockerham (Ed.), *New Blackwell companion to medical sociology* (pp. 312–333). Wiley-Blackwell.
Ciambrone, D. (2001). Illness and other assaults on self: The relative impact of HIV/AIDS on women's lives. *Sociology of Health & Illness, 23*, 517–540.
Clare, L., Rowlands, J., Burce, E., Surr, C., & Downs, M. (2008). 'I don't do like I used to do': A grounded theory approach to conceptualizing awareness in people with moderate to severe dementia living in long-term care. *Social Science and Medicine, 66*, 2366–2377.
Clarke, A. E. (1998). *Disciplining reproduction: Modernity, American life sciences and the 'problem of sex'*. University of California Press.
Clarke, A. E. (2005). *Situational analysis: Grounded theory after the postmodern turn*. Sage.
Clarke, A. E., & Fujimura, J. (1992). Introduction: What tools? Which jobs? Why right? In A. E. Clarke & J. Fujimura (Eds.), *The right tools for the job: At work in twentieth century life sciences* (pp. 3–44). Princeton University Press.
Clarke, A. E., & Montini, T. (1993). The many faces of RU486: Tales of situated knowledges and technological contestations. *Science, Technology and Human Values, 18*, 42–78.
Clarke, A. E., & Star, S. L. (2008). The social worlds framework: A theory/methods package. In M. Lynch, O. Amsterdamska, & E. Hackett (Eds.), *Handbook of science and technology studies* (pp. 113–137). MIT Press.
Cockerham, W. C. (2012). *Medical sociology* (12th ed.). Pearson Prentice-Hall.
Conrad, P. (1987). The experience of illness: Recent and new directions. *Research in the Sociology of Health Care: The Experience and Management of Chronic Illness, 6*, 1–32.
Corbin, J. M., & Strauss, A. (1984). Managing chronic illness at home: Three lines of work. *Qualitative Sociology, 8*, 224–247.
Corbin, J. M., & Strauss, A. (1987). Accompaniments of chronic illness: Changes in body, self, biography and biographical time. *Research in the Sociology of Health Care: The Experience and Management of Chronic Illness, 6*, 249–281.
Corbin, J. M., & Strauss, A. (1988). *Unending work and care: Managing chronic illness at home*. Jossey-Bass.
Crossley, N. (2004). The circuit trainer's habitus: Reflexive body techniques and the sociality of the workout. *Body and Society, 10*, 37–69.
Davies, C. (2003). Some of our concepts are missing: Reflections on the absence of a sociology of organisations. *Sociology of Health & Illness, 25*, 172–190.
Davis, M. S. (1973). *Living with multiple schlerosis: A social psychological analysis*. Charles C. Thomas.
Day, R., & Day, J. V. (1977). A review of the current state of negotiated order theory: An appreciation and a critique. *The Sociological Quarterly, 18*, 126–142.
Encandela, J. A. (1997). Social construction of pain and aging: Individual artfulness within interpretive structures. *Symbolic Interaction, 20*, 251–273.
Estes, C. L., Biggs, S., & Phillipson, C. (2003). *Social theory, social policy, and aging*. Open University Press.

Faircloth, C., Boylstein, C., Rittman, M., & Young, M. E. (2004a). Disrupted bodies: Experiencing the newly limited body in stroke. *Symbolic Interaction, 27*, 71–87.

Faircloth, C. A., Boylstein, C., Rittman, M., Young, M. E., & Gubrium, J. F. (2004b). Sudden illness and biographical flow in narratives of stroke recovery. *Sociology of Health & Illness, 26*, 242–261.

Foote-Ardah, C. E. (2003). The meaning of complementary and alternative medicine practices among people with HIV in the United States: Strategies for managing everyday life. *Sociology of Health & Illness, 25*, 481–500.

Freidson, E. (1961). *Patients' views of medical practice: A study of subscribers to a prepaid medical plan in the Bronx*. Russell Sage Foundation.

Gabe, J. (2005). Medicalization. In J. Gabe, M. Bury, & M. A. Elston (Eds.), *Key concepts in medical sociology* (pp. 59–73). Sage.

Galvin, R. D. (2005). Researching the disabled identity: Contextualising the identity transformations which accompany the onset of impairment. *Sociology of Health & Illness, 27*, 393–413.

Ghaziani, A. (2004). Anticipatory and actualized identities: A cultural analysis of the transition from AIDS disability to work. *Sociological Quarterly, 45*, 273–301.

Glaser, B. G., & Strauss, A. L. (1965). *Awareness of dying*. Aldine.

Glaser, B. G., & Strauss, A. L. (1968). *Time for dying*. Aldine.

Goffman, E. (1959). *The presentation of self in everyday life*. Doubleday.

Goffman, E. (1961). *Asylums*. Doubleday.

Goffman, E. (1963). *Stigma: Notes on the management of spoiled identity*. Prentice-Hall.

Griffiths, L. (2003). Making connections: Studies of the social organisation of healthcare. *Sociology of Health & Illness, 25*, 155–171.

Gubrium, J. (1986). *Oldtimers and Alzheimer's: The descriptive organization of senility*. JAI Press.

Haddow, G. (2005). The phenomenology of death, embodiment, and organ transplantation. *Sociology of Health & Illness, 27*(1), 92–113.

Haworth-Hoeppner, S., & Maines, D. (2005). A sociological account of the persistence of invalidated anorexic identities. *Symbolic Interaction, 28*, 1–23.

Hayes, J., Boylstein, C., & Zimmerman, M. K. (2009). Living and loving with dementia: Negotiating spousal and caregiver identity through narrative. *Journal of Aging Studies, 23*, 48–59.

Hewitt, J. (2000). *Self and society: A symbolic interactionist social psychology*. Allyn & Bacon.

Hinojosa, R., Boylstein, C., Rittman, M., Hinojosa, M. S., & Faircloth, C. A. (2008). Constructions of continuity after a stroke. *Symbolic Interaction, 31*, 205–224.

Holstein, J. A., & Gubrium, J. F. (2007). Constructionist perspectives on the life course. *Sociology Compass, 1*, 335–352.

Holstein, M. B., & Minkler, M. M. (2003). Self, society, and the 'new gerontology'. *The Gerontologist, 43*, 787–796.

Horowitz, R. (2011). Organic public sociology in the pragmatist perspective: A multifaceted approach. *Symbolic Interaction, 32*, 1–19.

Hubbard, G., Kidd, L., & Kearney, N. (2010). Disrupted lives and threats to identity: The experiences of people with colorectal cancer within the first year following diagnosis. *Health, 14*, 131–146.

Jones, I. R., & Higgs, P. F. (2010). The natural, the normal, and the normative: Contested terrains in ageing and old age. *Social Science and Medicine, 71*, 1513–1519.

Karner, T. X., & Bobbitt-Zeher, D. (2005). Losing selves: Dementia care as disruption and transformation. *Symbolic Interaction, 28*, 549–570.

Lawton, J. (2003). Lay experiences of health and illness: Past research and future agendas. *Sociology of Health & Illness, 25*, 23–40.

Link, B. G. (2003). The production of understanding. *Journal of Health and Social Behavior, 44*, 457–469.

Löfmark, U., & Hammarström, A. (2005). Older stroke patients' negotiations within the hierarchic medical context. *Qualitative Health Research, 15*, 778–790.

Lombardo, A. P. (2004). Anatomy of fear: Mead's theory of the past and the experience of the HIV/AIDS 'worried well'. *Symbolic Interaction, 27*, 531–548.

Lowton, K., & Gabe, J. (2003). Life on a slippery slope: Perceptions of health in adults with cystic fibrosis. *Sociology of Health & Illness, 5*, 289–319.

MacRae, H. (2010). Managing identity while living with Alzheimer's disease. *Qualitative Health Research, 20*, 293–305.

Maines, D. R., & Charlton, J. C. (1985). The negotiated order approach to the analysis of social organization. In H. A. Farberman & R. S. Perinbauayagam (Eds.), *Foundations of interpretive sociology: Original essays in symbolic interaction* (pp. 271–308). JAI Press.

Markens, S., Browner, C. H., & Mabel Preforan, H. (2010). Interrogating the dynamics between power, knowledge and pregnant bodies in amniocentesis decision making. *Sociology of Health & Illness, 32*, 37–56.

Mathieson, C., & Stam, H. (1995). Renegotiating identity: Cancer narratives. *Sociology of Health & Illness, 17*, 283–306.

McKenzie, H., & Crouch, M. (2004). Discordant feelings in the lifeworld of cancer survivors. *Health, 8*(2), 139–157.

Mead, G. H. (1932). *Philosophy of the present*. Open Court Press.

Mead, G. H. (1934). *Mind, self and society*. University of Chicago Press.

Miles, A., Curran, H. V., Pearce, S., & Allan, L. (2005). Managing constraint: The experience of people with chronic pain. *Social Science and Medicine, 61*, 431–441.

Murphy, R. F. (1987). *The body silent*. Henry Holt.

Nack, A. (2008). *Damaged goods? Women living with incurable sexually transmitted diseases*. Temple University Press.

Nadai, E., & Maeder, C. (2007). Negotiations at all points? Interaction and organization. *Forum Qualitative Sozialforschung/Forum: Qualitative Social Research*. http://www.qualitative-research.net/fqs-texte/1-08/08-1-32-e.htm

Nettleton, S., Burrows, R., & Watt, I. (2008). Regulating medical bodies? The consequences of the 'modernization' of the NHS and the disembodiment of clinical knowledge. *Sociology of Health & Illness, 30*, 333–348.

Parry, D. C. (2006). Women's lived experiences with pregnancy and midwifery in a medicalized and fetocentric context: Six short stories. *Qualitative Inquiry, 12*, 459–471.

Phoenix, C., & Sparkes, A. C. (2009). Being Fred: Big stories, small stories, and the accomplishment of a positive ageing identity. *Qualitative Research, 9*, 219–236.

Pierret, J. (2003). The illness experience: State of knowledge and perspectives for research. *Sociology of Health & Illness, 25*, 4–22.

Pierret, J. (2007). An analysis over time (1990–2000) of the experiences of living with HIV. *Social Science and Medicine, 65*, 1595–1605.

Robillard, A. B. (1999). *Meaning of a disability: The lived experience of paralysis*. Temple University Press.

Roth, J. A. (1963). *Timetables*. Bobbs-Merrill.

Sanders, C., Donovan, J., & Dieppe, P. (2002). The significance and consequences of having painful and disabled joints in older age: Co-existing accounts of normal and disrupted biographies. *Sociology of Health & Illness, 24*, 227–253.

Sandstrom, K. L. (1990). Confronting deadly disease: The drama of identity construction among gay men with AIDS. *Journal of Contemporary Ethnography, 19*, 271–294.

Sandstrom, K. L. (1998). Preserving a vital and valued self in the face of AIDS. *Sociological Inquiry, 68*, 354–371.

Shriver, T. E., & Waskul, D. D. (2006). Managing the uncertainties of Gulf war illness: The challenges of living with contested illness. *Symbolic Interaction, 29*, 465–486.

Sinding, C., & Wiernikowski, J. (2008). Disruption foreclosed: Older women's cancer narratives. *Health, 12*, 389–411.

Smith, B., & Sparkes, A. C. (2008). Hanging bodies, changing narratives and the consequences of tellability: A case study of becoming disabled through sport. *Sociology of Health & Illness, 30*, 217–236.
Snow, D. A. (2002). Extending and broadening Blumer's conceptualization of symbolic interactionsim. *Symbolic Interaction, 25*, 571–575.
Star, S. L. (1989). *Regions of the mind: Brain research and the quest for scientific certainty*. Stanford University Press.
Star, S. L. (1991). The sociology of the invisible: The primacy of work in the writings of Anselm Strauss. In D. R. Maines (Ed.), *Social organization and social process: Essays in honor of Anselm Strauss* (pp. 265–284). Aldine de Gruyter.
Star, S. L. (1993). Cooperation without consensus in scientific problem solving: Dynamics of closure in open systems. In S. Easterbrook (Ed.), *CSCW: Cooperation or conflict?* (pp. 93–105). Springer.
Star, S. L., & Griesemer, J. R. (1989). Institutional ecology, 'translations' and boundary objects: Amateurs and professionals in Berkeley's museum of vertebrate zoology, 1907–39. *Social Studies of Science, 19*, 387–420.
Stockl, A. (2007). Complex syndromes, ambivalent diagnosis, and existential uncertainty: The case of systemic lupus erythematosus (SLE). *Social Science and Medicine, 65*, 1549–1559.
Strauss, A. L. (1959). *Mirrors and masks: The search for identity*. Free Press.
Strauss, A. L. (1978a). *Negotiations, varieties, context, processes, and social order*. Jossey-Bass Publishers.
Strauss, A. L. (1978b). A social world perspective. *Studies in Symbolic Interaction, 1*, 119–128.
Strauss, A. L. (1982). Social worlds and legitimation processes. *Studies in Symbolic Interaction, 4*, 171–190.
Strauss, A. L. (1984). Social worlds and their segmentation processes. *Studies in Symbolic Interaction, 5*, 123–139.
Strauss, A. L. (1987). *Qualitative analysis for social scientists*. Cambridge University Press.
Strauss, A. L. (1993). *Continual permutations of action*. Aldine de Gruyter.
Strauss, A. L., & Glaser, B. (Eds.). (1975). *Chronic illness and the quality of life*. C.V. Mosby.
Strauss, A., Leonard, S., Danuta, E., Rue, B., & Melvin, S. (1963). The hospital and its negotiated order. In E. Freidson (Ed.), *The hospital in modern society*. Free Press.
Strauss, A. L., Fagerhaugh, S., Suczek, B., & Wiener, C. (1985). *Social organization of medical work*. University of Chicago Press.
Svensson, R. (1996). The interplay between doctors and nurses: A negotiated order perspective. *Sociology of Health & Illness, 18*, 379–414.
Turner, R. (1976). The real self: From institution to impulse. *American Journal of Sociology, 81*, 989–1016.
Turner, B. S., & Wainwright, S. P. (2003). Corps de ballet: The case of the injured ballet dancer. *Sociology of Health & Illness, 25*, 269–288.
Vittoria, A. K. (1999). 'Our own little language': Naming and the social construction of Alzheimer's disease. *Symbolic Interaction, 22*, 361–384.
Walsh, D. (2010). Childbirth embodiment: Problematic aspects of current understandings. *Sociology of Health & Illness, 32*, 486–501.
Warin, M., Turner, K., Moore, V., & Davis, M. (2008). Bodies, mothers and identities: Rethinking obesity and the BMI. *Sociology of Health & Illness, 30*, 97–111.
Waskul, D. D., & Vannini, P. (2006). Introduction: The body in symbolic interaction. In D. Waskul & P. Vannini (Eds.), *Body/embodiment: Symbolic interaction and the sociology of the body* (pp. 1–18). Ashgate.
Wiener, C. (1991). Arenas and careers: The complex interweaving of personal and organizational destiny. In D. Maines (Ed.), *Social organization and social process: Essays in honor of Anselm Strauss* (pp. 175–188). Aldine de Gruyter.
Wiener, C. (2000). *The elusive quest: Accountability in hospitals*. Aldine de Gruyter.
Williams, S. J. (2003). *Medicine and the body*. Sage.

Zola, I. K. (1972). Medicine as an institution of social control. *The Sociological Review, 20*, 487–504.
Zola, I. K. (1991). The medicalization of aging and disability. *Advances in Medical Sociology, 2*, 299–315.

Chapter 3
Social Construction and Health

Sigrún Ólafsdóttir

Social construction represents a major theme in sociology. Ever since Berger and Luckmann (1967) suggested that some of our most taken-for-granted assumptions about society are embedded in specific "realities", sociologists, across the board, have been interested in such processes and applied them to a wide array of topics. Social constructs are viewed as the by-products of countless human choices, rather than laws that result from divine will or nature. This approach stands in contrast to essentialism that considers specific phenomena as inherent and transhistorical essences independent of human actions and decisions (Burr, 1995). The theoretical contributions of medical sociologists within this perspective are shaped by the development of medical sociology itself. Early on, Straus (1957) pointed out the inherent tension between sociologists *in* medicine and sociologists *of* medicine. The former generally collaborate closely with medical doctors to solve practical problems in medicine, but the latter are committed to use issues of health, illness, and healing as a window to help us understand larger sociological questions. Increasingly, sociologists are interested in questions that simultaneously advance sociological theory and have implications for the well-being of populations and individuals. Not surprisingly, these questions often center on how social and cultural factors matter for the way in which we understand and respond to biological processes.

In many ways, issues of health, illness, and healing offer particularly interesting insights into our understanding of the social construction of reality. While almost all aspects of human society, from the largest organizational features to the smallest routine interactions are continually (re)constructed, our health has an "objective" biological component that individuals and societies respond to. A useful distinction emerged between disease (the social meaning of the condition), highlighting the importance of understanding every issue related to health and illness as shaped by

S. Ólafsdóttir (✉)
University of Iceland, Reykjavík, Iceland
e-mail: sigruno@hi.is

W. C. Cockerham (ed.), *Medical Sociology on the Move*,
https://doi.org/10.1007/978-3-031-92456-9_3

biological as well as social factors (Eisenberg, 1977). It is the case that social and cultural factors impact virtually every question that medical sociologists are interested in, including, how we understand the biological abnormalities in our bodies, how we respond to illness, how we interact with medical professionals, and how we deliver our health care. All these processes have been created and recreated in human interaction over an extended period of time. Consequently, issues of health, illness, and healing offer us an opportunity to examine the interplay of the biological and the social in our lives.

Although notions of social constructions are evident in the earliest sociological writings (e.g., Durkheim, Mannheim, and Thomas), the approach took off as a major theoretical perspective both in sociology and medical sociology in the 1960s. One strand of research emerged from those scholars interested in understanding the role of deviance in society. They pointed out the lack of a universal law guiding what is abnormal or deviant; rather, certain social behaviors become defined in such a way within a particular social context. Inevitably, this definition has a strong association with power, namely certain individuals and groups have the power to label the behavior of other individuals and groups as weird, criminal, deviant, or sick (Becker, 1963; Conrad & Schneider, 1992; Spector & Kitsuse, 1977; Zola, 1972). This was also a time where major sociological thinkers were considering how issues related to health, illness, and healing do not represent an actual reality. As an example, Goffman (1961, 1963) pointed out how the "moral career" involves both biological conditions as well as social experiences; Freidson (1970) illustrated how illness and disease are socially constructed in his important book on the *Profession of Medicine*, and Foucault (1965, 1973) showed how the medical profession, through its powerful position, was able to label what was normal and abnormal. And more recently, Pescosolido and Green (2024) argue for the importance of understanding the social construction of mental illness at three levels, the individual, within social networks and among professionals. Together, this body of work continues to inspire work in medical sociology, nicely captured by Conrad and Barker (2010: S69) as illustrating "how illness is shaped by social interactions, shared cultural traditions, shifting frameworks of knowledge, and relations of power."

Given the centrality of social construction within the sociology of health, illness, and healing, it would be impossible to count all the different ways in which medical sociologists engage with the approach. Consequently, I focus on a few major areas where important contributions have been made and consider: (1) The cultural meanings of illness; (2) The distinction between the normal and the abnormal; (3) How illness responses are embedded in the community; and (4) How medical knowledge itself is impacted by social factors. I then discuss the strengths and weaknesses of the approach and consider future directions that highlight how our world of health and illness is simultaneously impacted by biological realities, cultural traditions, historical trajectories, and institutional arrangements. To illustrate that point, I draw on a cross-national perspective and consider how it can increase our understanding of health, illness, and healing.

The Cultural Meanings of Illness

Historically, illnesses have represented reality to most people. They represent abnormal variations in our bodies and our responses are often considered rational and even the only way to respond. This reality has become so taken for granted that we fail to notice that it is embedded in specific social contexts and ideologies. Even in cases when there are biological abnormalities, there are social and cultural meanings attached to them. These meanings help us make sense of the illness and have consequences on patients and health care. As an example, Sontag (1978) argued that negative metaphorical meanings of cancer, as evil or repressive, are common in our society and significantly impact those afflicted with the disease. In many ways, the cultural understanding of cancer "and particularly breast cancer" has been altered through the survivor movement, which at first glance appears to be a positive development, as it empowers those suffering from it. However, research has shown that many women alter the meaning of survivorship or reject it all together. In particular, the "positive" survivor discourse alienates women who struggle with the threat of recurrence, who feel their cancer experience was not severe enough to merit this title, or who prefer to grapple with the disease more privately (Kaiser, 2008).

Although all illnesses have a cultural component, those with stigma attached to them illustrate this point particularly well. The concept of stigma, originally formulated by Goffman (1963) is an attribute that, according to prevailing social norms, is deeply discrediting, marks a person as tainted, and allows the target to be denigrated. Sociologists have pointed out several illnesses frequently stigmatized in societies, including epilepsy, cancer, mental illness, HIV/AIDS, and sexually transmitted diseases (Conrad & Barker, 2010). The reemergence of infectious disease, including COVID-19 has resulted in stigma across both low- and high-income countries (Rewerska-Juśko & Rejdak, 2022; Yuan et al., 2022). As COVID-19 became a worldwide pandemic, issues of stigma became particularly prevalent with stigma associated with the areas where the infection emerged (Xu et al., 2021).

Link and Phelan (2001) define stigma as the co-occurrence of its components: labeling, stereotyping, separation, status loss, and discrimination, and suggest that power must be exercised for stigmatization to take place. Many children, even before entering first grade have notions about what it means to be crazy and have ideas about what "those" people are like. These ideas have been created and recreated in social interaction but have become an inherent part of our cultural context, helping us to make sense of individuals who behave a strange way. However, what is considered strange is not equally determined across social groups as those in more powerful positions have greater power to define what constitutes such behavior.

The difference between illnesses that carry high versus low levels of stigma illustrates that there is nothing inherent in some conditions that naturally leads to stigma. Comparison across different types of physical and mental illness shows this clearly. It would seem that individuals and societies should view all types of cancer in a similar way, yet research has indicated that while some stigma may be associated with all types of cancer (Muzzin et al., 1994), those diagnosed with lung cancer experience particularly high levels of stigma, as the disease is strongly associated with smoking and therefore caused by the individuals in many people's minds (Godward et al., 2022). Further, those diagnosed with smoking-related cancers expressed higher levels of internalized stigma as compared to those not experiencing smoking-related cancers (Warner et al., 2022). This does, however, not apply exclusively to smokers but non-smokers felt stigmatized in the same way (Chapple et al., 2004).

And while mental illnesses are more likely to be stigmatized in general, some mental illnesses carry more stigma than others. For example, individuals are more likely to hold negative attitudes toward those with schizophrenia as compared to depression, and a key explanation is the link between violent behavior and schizophrenia (Martin et al., 2000). As we may be witnessing less stigma associated with some types of mental illness (e.g., depression in recent years), the stigma associated with more serious mental illnesses (e.g., schizophrenia) appear persistent and are found across contexts, including in Germany (Schomerus et al., 2022), Iceland (Olafsdottir, 2022) and the U.S. (Pescosolido et al., 2021). This difference across disorders has even been observed amongst children; for example, Americans are more likely to be willing to have a child with depression in the same class as their child, as compared to ADHD. Yet, the reverse happens when they are asked whether they would want their child to be friends with a hypothetical child with depression or ADHD (Martin et al., 2007).

History can serve as a powerful tool to better understand how meaning is created and recreated in social interaction. Research has shown that the meanings of behavior change over time and, in the US today, few would regard some illnesses of the past in such a way. For example, masturbation was once considered as an illness, as well as Drapetomani: a condition described by American physician Samuel A. Cartwright as a mental illness causing black slaves to flee captivity. The example that is perhaps best known is homosexuality—included in the Diagnosis and Statistical Manual (DSM) of the American Psychiatric Association (APA) as a disorder until 1973. It was removed largely due to efforts of the gay rights movement and general changes in the landscape of norms surrounding human rights issues. Despite the strong sentiment that homosexuality was not a disease, the APA refused to completely eliminate it and created a new disease, ego-dystonic homosexuality. Rather than considering all homosexuality as an illness, the disease was now limited to those who had homosexual feelings but wanted to be heterosexual. It was not until 1986 that homosexuality was completely removed from the DSM as a potential illness (Conrad & Schneider, 1992). These examples show that, in some cases, the label of an illness is closely related to the overarching cultural and political landscape of a society and, in many cases, has a moral component where more powerful groups view the behavior of less powerful groups as immoral and as something that society needs to respond to and control.

What Is Normal and Abnormal?

Tracing back to the 1960s and 1970s, sociologists have been interested in understanding how particular social behaviors become defined as deviant, especially within the subfields of criminology and medical sociology. These scholars pointed out that there was nothing inherently wrong in many of the behaviors we consider deviant; rather, these behaviors represent deviations from the social norms that guide our everyday life, and in particular deviate from the norms that more powerful groups consider important. Early on, Szasz (1961) argued that mental illnesses were nothing but a myth, as such "illness" lacked the characteristics that we normally require from illnesses—most importantly some form of biological deviation. He argued that mental illnesses simply represented problems in living and in some way reflect a normal response to an abnormal world. Within sociology, Scheff (1966) was the first to articulate the link between labeling and mental illness, arguing that we all, at one point or another, engage in deviant behavior. What matters is that some people become labeled as deviant whereas others can avoid the label. He points out that being mentally ill is in essence a social role and once the label is applied, others expect certain behavior from the "sick" individual that continues to perform as expected of him or her.

Rosenhan's (1973) study of *Being Sane in Insane Place* clearly illustrates the difficulties in distinguishing between the normal and the abnormal. In this study, eight pseudo-patients attempted to be admitted to a mental hospital with symptoms of schizophrenia, which proved successful in all cases. Upon admission, they acted like they normally would, yet were hospitalized for 7–52 days and all released with schizophrenia in remission. In addition, their behavior (e.g. taking notes) was interpreted as a reflection of the illness within the hospital walls. This highlights the inadequacy of the psychiatric diagnosis system, raising question of how we can distinguish between the normal and the abnormal.

Social constructionism and labeling quickly came under attack when some argued that mental illness did, in fact, represent real illness (Gove, 1970). This resulted in heated debates both on the role of labeling as steering an individual into treatment as well as whether the causes of rejection were associated with labeling and stigma or simply a response to the symptoms themselves (Gove, 1975; Scheff, 1974). The opposing views clash on the understanding of what mental illness is, particularly whether there is a reality to such illness beyond the label. To consolidate the two viewpoints, Link and his colleagues offered their modified labeling theory, using insights from the original labeling theory, but not arguing that labeling is a direct cause of mental illness (Link, 1982, 1987; Link et al., 1989). In this view, stereotypes of mental illnesses play a powerful role in limiting the opportunities of those experiencing mental illness, both concretely through a direct rejection but also more indirectly, since there is a general agreement that those experiencing mental illness are different from others. Specifically, they are often viewed as less reliable, less capable, and/or more dangerous than the average individual. Consequently, individuals who have been diagnosed with mental illness are confronted by the reality that the label of mental illness is now a part of them, resulting in a fear of rejection in a wide array of personal and professional situations. Regardless of what such labels play in causing mental illness in society, they continue to have important consequences for those living with mental illness, especially as many people have strong notions about what the mentally ill are like, even before they get to know someone who has experienced such illness.

Closely related to the labeling perspective are notions of medicalization. Like labeling, this perspective focuses on how some individuals and groups in society have the power to define and respond to "abnormal" behavior of other groups, often with less power. The key difference between the two perspectives is the focus of medicalization theories on the role of medicine as an institution of social control, holding power to define what is normal and what is abnormal. More specifically, the concept refers to a process in which medical authority has to a large degree replaced religious and legal authority systems (Conrad & Schneider, 1992; Zola, 1972) as the main agent with power to define and respond to deviant behavior. Social behaviors previously defined as a sin or as a crime are increasingly defined as an illness and the sinner and the criminal have been replaced by the patient. This trend has happened across a large number of conditions, ranging from abnormal behavior and processes to normal biological processes, to potential risk factors for disease and has been so large-scale that it has been labeled as one of the major social transformations in advanced, industrialized nations (Clarke et al., 2003).

It is important to consider that theories of medicalization are ultimately theories of power, specifically, who has the power to define, describe, and respond to variations in social behaviors, emotions, and feelings. In the original formulation, the power largely resided with the medical profession itself (Conrad, 1992), but as societies have changed other powerful agents of medicalization have emerged, including the pharmaceutical industry, consumers, and managed care (Conrad & Leiter, 2004). Countless examples from past research illustrate how power shapes our definitions of what is abnormal. For instance, historically, societies were more likely to medicalize women's problems. Of course, we might consider that women are simply in more need to be fixed with medical innovations, but a more plausible explanation is that an historically male-dominated medical profession tended to view issues pertaining to women as problematic. For example, the APA decided to include premenstrual syndrome (PMS) as a psychiatric disorder in its manual in 1986, which potentially meant that all women could have a mental illness. Regardless of whether PMS is real or not, the inclusion clearly corresponds to the cultural position of women in society and the meaning associated with the gender roles attached to men and women (Figert, 1996). It is however important to note that various problems associated with men and masculinity have become more likely to be medicalized, including sexual disfunction (Liu & Luo, 2024) and in the transition to manhood (Bröer & Agyekum, 2021).

At least since the beginning of the twenty-first century, the pharmaceutical industry impacts how we think about what is normal and abnormal. In fact, this has led some scholars to use pharmaceuticalization instead of or complementary to medicalization (Abraham, 2010; Bell & Figert, 2012). The beginning of this development is often illustrated by the introduction of Paxil to the market in the 1990s, when the drug company GloxoSmithKline faced the problem of not having enough potential buyers. While severe anxiety has long been known as a disabling condition, marketing to that limited population would not have been a particularly profitable endeavor. Instead, the solution was the now well-known strategy of simultaneously marketing milder versions of the condition and the drug to treat it. The ads implied that everyone who experiences any kind of anxiety throughout the day may, in fact, suffer from seasonal anxiety disorder and/or general anxiety disorder. Although the drug company was later charged for inappropriate and misleading marketing, the fact remains that both disorders are now a part of our social landscape (Moynihan & Cassels, 2005). More recently, the discussion of medicalization has pointed out how there is a certain danger associated with painting medicalization in too dark of a light (e.g., vaccination resistance), yet both processes of medicalization and pharmaceuticalization can pose threats to individual health and well-being (Kaczmarek, 2022) as well as taking our focus away from the social, political and economic factors that impact individual health (Lantz et al., 2023).

In sum, regardless of whether we approach the definitions of normality and abnormality through the perspective of labeling or medicalization, sociologists argue that definitions of what constitutes normal behavior is, at least in part, constructed within a specific social context with a specific power structure, where some groups have the power to define and others have little power to resist the definitions forced upon them.

Illness Responses Embedded in Cultural Context

Just as illness is often viewed from a pure biological standpoint, responses to illness are often considered logical responses to abnormal biological processes. That is, individuals consider their choices and make informed decisions based on these choices when they get sick. Yet, this is only a partial account as individuals look for clues about what is going on with them and what is most appropriate to do within their social environment. Decisions about responses are embedded in the social networks of individuals and fall in line with the cultural norms and expectations followed by those that matter to us (Manago et al., 2019; Olafsdottir & Pescosolido, 2009; Pescosolido, 1992; Pescosolido & Green, 2024).

Across disciplines, scholars have been concerned with the role of culture in responses to illness. Anthropologists have long highlighted that cultural beliefs impact what is perceived as an appropriate reaction to illness (Kleinman, 1980). They view culture as "located in the realm of expectations, values, ideas, and belief systems" (Jayasuriya, 1992: 41). In order to understand how people use services, psychologists have developed models conceptualizing health beliefs or intentions as important predictors of use (Fishbein & Ajzen, 1975; Rosenstock, 1966) and sociologists have focused on predisposing characteristics, such as race and gender, as proxies for cultural influences on utilization (Andersen, 1968, 1995). As far back as the 1960s, sociologists illustrated that the beliefs of the group mattered for illness behavior. In an early study, Kadushin (1966) identified a social circle of *friends and supporters of psychotherapy*. The individuals belonging to this group shared certain characteristics, including being more likely to know someone who had been in therapy, asking for a referral as well as being more likely to go to plays, concerts, and museums. He argues that those belonging to this circle are more likely to go to psychotherapy, not necessarily because they have more problems that require the attention of a therapist, but because they exist in a social context that encourages such a solution.

The social environment matters for what we do when we encounter illness in general, but it is particularly important when we encounter mental illness. The Network-Episode Model (NEM), originally proposed in 1991, is designed to better capture the experience of seeking treatment for mental illness. The NEM views help seeking behavior as a phenomenon assigned meaning within social networks. The model originally highlighted the dynamics of the illness career and the importance of social networks in shaping health care outcomes. Social interactions give the initial sources of normative meaning and individual reactions (Pescosolido, 1992, 2011). In the earlier conceptualization it was illustrated that individuals experience multiple pathways to mental health treatment, falling into the three broad categories of: (1) choice; (2) coercion; and (3) muddling through. The first two may be self-explanatory, individuals choose to enter treatment because they recognize a problem, or they are forced into treatment because those around them recognize a problem. The category of muddling through is less clear and refers to individuals who neither actively seek out treatment nor actively reject it, they simply somehow end up in treatment (Pescosolido et al., 1998a).

More recently, Pescosolido and Green (2024) have examined the convergence and divergence across the views and responses of the individual that experiences a mental health problem, the social network that the individual is embedded within and the professional diagnosis that is used within the U.S. context. The results show that almost 65% of people can be defined as "well" where assessments at all levels agree on an absence of a mental health problem and for about 7% all assessments agree that the individual is "sick." Yet, that leaves almost 30% of respondents with some divergence in opinion, e.g., they may view themselves as sick but not meet an official professional diagnosis. The different trajectories inspired by the Network-Episode Model illustrate that the interpretation of symptoms and what should be done about them is embedded in the community where both the individual experiencing the problem and those around him/her attempt to make sense of what is going on.

It is established that social networks matter for what we do when we encounter illness, yet research has found contradictory results. Some have shown that they accelerate entry into mental health treatment (Kadushin, 1966; McKinlay, 1972), while others show that they delay or deter use of such services (Horwitz, 1977). To better understand how social networks matter, the Network Episode Model highlights not only the importance of the size and structure of social networks, but also the cultural context of the networks themselves. That is, to fully understand how and why social networks matter, we must understand the ideas, beliefs, and values that individuals connected through networks hold about issues of health, illness and healing. To test this idea, Pescosolido et al. (1998b) looked at the impact of large social networks on utilization of mental health services in Puerto Rico and found that larger networks delayed or deterred help-seeking. This finding can only be understood through knowledge of the cultural context of Puerto Rico. The population consists of lower-class individuals of an ethnic minority, characteristics often related to less positive views about mental health services. Therefore, it is not surprising that knowing many individuals that hold such attitudes and beliefs results in a lower likelihood of entering services, as treatment is not considered a logical response to the situation.

Despite these early insights about the importance of the cultural context to understand illness behavior, researchers have only recently begun to unpack what culture means within utilization research. While this has long been of interest to medical sociologists, they usually focus on major social categories (e.g. race/ethnicity) as proxies for culture. Here, researchers point to language as a "carrier of culture" (Bernal et al., 1995) and argue that ethnicity and language, at least in part, capture cultural characteristics (Takeuchi et al., 1999). For example, language and cultural issues of "face" predict utilization for Filipino Americans (Gong et al., 2003) and adherence to Asian cultural values decreases likelihood of using counseling (Kim & Omizo, 2003; Lau & Takeuchi, 2001). Along similar lines, research has shown demographic factors matter for whether there is a convergence in agreement across the individual, the social network and professional assessment. For example, both the individual and the social network is less likely to see a problem for less educated individuals even when a professional assessment would detect a problem (Pescosolido & Green, 2024). While this research has provided us with important insights into how social construction and culture shape responses to illness, it does not consider the larger cultural systems that impact such responses.

In response and following the "cultural turn" in sociology, researchers have reframed the key theoretical and methodological issues in health care utilization research (Olafsdottir & Pescosolido, 2009; Pescosolido, 2011; Pescosolido & Olafsdottir, 2010). We argue that individuals use cultural maps to make sense of their health care choices and that we need to consider whole cultural systems of beliefs, attitudes, and values to understand how and why individuals use or do not use services. Individuals mentally evoke different options when they are faced, directly (self) or indirectly (others), with a health problem. While some have multiple locations on their maps (e.g. counselor, medical, doctor and psychiatrist), others have few, or even only one (e.g. doctor). The concept of cultural mapping identifies cultural boundaries by showing how individuals discriminate between different providers in the medical marketplace. The focus has therefore shifted from simply understanding whether individuals endorse particular provider to how they discriminate across culturally "legitimate" sources of care (Olafsdottir & Pescosolido, 2009).

Thinking about the relationship between culture and illness responses in this way shows that individuals endorse multiple options simultaneously as would be expected by the Network Episode Model. However, they also clearly discriminate among them and they do so based on cultural attitudes, their evaluation of the situation, and occasionally on their social location. As an example, how serious the situation is perceived does not only provide a clue that treatment is needed, but it results in discrimination where the mental health system is preferred over the general medical system. Counseling may represent the clearest line on the public's cultural map. When situations are attributed to stressful circumstances, Americans prefer counselors over other options. Finally, the public draws a clear line if violence is anticipated, endorsing psychiatrists over doctors and counselors, and they express the rare cultural preference for hospitalization over visits to psychiatrist when the person may be dangerous toward others (Olafsdottir & Pescosolido, 2009).

To conclude, sociologists have been interested in responses to illness for at least the past 70 years and have powerfully demonstrated that culture matters for what we do when we encounter physical and especially mental abnormalities. Our responses are therefore not based on a notion of the "correct" response to illness but are shaped in the community and influenced by the cultural context of those communities.

The Social Construction of Medical Knowledge

A final theme considered is the social construction of knowledge. Again, it is possible to consider medical knowledge to be neutral and simply reflecting reality. Along those lines, changes in how we think about health and illness as well as treatment simply reflect scientific processes, and if they change over time it is because we know more now than we did in the past. However, when these statements are examined through a critical lens, it becomes clear that this is far from the truth. Just as the world is socially constructed, so is the world of medical knowledge. Freidson (1970) was probably the first medical sociologist to articulate how medical knowledge is embedded within particular social and political context (Conrad & Barker, 2010). He showed how the medical profession has a set of assumptions about what illness is, partly reflecting biological realities but also the social world. There are multiple interpretations of illness and professional understandings are often at odds with lay understanding of illness (Pescosolido & Green, 2024). By acknowledging the existence of multiple knowledge systems, it is possible to consider that our definitions of health and illness have components that may have less to do with scientific norms than with various cultural and political agendas.

While medical and lay diagnosis represent two different knowledge system, both have an important impact on how knowledge about health and illness is constructed (Olafsdottir & Pescosolido, 2011). Lay impressions of illness are embedded in a broader social context, and rather than representing a concrete disease experience, they allow individuals to make sense of deviations from usual health status in themselves and others (Freidson, 1970; Olafsdottir & Pescosolido, 2009; Pescosolido, 1992, 2011). Or as Jutel (2010, p. 1084) notes, the lay counterpart represents a first step in whether individuals cast "life's experiences as medical in nature". The consideration of lay beliefs allows for an understanding of how medical knowledge is constructed, both formally within the medical system as well as informally in the community. This is particularly important, as lay beliefs may vary systematically from professional scripts and categorizations of physical and mental illness. For example, research has shown that cancer beliefs held by African American women, regarding effectiveness of treatment, are significantly different than those held by physicians (Gregg & Curry, 1994). Feminist scholars have also pointed out how medical realities are shaped by the fact that only one gender has historically had power to define what is normal or abnormal. They suggest that medical discourses and practices may have more to do with existing gender norms than biological realities (Clarke, 1998; Ehrenreich & English, 1978; Lorber, 1997). For example, ideas about women's "proper" place in society are clearly a part of the medical discourse on various health "problems" associated with women, including pregnancy, PMS, childbirth, and menopause (Conrad & Barker, 2010).

The notion of gender stereotypes has been found to have profound impact in medical care, resulting in inferior treatment for women when they encounter certain illnesses. McKinlay (1996) provides a powerful example here by showing that the "fact" that women did not experience heart disease until menopause was accepted knowledge within the medical community. He showed that gender differences in heart disease were an artifact of incorrect medical observations. The symptoms that heart disease produced among women were different than in men, leading to a dismissal of it as the explanation and instead attributing the symptoms to stomach problems or even emotional problems. As a consequence of this medical practice, the rates that doctors use to guide their diagnosis process were based on wrong assumptions that then resulted in a wrong diagnosis that continued to support the socially constructed gender rates. Using the sociological imagination, McKinlay changed how medicine viewed gender differences in heart disease by distinguishing between the personal trouble of an individual woman being misdiagnosed and a social issue where we witnessed thousands of women being systematically misdiagnosed due to socially constructed rates that were, at least in part, grounded in a gendered ideology related to medicine where the male body was traditionally viewed as the norm and the female body as deviation from the normal.

Scholars at the intersection of medical sociology and science studies have pointed out the relationship between medical knowledge and the social context in which it is embedded (Conrad & Barker, 2010). They point out that our notions of biological disease or biomedical evidence are negotiated and interpreted within a specific social context (Joyce, 2008; Timmermans, 2007). More specifically, it has been pointed out that the mid-1980s witnessed the birth of a new paradigm, where an inclusion of previously excluded groups (e.g., based on gender and/or race) became important in any medical research. This represented change in medical thinking away from the assumption that it is possible to understand all bodies in the same manner, highlighting the possibility of different disease processes and treatment outcomes across major fault lines in society. While certainly an important step forward, Epstein (2007) shows that this inclusion has the unintended consequence of grounding social categories even more firmly as rooted in biological differences.

Through an examination of the process of how this happened, he shows that the knowledge that is produced about race and gender has as much to do with social and political conflicts and negotiations, as true differences based on biology.

In sum, studies on medical knowledge illustrate that the construction of such knowledge is embedded within specific social context where certain groups have power to define what is an illness and how it should be treated, whereas other groups are largely or exclusively the subject of the medical gaze (Foucault, 1973). Importantly, they underscore that different knowledge systems often clash in the interpretation of disease which has implications for how we understand and respond to health problems in societies.

The Strengths and Weaknesses of Social Constructionism

As a conceptual framework, social constructionism has made important contributions to our understanding of health and illness, and it provides an important counterpoint to the largely deterministic approach that medicine has toward disease and illness (Conrad & Barker, 2010). While processes of rationality and scientific advancement have provided important contributions to human lives through the past centuries, they have been coupled with a darker side that often goes unnoticed, simply because we have taken for granted that medical innovations represent neutral knowledge and progress for mankind. Yet, we have evidence that some of the major advancement in human health during the nineteenth century had as much to do with improvements in social conditions, as with innovations in medicine (McKeown, 1979; McKinlay, 1981). History, however, has often been constructed in a way that gives more credit to medicine and has resulted in a view of medicine as neutral, and medical doctors as scientists committed to solve mysteries related to health and illness.

It can be argued that this has become even more important as the medical landscape has changed. Earlier, it was largely the medical profession who held the power to define and respond to issues of health and illness, although of course the lay referral system has always been an important force shaping people's ideas (Freidson, 1970). This was also an era where health problems were less complex, and physicians frequently responded to acute, infectious diseases using medical solutions proven effective. Two changes have made it even more important to understand how our ideas about health and illness are embedded within a specific social context. First, there are more stakeholders that attempt to impact our understanding of what health problems are, many who have direct interest in making us believe that our experiences are problematic in one way or another. The pharmaceutical companies provide a key example. Just as the medical profession was simply providing us with better solutions to the physical problems of the past, many view the pharmaceutical companies as simply providing us with better solutions to a wide array of physical and mental health problems. And more recent examples show how politics have become more important in defining health and illness, with politicians denying the seriousness of a worldwide pandemic, openly disagreeing with public health experts (Rutledge, 2020). The perspective of social construction helps us understand that while the pharmaceutical companies provide medicine that improve health, they also have a direct interest in selling more of their medication, which shapes the reality that they are invested in protecting and even in some cases creating. Second, the potential health problems that we currently suffer from are more complex than ever before, and some have argued that everything is a potential disease in modern societies. Third, the return of infectious diseases at a large global scale show an ongoing construction of illness definitions, threats associated with the illness and potential responses. This reality makes a counterpoint to the medical/pharmaceutical perspective more crucial than ever before.

Finally, it has perhaps never been more critical, yet difficult to get our points across to policymakers, at least in some contexts. Conrad and Barker (2010) illustrate how each domain of the cultural meaning of illness, the illness experience as socially constructed, and medical knowledge as constructed has important policy implications. For example, it can make policymakers realize that the "facts" that are presented to them do not present a concrete reality or even the "best" reality. It remains true that the stakeholders in the health field do not hold equal power in the policy process and claims by some are taken more seriously than others. Medical doctors have often been able to put their perspective forward as the way the world really is, often ignoring the perspective of other professions involved in the same jurisdiction as well as the important perspective of those who are suffering. However, it is more recent that expertise from virtually all professions is questions and even denied (Woolhandler et al., 2021). In addition, an understanding of the world as socially constructed allows us to envision a reality where issues of health, illness, and healing can be understood differently. It is possible to individualize various "problems," but it is equally possible to view them as a reflection of a larger social problem. For example, we can view the existence of ADHD as a reflection of that some kids are flawed, as bad kids or biologically damaged product, or we can view our school system as flawed in ways that does not allow all children to succeed within the classroom. The way in which this is constructed clearly guides policies on this issue and has more general implications.

With every strength comes a weakness and as powerful the perspective of social construction is, it is not without limitations. The most general is perhaps the issue of why we should care that the world is socially constructed? What have we learned if we do not move further to understand and explain how it impacts the actual life of individuals and broader social processes, such as inequality? Within sociology, we are often content to show that certain phenomenon are socially constructed, but fail to address why and how it matters. As an example, numerous studies have provided important insights into how and why particular conditions were medicalized and pointed out the specific forces involved in the medicalization process, but less is known about how this matters for individuals and societies. For example, is medicalization likely to increase or decrease health inequalities? Does medicalization reduce stigma of mental illness? Insights from research that are not particularly focused on social construction can provide some cues into how this may matter. For example, the perspective of fundamental causes of health disparities shows us that those who have more resources can repeatedly transfer them into better health outcomes and services (Clouston & Link, 2021; Link & Phelan, 1995). This is partly due to their capabilities of taking advantage of medical solutions as they become available. This has been supported by showing that more diseases with more preventable causes are more strongly related to socioeconomic status (Phelan et al., 2004) Yet, as highlighted by medicalization scholars, the process is not always one that results in better health for individuals. An attempt to link together medicalization and health inequalities and outcomes would provide a strong statement for how the construction of what constitutes a health problem has an impact on key outcomes of interest to sociologists.

Similarly, it is possible to consider whether the way in which mental health problems are constructed matter for individuals experiencing such problems. In contrast to the psychiatric perspective, sociology has the power to unveil how our understanding of mental health problems does not simply follow a scientific process but is embedded in a particular context where interests play as large of a role (Kirk & Kutchins, 1992). As a result, we know that certain professions may have more investment in highlighting the biological and/or genetic approach to mental illness. But we also know that many mental health problems are rooted in the social environment and the public endorses a wide array of social, biological, and individual causes of mental illness (Martin et al., 2000). However, we have witnessed an increase in user involvement in their mental health treatment, with the focus changing from one on management of symptoms to recovery and empowerment (Pilgrim & McCranie, 2013).

While it is important to understand the multiple understandings of mental illness across professionals and the lay public, as well as how these understandings are shaped by interest, we also want to know how these attributes translate into the lives of individuals. An important study by Phelan (2005) provides evidence that public understanding of what mental illness is matters for stigma. In particular, those individuals who believe that mental illness are caused by genes are more likely to stigmatize the sibling of the individual, indicating that such attribution may move us away from a model where something is not only problematic with the individual experiencing mental illness, but also close family members. Research that pushes us to not only show that many of our taken-for-granted assumptions are viewed in such a way because a particular group of individuals have believed them for a long time but that they have consequences for individuals and societies, are all the more powerful than research that simply points out that a wide array of things we take for granted are socially constructed.

Finally, while the perspective of social construction provides an important correction to biological essentialism, it is important that we do not embrace a similarly narrow social essentialism. The debate of nature versus nurture has largely been settled with many agreeing that we need to think about nature and nurture as complementary (Pescosolido et al., 2008), yet some sociologists continue to be skeptical of too close a collaboration with medical doctors and natural scientists focusing on biological roots of illness. While decreasing due to increased emphasis on interdisciplinary approaches both within universities and funding agencies, this standpoint can be dangerous to the field of medical sociology, as cutting-edge research across multiple fields (e.g. medicine, sociology, public health) shows that a large proportion of the dominant illnesses are rooted simultaneously in social, psychological, and biological factors. This provides a unique opportunity as those interested in health and illness from a biological standpoint cannot ignore the importance of social factors, but without direct participation we allow them to trivialize it and rely on faulty measures, as their training is not in understanding the social world. Consequently, it is important for sociologists to continue to step up to the plate and show the power of social factors in shaping our understandings of health, illness, and healing. Current realities do not allow us to do that from a pure social constructionist standpoint, rather we must take into account current knowledge about the complex realities of health and illness in advanced, industrialized nations, such as the United States.

Illustrating Social Construction: The Power of Cross-National Comparisons

As originally pointed out by Berger and Luckmann (1967), the way in which societies are organized and social life is understood quickly becomes a part of who the individual is and how he or she understands the world. That is, even though certain actions and decisions by individuals originally determine how we understand a wide array of social phenomenon and how we provide and organize major social institutions (e.g. education, health care, correctional facilities), this "reality" becomes taken for granted overtime in a way that any other understanding or arrangements seem impossible. While there are many ways to illustrate that other realities are possible, a cross-national perspective is especially powerful in showing how ideas and responses within one cultural context appear strange or even impossible in another cultural context. Yet, individuals happily go about their daily business in both contexts, never wondering if the world could somehow be better, or even different. Issues of health, illness, and healing are no exception as they simultaneously reflect biological and scientific realities and cultural adaptations and understandings.

A cross-national perspective clearly illustrates the power of cultural meanings of illness and perhaps especially mental illness. Depression can serve as an example here, as one of the conditions that has greatly increased in prevalence overtime and has been declared as one of the leading global causes of disability (Murray & Lopez, 1996). This development can partly be explained as Western, biomedical criteria (especially DSM III) are applied to multiple contexts. Therefore, new understandings of depression within a context may have more to do with how mental health is understood within a specific scientific community, as compared to changes where a larger proportion of the population across countries is biologically vulnerable to depression. Here, Lutz (1985) has pointed out that Western psychologists often view the failure to look for happiness as a symptom of depression, yet the desire for happiness is not natural, but a culturally constructed goal. Further what constitutes happiness is likely to vary across the life course as people emphasize different things at different points in time (Buijs et al., 2021). Similarly, Kleinman and Good (1985) argue that a universal experience of depression is unfounded. While some work has indicated that ideas about depression (and other illnesses) travel across national boundaries, research focusing on how global biomedical models of illness are adopted, rejected, or modified at the local level can give us insights into the relationship between medical knowledge and cultural understandings of illness.

What is considered normal and abnormal is different across groups and places within a single society, but a comparison across nations can illustrate this even more profoundly. For example, we can ask whether specific social behaviors and emotions are constructed in the same manner across societies and attempt to explain the variations in understanding across nations. In addition, a cross-national perspective adds to our understanding of labeling and stigma by considering how these processes may operate similarly or differently across context. For example, Olafsdottir (2011) shows that the cultural images associated with mental illness vary systematically across the U.S., Germany, and Iceland. As expected, and often discussed, the overarching picture provided in the U.S. is that individuals experiencing mental illness are dangerous and to be feared. A single society examination may lead to the conclusion that mental health problems are strongly embedded in a culture of fear, yet the analysis from the other two countries shows a different picture. At least partly reflecting the social organization of welfare, the Icelandic context illustrates a culture of solidarity, where mental illness is social in nature and it is the responsibility of society to do something about them both in terms of providing solutions as well as creating society that is more beneficial to mental health. Similarly, the German context is embedded in a specific historical trajectory where the events of World War II have constructed a careful discourse that avoids blame making and highlights the importance of learning from history and never go back to the cruel realities of that period. Research has shown that this overall cultural landscape may contribute to variations in stigma across the three countries by showing that stigmatizing responses correspond to the cultural climate surrounding mental illness (Manago et al., 2019).

Turning to responses to illness, not surprisingly they are embedded within a specific cultural context. An examination of public attitudes in countries that all adhere to similar biomedical understanding of schizophrenia shows that public responses vary, both in terms of lay recognition of schizophrenia as well as appropriate responses. The public, in this sample of advanced, industrialized nations, largely recognizes schizophrenia as mental illness in general, but not schizophrenia in particular and the level of recognition varies drastically (Olafsdottir & Pescosolido, 2011). Similarly, there is a cultural variation in what the public believes should be done about the problem and how effective treatment would be. Importantly, cross-national differences do not only reflect different responses in terms of what individuals do when they encounter illness, but also in what kind of treatment is provided and importantly paid for. Sociologists have pointed out how changes in the reimbursement system within the U.S., impacts what choices are available to doctors when they treat patients (McKinlay, 1996) and this is likely to be even more prominent when examined in a cross-national perspective. Research focusing on what kind of treatments are provided and reimbursed across different societies, in addition to an understanding of how individuals use services and conceptualize the problem, has the potential to add to our understanding of the relationship between culture and responses to illness.

Finally, there is a relationship between culture and medical knowledge. The obvious differences are across what often is labeled as alternative and scientific medicine, but even among nations that adhere to the same biomedical model, differences are observed. As an example, how frequently women are expected to have a cervical cytology varies across countries, as do norms of whether screening for prostate cancer represent a useful strategy to improve men's health at the population level. Of course, it can be argued that countries with more extensive screening are doing a better job, yet that does not translate into population health. In many cases, screening is more frequent in the United States, where health outcomes are still lagging behind most advanced, industrialized nations. And contrasting the United States and Japan, where the latter would have a greater reliance of alternative sources of care, reveals that the Japanese do better on various health outcomes, including life expectancy, that are among the highest in the world. Research that can trace how the cultural context of medical knowledge varies across context, with an attention of how it matters for the health profile of populations is especially valuable to understand the social realities of medicine and how medical knowledge does not merely reflect superior scientific knowledge.

Conclusion

Sociology has an important role in providing a counterpoint to the predominant biological and medical approaches to health and illness. As this chapter has illustrated, the social matters for virtually every aspect of health, illness, and healing. Our understandings of illness and responses are embedded in the community and knowledge is created by individuals with specific background, orientation, and interest, highlighting that social factors play not simply a complementary, but a critical role. This role has perhaps never been more important, as the disease profile of societies has become more complex, and it is impossible to respond to health problems without a serious consideration of how they are embedded within specific cultural contexts. In addition, sociologists have brought issues such as power and interest to the forefront of how we understand and respond to health problems, acknowledging the important role that medicine and the pharmaceutical industry play in responding to illness, while pointing out the dangers associated with too much reliance on professions and corporations, that in the end, have enormous gains associated with a specific understanding of health and illness in contemporary societies. Consequently, the sociological imagination that allows us to connect the society to the individual has perhaps never been more important and holds a power to provide a crucial counterpoint to the biological approach, often assuming that there is an concrete "reality" to our illness and responses to it.

References

Abraham, J. (2010). Pharmaceuticalization of society in context: Theoretical, empirical and health dimensions. *Sociology, 44*(4), 603–622.

Andersen, R. (1968). *Behavioral model of families' use of health services. Center for Health Administration*. University of Chicago.

Andersen, R. (1995). Revisiting the behavioral model and access to medical care: Does it matter? *Journal of Health and Social Behavior, 36*, 1–10.

Becker, H. (1963). *Outsiders: Studies in the sociology of deviance*. Free Press.

Bell, S. E., & Figert, A. E. (2012). Medicalization and pharmaceuticalization at the intersections: Looking backward, sideways and forward. *Social Science & Medicine, 75*(5), 775–783.

Berger, P. L., & Luckmann, T. (1967). *The social construction of reality: A treatise in the sociology of knowledge*. Doubleday.

Bernal, G., Bonilla, J., & Bellido, C. (1995). Ecological validity and cultural sensitivity for outcome research: Issues for the cultural adaptation and development of psychosocial treatments with Hispanics. *Journal of Abnormal Child Psychology, 23*, 67–82.

Bröer, C., & Agyekum, H. A. (2021). Medicalization and manhood: Is an ADHD diagnosis emerging for allegedly troublesome boys in Accra, Ghana? *Social Science & Medicine, 291*, 114465.

Buijs, V. L., Jeronimus, B. F., Lodder, G. M., Steverink, N., & de Jonge, P. (2021). Social needs and happiness: A life course perspective. *Journal of Happiness Studies, 22*(4), 1953–1978.

Burr, V. (1995). *Social constructionism*. Routledge.

Chapple, A., Ziebland, S., & McPherson, A. (2004). Stigma, shame, and blame experienced by patients with lung cancer: Qualitative study. *BMJ*. https://doi.org/10.1136/bmj.38111.639734.7C. (Published 11 June 2004).

Clarke, A. E. (1998). *Disciplining reproduction: Modernity, American life sciences, and "The Problems of Sex"*. University of California Press.

Clarke, A. E., Mamo, L., Fishman, J. R., Shim, J. K., & Fosket, J. R. (2003). Biomedicalization: Technoscientific transformations of health, illness, and U.S. biomedicine. *American Sociological Review, 68*, 161–194.

Clouston, S. A., & Link, B. G. (2021). A retrospective on fundamental cause theory: State of the literature and goals for the future. *Annual Review of Sociology, 47*(1), 131–156.

Conrad, P. (1992). Medicalization and social control. *Annual Review of Sociology, 18*, 209–232.

Conrad, P., & Barker, K. K. (2010). The social construction of illness: Key insights and policy implications. *Journal of Health and Social Behavior, 51*, S50–S79.

Conrad, P., & Leiter, V. (2004). Medicalization, markets and consumers. *Journal of Health and Social Behavior, 45*, 158–176.

Conrad, P., & Schneider, J. W. (1992). *Deviance and medicalization: From badness to sickness*. Temple University Press.

Ehrenreich, B., & English, D. (1978). *For her own good: 150 years of the experts' advice to women*. Doubleday.

Eisenberg, L. (1977). Disease and illness: Distinctions between professional and popular ideas of sickness. *Culture, Medicine and Psychiatry, 1*, 9–23.

Epstein, S. (2007). *Inclusion: The politics of difference in medical research*. The University of Chicago Press.

Figert, A. E. (1996). *Women and the ownership of PMS: The structuring of a psychiatric disorder*. Aldine De Gruyter.

Fishbein, M., & Ajzen, I. (1975). *Belief, attitude, intention, and behavior: An introduction to theory and research*. Addison-Wesley.

Foucault, M. (1965). *Madness and civilization: A history of insanity in the age of reason*. Pantheon Books.

Foucault, M. (1973). *The birth of the clinic: An archaeology of medical perception*. Vintage Books.

Freidson, E. (1970). *Profession of medicine: A study of the sociology of applied knowledge*. Harper & Row.

Godward, J., Riordan, B. C., Winter, T., Ashton, J. C., Hunter, J., & Scarf, D. (2022). Lung cancer attracts greater stigma than other cancer types in Aotearoa New Zealand. *Journal of Oncology, 2022*(1), 2183055–2183056.

Goffman, E. (1961). *Asylums: Essays on the social situation of mental patients and other inmates*. Doubleday.

Goffman, E. (1963). *Stigma: Notes on the management of spoiled identity*. Prentice Hall.

Gong, F., Gage, S.-J., & Tacada, L. A. (2003). Help-seeking behavior among Filipino Americans: A cultural analysis of face and language. *Journal of Community Psychology, 31*, 469–488.

Gove, W. R. (1970). Societal reactions as an explanation of mental illness: An evaluation. *American Sociological Review, 35*, 873–884.

Gove, W. R. (1975). Labeling and mental illness. In W. Gove (Ed.), *The labeling of deviance: Evaluating a perspective* (pp. 35–81). Halsted.

Gregg, J., & Curry, R. H. (1994). Explanatory models for cancer among African-American women at two Atlanta neighborhood health centers: The implications for a cancer screening program. *Social Science and Medicine, 39*, 519–526.

Horwitz, A. (1977). Social networks and pathways to psychiatric treatment. *Social Forces, 56*, 86–105.

Jayasuriya, L. (1992). The problematic of culture and identity in social functioning. *Journal of Multicultural Social Work, 2*, 37–58.

Joyce, K. (2008). *Magnetic appeal: MRI and the myth of transparency*. Cornell University Press.

Jutel, A. (2010). Framing disease: The example of female hypoactive sexual desire disorder. *Social Science and Medicine, 70*, 1084–1090.

Kaczmarek, E. (2022). Promoting diseases to promote drugs: The role of the pharmaceutical industry in fostering good and bad medicalization. *British Journal of Clinical Pharmacology, 88*(1), 34–39.

Kadushin, C. (1966). The friends and supporters of psychotherapy: On social circles in urban life. *American Sociological Review, 31*, 786–802.

Kaiser, K. (2008). The meaning of the survivor identity for women with breast cancer. *Social Science and Medicine, 67*, 79–87.

Kim, B. S. K., & Omizo, M. M. (2003). Asian cultural values, attitudes toward seeking professional psychological help, and willingness to see a counselor. *The Counseling Psychologist, 31*, 343–361.

Kirk, S. A., & Kutchins, H. (1992). *The selling of DSM: The rhetoric of science in psychiatry*. Aldine de Gruyter.

Kleinman, A. (1980). *Patients and healers in the context of culture: An exploration of the borderland between anthropology, medicine, and psychiatry*. University of California Press.

Kleinman, A., & Good, B. J. (Eds.). (1985). *Culture and depression: Studies in the anthropology and cross-cultural psychiatry of affect and disorder*. University of California Press.

Lantz, P. M., Goldberg, D. S., & Gollust, S. E. (2023). The perils of medicalization for population health and health equity. *The Milbank Quarterly, 101*(Suppl 1), 61–82.

Lau, A., & Takeuchi, D. T. (2001). Cultural values in help-seeking for child behavior problems: Value orientation, affective responding, and severity appraisals among Chinese American parents. *Journal of Community Psychology, 29*, 675–692.

Link, B. G. (1982). Mental patient status, work, and income: An examination of the effects of a psychiatric label. *American Sociological Review, 47*, 202–215.

Link, B. G. (1987). Understanding labeling effects in the area of mental disorders: An assessment of the effects of expectations of rejection. *American Sociological Review, 52*, 96–112.

Link, B. G., & Phelan, J. C. (1995). Social conditions as fundamental causes of diseases. *Journal of Health and Social Behavior, 36*(Extra issue), 80–94.

Link, B. G., & Phelan, J. C. (2001). Conceptualizing stigma. *Annual Review of Sociology, 27*, 363–385.

Link, B. G., Cullen, F. T., Struening, E., Shrout, P., & Dohrenwend, B. P. (1989). A modified labeling theory approach in the area of mental disorders: An empirical assessment. *American Sociological Review, 54*, 400–423.

Liu, X., & Luo, Z. (2024). Communicating male sexual dysfunction: The medicalization and psychologization of sexual experiences in Chinese online medical consultations. *Social Science & Medicine, 350*, 116927.

Lorber, J. (1997). *Gender and the social construction of illness*. Sage.

Lutz, C. (1985). Depression and the translation of emotional worlds. In A. Kleinman & B. J. Good (Eds.), *Culture and depression: Studies in the anthropology and cross-cultural psychiatry of affect and disorder* (pp. 63–100). University of California Press.

Manago, B., Pescosolido, B. A., & Olafsdottir, S. (2019). Icelandic inclusion, German hesitation and American fear: A cross-cultural comparison of mental-health stigma and the media. *Scandinavian Journal of Public Health, 47*(2), 90–98.

Martin, J. K., Pescosolido, B. A., & Tuch, S. A. (2000). Of fear and loathing: The role of 'disturbing behavior', labels, and causal attributions in shaping public attitudes toward persons with mental illness. *Journal of Health and Social Behavior, 41*, 208–223.

Martin, J. K., Pescosolido, B. A., Olafsdottir, S., & McLeod, J. D. (2007). The construction of fear: Americans' preferences for social distance from children and adolescents with mental health problems. *Journal of Health and Social Behavior, 48*, 50–67.

McKeown, T. (1979). *The role of medicine: Dream, mirage, or nemesis?* Princeton University Press.

McKinlay, J. B. (1972). Some approaches and problems in the study of the use of services—An overview. *Journal of Health and Social Behavior, 13*, 115–152.

McKinlay, J. B. (1981). Refocusing upstream. In P. Conrad & R. Kern (Eds.), *The sociology of health and illness*. St. Martin's Press.

McKinlay, J. B. (1996). Some contributions from the social system to gender inequalities in heart disease. *Journal of Health and Social Behavior, 37*, 1–26.

Moynihan, R., & Cassels, A. (2005). *Selling sickness: How the world's biggest pharmaceutical companies are turning us all into patients*. Nation Books.

Murray, C. J. L., & Lopez, A. D. (Eds.). (1996). *The global burden of disease*. World Health Organization.

Muzzin, L. J., Anderson, N. J., Figueredo, A. T., & Gudelis, S. O. (1994). The experience of cancer. *Social Science and Medicine, 38*, 1201–1208.

Olafsdottir, S. (2011). Medicalization and mental health: The critique of medical expansion, and a consideration of how National States, markets, and citizens matter. In D. Pilgrim, A. Rogers, & B. A. Pescosolido (Eds.), *The SAGE handbook of mental health and illness* (pp. 239–260). Sage Publications.

Olafsdottir, S. (2022). *Trends in Stigma in Iceland*. Geðhjálp.

Olafsdottir, S., & Pescosolido, B. A. (2009). Drawing the line: The cultural cartography of utilization recommendations for mental health problems. *Journal of Health and Social Behavior, 50*, 228–244.

Olafsdottir, S., & Pescosolido, B. A. (2011). Constructing illness: How the public in eight western Nations responds to a clinical description of Schizophrenia. *Social Science and Medicine, 73*, 929–938.

Pescosolido, B. A. (1992). Beyond rational choice: The social dynamics of how people seek help. *American Journal of Sociology, 97*, 1096–1138.

Pescosolido, B. A. (2011). Organizing the sociological landscape for the next decades of health and health care research: The network episode model III-R as cartographic subfield guide. In

B. A. Pescosolido, J. K. Martin, J. D. McLeod, & A. Rogers (Eds.), *Handbook of the sociology of health, illness, and healing: A blueprint for the 21st century* (pp. 39–66). Springer.
Pescosolido, B. A., & Green, H. D., Jr. (2024). Who has mental health problems? Comparing individual, social and psychiatric constructions of mental health. *Social Psychiatry and Psychiatric Epidemiology, 59*(3), 443–453.
Pescosolido, B., & Olafsdottir, S. (2010). The cultural turn in sociology: Can it help us resolve an age-old problem in understanding decision-making for health care? *Sociological Forum, 25*, 655–676.
Pescosolido, B. A., Brooks-Gardner, C., & Lubell, K. M. (1998a). How people get into mental health services: Stories of choice, coercion and 'muddling through' from 'first-timers'. *Social Science and Medicine, 46*, 275–286.
Pescosolido, B. A., Wright, E. R., Alegria, M., & Vera, M. (1998b). Social networks and patterns of use among the poor with mental health problems in Puerto Rico. *Medical Care, 36*, 1057–1072.
Pescosolido, B. A., Perry, B. L., Scott Long, J., Martin, J. K., Nurnberger, J. I., Jr., & Hesselbrock, V. (2008). Under the influence of genetics: How transdisciplinarity leads us to rethink social pathways to illness. *American Journal of Sociology, 114*, S171–S201.
Pescosolido, B. A., Halpern-Manners, A., Luo, L., & Perry, B. (2021). Trends in public stigma of mental illness in the US, 1996-2018. *JAMA Network Open, 4*(12), e2140202–e2140202.
Phelan, J. C. (2005). Geneticization of deviant behavior and consequences for stigma: The case of mental illness. *Journal of Health and Social Behavior, 46*, 307–322.
Phelan, J. C., Link, B. G., Diez-Roux, A., Kawachi, I., & Levin, B. (2004). "Fundamental causes" of social inequalities in mortality: A test of the theory. *Journal of Health and Social Behavior, 45*(3), 265–285.
Pilgrim, D., & McCranie, A. (2013). *Recovery and mental health: A critical sociological account*. Bloomsbury Publishing.
Rewerska-Juśko, M., & Rejdak, K. (2022, February). Social stigma of patients suffering from COVID-19: Challenges for health care system. *Healthcare, 10*(2), 292. MDPI.
Rosenhan, D. L. (1973). On being sane in insane places. *Science, 179*, 250–258.
Rosenstock, I. M. (1966). Why people use health services. *Milbank Memorial Fund Quarterly, 44*, 94–106.
Rutledge, P. E. (2020). Trump, COVID-19, and the war on expertise. *The American Review of Public Administration, 50*(6–7), 505–511.
Scheff, T. J. (1966). *Being mentally ill: A sociological theory*. Aldine Publishing Company.
Scheff, T. J. (1974). The labeling theory of mental illness. *American Sociological Review, 39*, 444–452.
Schomerus, G., Schindler, S., Sander, C., Baumann, E., & Angermeyer, M. C. (2022). Changes in mental illness stigma over 30 years–Improvement, persistence, or deterioration? *European Psychiatry, 65*(1), e78.
Sontag, S. (1978). *Illness as a metaphor*. Farrar, Straus and Giroux.
Spector, M., & Kitsuse, J. (1977). *Constructing social problems*. Cummings.
Straus, R. (1957). The nature and status of medical sociology. *American Sociological Review, 22*, 200–204.
Szasz, T. S. (1961). *The myth of mental illness: Foundations of a theory of personal conduct*. Dell Publishing Company.
Takeuchi, D. T., Edwina, S. U., & Maramba, G. (1999). Cultural diversity and mental health treatment. In A. V. Horwitz & T. L. Scheid (Eds.), *The sociology of mental health and illness* (pp. 550–565). Cambridge University Press.
Timmermans, S. (2007). *Postmortem: How medical examiners explain suspicious deaths*. The University of Chicago Press.
Warner, E. T., Park, E. R., Luberto, C. M., Rabin, J., Perez, G. K., & Ostroff, J. S. (2022). Internalized stigma among cancer patients enrolled in a smoking cessation trial: The role of cancer type and associations with psychological distress. *Psycho-Oncology, 31*(5), 753–760.

Woolhandler, S., Himmelstein, D. U., Ahmed, S., Bailey, Z., Bassett, M. T., Bird, M., et al. (2021). Public policy and health in the Trump era. *The Lancet, 397*(10275), 705–753.

Xu, J., Sun, G., Cao, W., Fan, W., Pan, Z., Yao, Z., & Li, H. (2021). Stigma, discrimination, and hate crimes in Chinese-speaking world amid Covid-19 pandemic. *Asian Journal of Criminology, 16*(1), 51–74.

Yuan, K., Huang, X. L., Yan, W., Zhang, Y. X., Gong, Y. M., Su, S. Z., et al. (2022). A systematic review and meta-analysis on the prevalence of stigma in infectious diseases, including COVID-19: A call to action. *Molecular Psychiatry, 27*(1), 19–33.

Zola, I. K. (1972). Medicine as an institution of social control. *The Sociological Review, 20*, 487–450.

Chapter 4
Fundamental-Cause Theory

Bruce G. Link and Jo C. Phelan

A stark and very commonly observed fact is evident when rates of morbidity and mortality are arrayed by socioeconomic status (SES), race/ethnicity, or stigmatized identity. All too often, these facts show that society's poorer members, those disadvantaged by racial hierarchies, and those resident in the stigmatized side of an us-them divide live in worse health and die younger than their counterparts. For example, concerning socioeconomic status, evidence suggests an enduring and perhaps even growing association between indicators of socioeconomic status and mortality (Sasson & Hayward, 2019) that is also evident in multiple European countries (Mackenbach et al., 2015). Evidence concerning mortality by race shows that inequalities between Black people and White people were reduced between 1999 and 2011 but then plateaued at an unequal level through 2019 and increased dramatically in 2020 (Caraballo et al., 2023). Evidence focused on disability-free life expectancy rather than mortality shows large gaps favoring non-Hispanic White people compared to both non-Hispanic Black and Hispanic people (Bauldry et al., 2023). Groups that experience societal stigma also frequently experience a mortality disadvantage. There is evidence, for example, of a mortality disadvantage for people who identify as sexual minorities (Hatzenbuehler et al., 2020) people with mental illnesses (Walker et al., 2015), people who have been incarcerated (Fernandez et al., 2022), and people with disabilities (Landes, 2024). Health inequalities like these are not only very common in modern times but have existed at similar levels for quite some time (Antonovsky, 1967). The evidence also indicates that the inequalities are not just evident in particular situations but are found for example in every state in the United States (Montez et al., 2019) and in multiple countries in

B. G. Link (✉)
University of California, Riverside, Riverside, CA, USA
e-mail: brucel@ucr.edu

J. C. Phelan
Columbia University, New York, NY, USA

W. C. Cockerham (ed.), *Medical Sociology on the Move*,
https://doi.org/10.1007/978-3-031-92456-9_4

Europe (Mackenbach et al., 2015). Additionally, across all these circumstances, from disadvantages as different as low socioeconomic status and the experience of a mental illness, the facts show that the health inequalities are not segregated to one particular type of disease but rather extend to many different diseases. The existence of health inequalities across time and place and the nature of the social disadvantage experienced pose a critical problem of explanation. What makes such a variety of health inequalities emerge with such regularity? The regularity is even more puzzling when we consider that the major diseases and risk factors that appeared to account for the inequalities seen in earlier periods, i.e. deadly infectious diseases such as diphtheria, measles, typhoid fever, and tuberculosis fueled by over-crowding and poor sanitation in low socioeconomic status (SES) homes and communities, have been virtually eradicated in the developed world. Rather than disappearing, health inequalities in mortality have persisted and now reflect new major causes of death including cancers and cardiovascular illness, fueled by sometimes newly identified risk and protective factors (Phelan et al., 2010).

It is the existence of health inequalities across such a broad array of disadvantaged circumstances along with their *persistence across time* that the theory of fundamental causes seeks to explain (Link & Phelan, 1995, Phelan et al., 2010, Hatzenbuehler et al., 2013, Clouston & Link, 2021). The theory proposes that we cannot claim to understand why health inequalities exist if we cannot explain why they occur across so many disadvantaged circumstances and persist under conditions that should eliminate or reduce them. Additionally, we reasoned that if we can understand why they persist in so many disadvantaged circumstances, it may provide clues to the more general problem of the causes of health inequalities. That is, the puzzling breadth and persistence of health inequalities may provide a lever for understanding the more general fact of their existence.

In this paper, we will explicate the theory as it has developed since its introduction in 1995, report some of the ways it has been elaborated and extended, indicate how the theory has been tested, and present its implications for efforts to reduce health inequalities.

Original Statement of the Theory

The theory of fundamental causes is rooted in Lieberson's (1985) concept of basic causes, which was first applied to the association between SES and mortality by House and colleagues (House et al., 1990, 1994). The theory has been developed primarily by Link and Phelan (Link & Phelan, 1995, Phelan et al., 2004, Link & Phelan, 2010; Phelan et al., 2010, Phelan & Link, 2015) with significant elaboration and extension by Lutfey and Freese (Lutfey & Freese, 2005; Freese & Lutfey, 2011), Clouston et al. (2016), Hatzenbuehler et al. (2013), and Clouston and Link (2021). The initial statement of the theory focused mainly on socioeconomic health inequalities, with subsequent extensions to racism (Phelan & Link, 2015) and stigmatized statuses more generally (Hatzenbuehler et al., 2013)

Writing in 1995 Link and Phelan (1995) indicated that a fundamental social cause of health inequalities has four essential features: First, it influences multiple disease outcomes, meaning that it is not limited to only one or a few diseases or health problems. Second, it affects these disease outcomes through multiple risk and protective factors. Third, fundamental social causes involve access to resources that can be used to avoid risks or to minimize the consequences of disease once it occurs. Finally, the association between a fundamental cause and health is reproduced overtime via the replacement of intervening mechanisms. It is their persistent effect on overall health in the face of dramatic changes in mechanisms that led Link and Phelan to call them "fundamental."

Mechanism Generators

Embedded within this statement of the essential features of a fundamental cause lies a provocative question. What causes the mechanisms to be replaced? Is it diabolical magic? Some malevolent force that reliably ensures that those at the bottom of whatever disadvantaged circumstance we consider experience inferior health outcomes? Clearly, this is a critical question that fundamental-cause theory needs to address. As a result, we now propose an additional requirement for the identification of a fundamental cause and that is a specification of what it is that leads to the replacement of mechanisms linking a fundamental cause to disease. A "mechanism generator" needs to be specified.

Flexible Resources as a Mechanism Generator

According to the theory of fundamental causes, one reason that SES is related to multiple disease outcomes through multiple pathways that change over time is that individuals and groups deploy resources to avoid risks and adopt protective strategies. Key resources such as knowledge, money, power, prestige, and beneficial social connections can be used no matter what the risk and protective factors are in a given circumstance. Consequently, fundamental causes affect health even when the profile of risk and protective factors and diseases changes radically. If the problem is cholera, for example, a person with greater resources is better able to avoid areas where the disease is rampant. If the problem is heart disease, a person with greater resources is better able to maintain a heart-healthy lifestyle and get the best medical treatment available. Because the sources involved can be used in different ways in different situations, we call them flexible resources.

To understand how flexible resources might facilitate the creation of new mechanisms linking SES and health, consider the following example. Screening for several deadly cancers has become possible over the past few decades, making it feasible to detect cancer or its precursors earlier, thereby helping to prevent mortality from these cancers. Since the screening procedures represent relatively recent technological advances, one can imagine a time before the procedures existed, when resources had no bearing on access to cancer screening because the procedures did not exist. There was no SES → Access to Screening → Health mechanism. After the screening procedures were developed, people with more resources could use those resources to gain access to the life-saving screens (Link et al., 1998; Clouston et al., 2020).

The flexible resources that are central to fundamental-cause theory operate at both individual and contextual levels. At the individual level, flexible resources can be conceptualized as the "causes of causes" or "risks of risk" that shape individual health behaviors by influencing whether people know about, have access to, can afford, and receive social support for their efforts to engage in health-enhancing or health-protective behaviors. In addition, resources shape access to broad contexts that vary dramatically in associated risk profiles and protective factors. For example, a person with many resources can afford to live in a high SES neighborhood where neighbors are also of high status and where, collectively, enormous clout is exerted to ensure that crime, noise, violence, pollution, traffic, and vermin are kept at a minimum and that the best health-care facilities, parks, playgrounds, and food stores are located nearby. Once a person has used SES-related resources to locate in an advantaged neighborhood, a host of health-enhancing circumstances comes along as a "package deal." Similarly, a person who uses educational credentials to procure a high-status occupation inherits a package deal that is more likely to include excellent health benefits and less likely to involve dangerous conditions and toxic exposures. Similarly, Cockerham (2005) describes how health lifestyles are shaped by one's status group. According to Cockerham, social norms and other social supports such as the health-product industry reinforce distinctive health lifestyles in different status groups, and the lifestyles of high SES groups are particularly healthful ones. In these circumstances, the person benefits in numerous ways that do not depend on his/her initiative or ability to personally construct a healthy situation—it is an "add-on" benefit operative at the contextual level. The same sort of add-on benefit can be enjoyed in other important contexts such as social networks, families, and marriages.

The Motivation to Keep People Down, In, or Away as a Mechanism Generator

A second mechanism generator was identified in extensions of FTC to racism (Phelan & Link, 2015) and stigma (Hatzenbuehler et al., 2013). Here the observation was that stigma can be used to achieve the desired ends of keeping people "down" to exploit or dominate them, "in" to control them, or "away" to exclude or segregate them (Phelan et al., 2008). Concerning *keeping people down,* high social status can be attained by a powerful group when that group successfully dominates or exploits another. Stigmatization helps create, legitimate, and perpetuate these inequalities as the stigmatized group is deemed to be inferior in terms of intelligence, character, competence, and the basic human qualities of worthiness and value (Phelan et al., 2008). Classic examples are the racial stigmatization of Black people beginning in the era of slavery, the Europeans' colonization of countries around the globe, and U.S. Whites' expropriation of the lands of American Indians (Feagin, 2010).

Concerning *keeping people in,* stigma can be used to enforce social norms so as to control people. Stigma is useful because it confers the painful cost of social disapproval that aims to make subsequent non-normative behavior less likely. But individually experienced social disapproval is not the only way stigma can be used to keep people in, as the people around the norm violator are also kept in by learning the boundaries of acceptable behavior and by observing what happens to someone who goes beyond those boundaries (Erikson, 1966). Concerning *keeping people away*, stigma can be effectively used to exclude people as stigma-related stereotypes are deployed to justify discrimination in jobs, housing, education, or medical care.

When people have an interest in keeping other people down, in, or away, stigma is a resource that allows them to obtain the ends they desire. Link and Phelan (2014) called this resource "stigma power" and used the term to refer to instances in which stigma processes achieve the aims of stigmatizers with respect to the exploitation, control, or exclusion of others. If a motivation to stigmatize remains, then as one mechanism for keeping people down, in, or away is blocked, another will take its place as those who benefit from stigmatizing others seek new ways to achieve desired ends. In addition to an enduring motivation, an additional required element for mechanism replacement is the existence of alternative mechanisms. In this regard, ever since Goffman (1963) began to unravel all the ways in which stigma can be enacted, it is clear that a "massive multiplicity" (Lutfey & Freese, 2005) of alternative mechanisms are available for use. There are just so many ways to exclude, disrespect and shame, so many possibilities to treat people in ways that indicate that they do not belong, are of lesser value, or are undeserving of basic human dignity, that finding alternative mechanisms can be easily achieved. Thus, in our formulation stigmatization/racism can be conceptualized as a mechanism generator that persistently separates the health fortunes of people who are exposed to stigma from those who are not. The addition of this second mechanism-generator is important for FCT because it allows the theory to account for persistent health inequalities that go beyond SES and that result from racism and stigmatization.

Testing Fundamental-Cause Theory

Is it possible to test FCT? FCT's proposition that a fundamental cause is related to multiple disease outcomes through multiple replaceable mechanisms demands that some empirical regularities need to be observed for the theory to have some relevance. As our brief recounting (see above) of recent facts regarding descriptive patterns of disease and death by SES, race/ethnicity, and some stigmatized statuses indicates, existing patterns continue to reflect the possibility that fundamental causes may be at work. It is possible that these descriptive facts could have changed since the theory was originally proposed 30 years ago but this is not something that has occurred. These enduring patterns of health inequality are a modest historical test of the ideas underlying FCT. However skeptical consumers may want and are entitled to more stringent testing.

The strongest tests of FCT make novel predictions—*ones that other theories would not make*. To the extent that predictions like these are supported by evidence, FCT gains credence and to the extent that such predictions fail, the theory loses credibility. Following this line of reasoning, Clouston and Link (2021) identified three approaches to testing FTC. The key feature of each of these tests involves identifying circumstances in which flexible resources can be more or less effective in garnering a health advantage.

The first approach is what they call **disease preventability** (Clouston & Link, 2021). Pioneered by Phelan et al. (2004) this approach examines the association between SES and mortality across multiple disease outcomes that vary in the preventability of death. Because FCT claims that SES associations emerge when people use flexible resources to garner a health advantage, it follows that if people are less able to use such resources to protect themselves (low preventability diseases), SES associations with mortality should be smaller than for diseases in which resources can be effectively deployed (high preventability disease). If we know little about how to prevent or cure a disease, resources are less useful for protecting oneself or those in one's circle of caring. If on the other hand, ways to avoid a disease or mitigate its consequences exist, then resources can be effectively used to protect health.

A second approach involves **preventability shifts** (Clouston & Link, 2021). In this approach, one tests the theory by focusing on particular diseases over time, before and after changes occurred in our capacity to address mortality from that particular disease. FCT predicts that when new knowledge or technology becomes available, people of higher SES are more able to benefit and SES associations with the disease will emerge or grow stronger.

The third approach is what Clouston and Link (2021) called **manipulated preventability**. In this approach, one examines whether inequalities by SES and/or race/ethnicity emerge during controlled trials where the interventions are randomly assigned. In this instance, the FCT prediction is that when effective interventions are randomly assigned but require resources to be effectively implemented, inequalities will emerge in the active treatment arm because higher SES individuals can use flexible resources to extract maximum benefit from the intervention whereas lower SES individuals are impeded in their capacity to do so. In a placebo group or no treatment control where the beneficial treatment is not available, the same flexible resources have little utility because the active treatment is not available to this group. SES inequalities are expected in the treatment but not the control arm of the experiment.

Clouston & Link, 2021 identified two reasons these approaches to testing FTC are effective. First, the predictions are directly derived from the idea of flexible resources and therefore seek instances in which such resources vary in whether they can or cannot be used to achieve a health advantage. When such circumstances can be identified, a very specific FCT-derived prediction about when SES-disease associations should be stronger or weaker is possible. Second, the predictions are novel in the sense that other theories or explanations for SES-disease associations would not make these predictions. For example, stress theory would have no reason to predict that SES-related stress happens to be greater for diseases that are more as opposed to less preventable. Similarly, if stress were the key driver of SES-disease outcomes one would expect such stress to operate both before and after the implementation of new knowledge or technology, creating a constant SES-disease association over time. Similarly, selection theories invoking reverse causation or confounding due to a common cause (e.g. genetic differences) would have no reason to predict that disability or genetic differences would work more strongly for preventable than non-preventable disease. And for the instances in which inverse associations emerge after the implementation of life-saving knowledge or technology becomes available, it is difficult from a selection theory point of view to explain why the selection processes did not operate before the new knowledge or technology emerged. Because FTC makes predictions for SES-mortality associations that other theories would not make in these circumstances, evidence about the outcome of these tests carry evidence about the utility of FCT.

Evidence from Tests

Having identified the three approaches to testing FCT, Clouston and Link (2021) presented evidence from 21 studies that used one of the three approaches to testing—12 labeled disease preventability, 5 preventability shifts, and 4 manipulated preventability. Using the authors' conclusions as a basis, Clouston and Link (2021) found that in general, the studies supported predictions of FCT. None of the studies reviewed claimed to strongly disconfirm the theory.

Additional evidence from tests of FTC has accrued since the Clouston and Link review (2021). One particularly salient test used the preventability-shift approach to understand the spread of Covid 19. In the early phase of the pandemic, the virus entered the U.S. through international travel, primarily carried by world-traveling affluent individuals. Early outbreaks emerged in locations like cruise ships and ski resorts, spreading undetected among travelers due to limited awareness of the disease's extent. The lack of knowledge at this stage hindered an effective response, constituting a stage of low preventability. However, as understanding of the virus improved, people with more resources were able to use those resources to arrange to work at home, avoid crowded circumstances, and even have others shop for groceries for them. These precautions enabled wealthier populations to limit within-community transmission and protect themselves. Meanwhile, people with fewer resources were disproportionately classified as essential workers or lived in crowded family conditions that did not allow social distancing. Consistent with these possibilities, evidence about the pandemic spread showed that rates were initially higher in higher SES counties in the United States (where world travelers were more common) but then shifted dramatically over time to affect lower SES counties more strongly (Clouston et al., 2021).

A study by Schmitz et al. (2024) proposes a new approach to testing fundamental-cause theory. It seeks to identify the unusual but theoretically enlightening circumstance in which people from different socioeconomic positions reside in largely standardized living conditions. While this is very rarely the case, Schmitz et al. (2024) identify such a circumstance in the life circumstances of monks who are distinguished as high SES if they are "padres" and low SES if they are "brothers." The interesting fact is that though distinguished by SES, the padres and brothers live in very similar standardized circumstances. Padres are not able to use SES-based flexible resources to garner an advantage over brothers because the conditions of life are largely standardized. Under this circumstance, FCT with its emphasis on the use of flexible resources predicts no SES association. This is what Schmitz et al. (2024) find across multiple cohorts of data about the longevity of the monks.

In the context of this general support for FCT, studies also find instances in which there are anomalies. For example, a study by Mackenbach et al. (2015) implemented a test using the disease-preventability approach in 19 settings in Europe and found that in the vast majority of tests, the FCT hypotheses were supported for both men and women but in a very few it was not. In other instances, elaborations of FTC were needed to fully account for the pattern of results (e.g. Zapata-Moya et al., 2019). In sum, the evidence signals substantial support for FCT but also, as Mackenbach et al. note, "other mechanisms than the theory implies also play a role" (2017, p. 1117). In keeping with this latter observation, we take up some potential elaborations of the theory that might broaden explanatory power and also present FCT as a "theory of the middle range" that needs to join other theories to achieve a more comprehensive explanation.

Elaborations of Fundamental-Cause Theory

Metamechanisms

Lutfey and Freese (2005) introduced the concept of "*metamechanism*" to indicate that a fundamental cause is "responsible for how specific and varied mechanisms are continuously generated over historical time in such a way that the direction of the enduring association is preserved…" (1327–1328). In a subsequent elaboration of the concept Freese and Lutfey (2011) propose three metamechanisms—***spillovers***, ***habitus***, and ***institutional processing***—as complements to individually-based resources. The major goal of their proposal was to account for situations in which higher SES people benefit without directly identifying a health-enhancing action or choice to use resources.

"Spillovers" occur when people use their resources to benefit themselves but in doing so, produce health benefits for other individuals they are connected to via social networks or neighborhood residence. A second metamechanism, "habitus," draws on work by Cockerham (2005) on health-lifestyle theory. In this metamechanism, different norms, dispositions, and lifestyles develop among different social-class groups, with those of higher status groups being more beneficial to health. For example, Bourdieu (1984) found that French working-class people preferred foods that were cheap and nutritious, whereas professionals preferred a diet that was tasty, healthful, light, and low in calories. In the case of habitus, unlike spillovers, the individual's health-related behavior does play a role in their health outcomes, but instead of being purposefully used to enhance health, these ways of being are not consciously aimed at improving one's health. Rather, they are preferences resulting from differential class-related socialization. "Institutions" as a third metamechanism refers to the agentic, dynamic action of institutions that end up treating people differentially according to their SES in a way that affects health inequalities. For example, Lutfey and Freese (2005) found that two diabetes clinics serving higher- vs. lower-SES patients differed in many aspects of medical care and educational resources that would be expected to contribute to SES differences in diabetes outcomes.

One contribution of Freese and Lutfey's delineation of metamechanisms is to extend the set of processes linking fundamental causes to health inequalities. The introduction of these concepts allows researchers to more fully and precisely identify these processes and the distinctions between them. They are particularly valuable in showing that some large part of the action derives from an individual's embeddedness in a context and that these contextual factors are part of how fundamental causality is realized. At the same time, in our view, individual resources remain vital in meta-mechanisms and should maintain a central place in fundamental-cause theory. People are not accidentally situated in neighborhoods or networks where spillovers occur, in social contexts where healthy dispositions (habitus) can be developed, or in institutions that can be expected to differentially process them. They may not nestle themselves into circumstances like these because of health concerns but they do regularly use resources to enhance their location in these respects. For these reasons, we argue that resources should retain a primary position in FCT.

Mechanism Demise and Death

Whereas, understandably, more attention has been given to the creation of mechanisms that produce health inequalities, fundamental-cause theory is predicated on the idea that mechanisms are *replaced*. Replacement implies that older mechanisms wane in importance over time. In fact, the theory emerged in part *because* prominent risk-factor mechanisms associated with vicious infectious diseases declined in significance as germ theory, improved sanitation, and vaccination came into existence. Thus, understanding the demise and death of mechanisms linking flexible resources to disease is an important area that needs more development and testing. We offer two examples. Salk's discovery of the polio vaccine is an example of a mechanism that was very short-lived. Before his discovery, people of all resource levels were afflicted, including, for example, President Franklin Roosevelt. After the discovery, resource-rich individuals were more likely to receive the vaccine and be protected (Glasser, 1958). A mechanism linking resources to health existed, but only for a short time. The vaccine was quickly approved for widespread dissemination to the United States population, and polio was virtually eradicated here. Other mechanisms remain potent for a very long time. For example, the discovery of the Pap test for the early detection and prevention of cervical cancer has existed since the 1940s. Early on, access to the test was shaped by flexible resources, creating an inequality in the use of this life-saving screen that remains prominent today (Asare et al., 2024). As these examples suggest, some mechanisms become long-lasting while others have short lives. If we can understand what leads to the demise of mechanisms and especially how that decline is related to flexible resources, we may open avenues to speed such a demise and reduce health inequalities. Indeed, much of the public health significance of fundamental-cause theory may reside in understanding how the link between flexible resources and health-relevant risk and protective factors has been broken.

Clouston et al. (2016) further elaborate and systematize the idea of mechanism demise and death by suggesting that social inequalities in health rise and fall according to a predictable dynamic process, which they call the "unnatural history of disease." Clouston et al. (2016) characterize the history of disease as falling into four stages: (1) The Natural Mortality stage is characterized by a lack of knowledge about prevention or effective treatment. Diseases in this stage are either randomly distributed across cleavages of advantage or are distributed non-randomly due to differential exposures to unknown causes of the disease. Consequently, diseases in this stage sometimes favor advantaged groups, other times favor disadvantaged ones, and still other times show no association with advantage. (2) In the stage of Producing Inequalities, populations develop new capacities to reduce the mortality burden of a disease, and the benefits of this capacity are unevenly distributed among SES groups, producing health inequalities. Fundamental-cause theory and its tests have focused largely on the transition from the first to the second stage. (3) To the extent that health-beneficial innovations become more universal and evenly distributed throughout the population, Clouston et al. (2016) predict a decrease in social inequalities in the Reducing Inequalities stage. This can occur if the innovation saturates the advantaged group, making further reduction impossible, or if diffusion efforts are sufficiently focused and the innovation is made widely accessible. In this situation, inequalities will stabilize or even shrink. (4) In the Reduced Mortality and Disease Death stage, a specific health innovation becomes universal, and no more gains can be made, regardless of socioeconomic status. This asymptote may be determined either by the effectiveness of the treatment (Reduced Mortality) or by the eradication of the disease itself (Disease Death).

Whether and when a disease moves from one stage to another will be influenced by social factors such as political and social efforts to reduce mortality in disadvantaged groups and biological factors such as the long incubation periods for some diseases such as lung cancer.

Paradoxes

Some descriptive epidemiological patterns of mortality run counter to expectations based on FCT and other SES-related theories. One of the most prominent of these has been called the "Latinx paradox" due to the finding that people of Latinx origin tend to live longer than their White counterparts despite being substantially disadvantaged in education, income, wealth, and exposure to discrimination (Markides & Coreil, 1986; Hummer & Hamilton, 2019). Similarly, women generally live longer than men despite differences that disadvantage women in terms of income and power. These descriptive patterns suggest that something other than resource utilization is at work, thereby posing a potential "paradox" for FCT. At the same time, as referenced in the introduction, findings focused on so-called disability-free years instead of mortality show patterns for Latinx groups that are consistent with FCT. Using large US data sets, Bauldry and colleagues define dual-function disability-free years as time spent living without significant physical or cognitive impairment. They show that when this metric is employed, there is a substantial gap favoring non-Hispanic White men and women over both foreign and US-born Hispanic men and women.

Beyond potentially paradoxical examples of epidemiological patterns, Clouston and Link (2021) identified two sets of processes that are likely to produce "paradoxical results" from an FCT vantage point: giving greater value to ends other than health, and exposure to constrained choices. Following Lutfey and Freese (2005) we call these "countervailing processes" as they push away from associations predicted by FCT.

Competing Valuations

An important assumption in fundamental-cause theory (FCT) is that when allowed to improve survival, individuals and communities will prioritize actions that enhance their health (Clouston & Link, 2021). While this assumption is generally valid, research suggests that it does not always hold. In some cases, concerns about long-term survival may be outweighed by competing priorities that individuals perceive as more essential to their identity, core values, or financial circumstances. For instance, engaging in known risky behaviors may provide individuals with benefits they deem valuable. Examples include activities traditionally associated with masculinity, such as playing professional football, serving in combat, or heroically rushing into burning buildings as a first responder—actions that confer social status or financial rewards despite posing significant health risks (Courtenay, 2000). This kind of prioritizing of status-conferring but dangerous activities and behaviors by men may be one reason for gender differences in mortality that run counter to FCT predictions. But beyond issues of gender, it is important to be reminded that individuals may choose to overlook the long-term consequences of risky behaviors in favor of their immediate social or personal benefits, such as inclusion in cultural groups, heightened social status, or a sense of control. However, despite these exceptions, health remains a widely valued priority in most cases and when it does we can expect FCT processes to operate.

Choice Constraint

A second assumption of fundamental-cause theory (FCT) is that individuals, whether acting alone or collectively, can effectively use flexible resources to enhance their health and survival. However, Bird and Rieker (2008) famously argued that these choices are often constrained by factors operating at multiple levels, including (1) the workplace and family, (2) community contexts, and (3) social policy structures. At each of these levels, norms, policies, and institutional practices can either facilitate or obstruct individuals' ability to pursue health-promoting behaviors (Bird & Rieker, 2008).

For instance, systemic racism limits the ability of racial and ethnic minorities to leverage flexible resources for health. Demonstrating this, Colen et al. (2018) analyzed 20 years of longitudinal data and found that Black individuals who experienced upward class mobility received fewer health benefits from that mobility compared to Whites. Other research supports this finding as it shows that protective effects of education and employment status tend to be more pronounced in privileged populations—such as highly educated White men—while offering fewer health advantages to others (Assari & Lankarani, 2016; Assari, 2018). This suggests that even when resources are ostensibly available to Black individuals, institutional racism limits their ability to translate these resources into health gains (Clouston & Link, 2021).

While these countervailing processes may sometimes challenge the assumptions of FCT, they do not eliminate the broader pattern of health inequalities by race and socioeconomic status, which remain consistently observed. Recognizing these constraints is crucial, as they help explain variations in the magnitude of health inequalities across different contexts. Moreover, as Phelan et al. (2010) suggest, identifying these constraints in advance can strengthen the testing of FCT. These constraints either arise because individuals prioritize other values over health or because structural conditions prevent the effective use of flexible resources. If the expected relationship between resource access and health outcomes weakens in settings where resource use is blocked, it reinforces the idea that such resources are indeed central to health advantage when they are accessible.

Fundamental Causality as a "Theory of the Middle Range"

Despite the ambitious name that Link and Phelan affixed to the theory (for reasons indicated above), fundamental-cause theory is best characterized as a theory of the middle range. In explicating his concept of middle-range theory Merton (1949, p. 5) proposed the need for theories "intermediate to the minor working hypotheses evolved in abundance during the day-by-day routine of research, and the all-inclusive speculations comprising a master conceptual scheme." For Merton, the day-to-day hypotheses fell short in their ability to produce robust synthetic explanations, whereas grand theories were too speculative and too far removed from the possibility of empirical testing to be useful. Fundamental-cause theory is a middle-range theory in that it resides above day-to-day hypotheses such as: Is SES causally related to disease x, to disease y, or disease z?; or is SES linked to disease x through risk factors a, b, or c? Instead, fundamental-cause theory explains why SES might be related to many diseases and why such an association might be reproduced in multiple contexts and at different times. At the same time, fundamental-cause theory resides below 'grand theory' in that it identifies a relatively specific phenomenon it seeks to explain—connections between health and social factors like SES and discrimination. Further unlike the prototype of grand theory that Merton describes, fundamental-cause theory generates, as we have shown above, empirical predictions that can yield evidence bearing on the theory's truth value.

Implicit in the idea that fundamental-cause theory is a theory of the middle range is that it must join with other theories to account for the social distribution of health and illness. Within medical sociology, other middle-range theories that need to be engaged are social-stress theory, a theory concerning health lifestyles, and an emerging sociological theory of health selection, among others. At the same time, there exists substantial evidence to indicate that other middle-range theories in medical sociology need to embrace fundamental-cause theory to account for some empirical findings that have not been adequately explained by those theories. Much of the evidence for fundamental-cause theory is presented above, but two sets of facts speak to the necessity of the perspective, because these facts are consistent with fundamental-cause theory but have not been explained by other middle-range theories in medical sociology. As indicated in the section on testing FCT, some of the predictions that the theory makes are novel in that other theories would not make them. The most comprehensive explanation is likely to be built around multiple intersecting medical-sociological theories.

Implications for Health Policy

FCT leads to very different policies for addressing health inequalities than does an individually oriented risk-factor approach. The latter asks us to locate modifiable risk factors that lie between distal causes (such as SES) and disease and to intervene in those risk factors. By addressing intervening factors, the logic goes, we will eliminate health disparities.

FCT points to pitfalls in this logic. The pitfall resides in the fact that lying behind individual risk and protective factors are fundamental causes that involve what we have called "mechanism generators." Unless addressed in and of themselves, these fundamental causes will recreate health inequalities by socioeconomic status, race/ethnicity, and multiple stigmatized circumstances. As described above, one of the mechanism generators encompasses SES-related flexible resources that can be used to avoid risks and adopt protective factors no matter what those factors are in a given place or time. The second mechanism generator is a motivation to keep other people "down" to exploit them, "in" to control them, or "away" to exclude them. As long as the motivation endures and people have the power to act on their inclinations, we expect them to creatively identify mechanisms that will allow them to achieve the ends they desire. The recipients of being kept down, in, or away are harmed not only by the resource depletion it brings but also by the process of stigmatization and the resulting minority stress it entails. One set of policy implications involves addressing the fundamental causes themselves.

Policies that Directly Address Fundamental Causes

While outside the domain of health policy per se, one of the most direct policy implications of FCT is that, if we redistribute resources in the population to reduce the degree of resource inequality, inequalities in health should also decline. Policies relevant to fundamental causes of disease form a major part of the national agenda, whether this involves the minimum wage, housing for unhoused people, capital gains and estate taxes, parenting leave, social security, head-start programs, college-admission policies, regulation of lending practices, or other initiatives of this type. We argue, consistent with the health-in-all-policies framework (Amdam, 2025) that all these policies are health-relevant policies and that understanding how they are should be claimed as an essential part of the domain of medical sociology.

The extension of FCT to include racism and stigmatization policies and interventions that directly address these factors are expected to impact health inequalities. Accumulating evidence focused on the concept of "structural stigma" has shown that LGBTQ+ individuals exposed to adverse structural conditions experience harm to their health (Hatzenbuehler et al., 2024). What the evidence also seems to show is that policies can enact stigma and harm health or mitigate stigma and improve health depending on the valence of the structural intervention (Link & Hatzenbuehler,

2016). Thus, the evidence suggests that fundamental causes stemming from racism and stigmatization can be altered by policy at the structural level, but so far, the structural interventions implemented have just as often harmed as helped.

Other Strategies to Reduce Health Inequalities

Short of addressing the fundamental causes themselves, we suggest public health approaches that either reduce the importance of resources in obtaining benefits (or avoiding risks) or are delivered to entire contexts benefiting everyone independent of their level of resources. Adopting approaches like these may not entirely eliminate health inequalities by socioeconomic status, race/ethnicity, and stigmatized statuses, but they could help to reduce them.

Contextualize risk and protective factors. Potential interventions that seek to change individual risk profiles should first analyze factors that put people at risk of risks. If, for example, the issue is gaining access to a beneficial health screen, the factors that block access should be identified and then interventions constructed that simultaneously address the specific behavior and the contextual factors surrounding that behavior. If such a contextualized approach is adopted, it will reduce the salience of resource differences that otherwise would have been expressed in the outcome.

Prioritize the development of interventions that do not entail the use of resources or that minimize the relevance of resources. As we seek to create interventions to improve health, we need to ask if an intervention is something that anyone can potentially adopt, or whether the benefit will only be available to people with the requisite resources. Fundamental-cause theory suggests that health inequalities based on SES can be reduced by instituting health interventions that automatically benefit individuals irrespective of their own resources or behaviors. Examples are the manufacture of automobiles with airbags in addition to seat belts; providing health screenings in schools, workplaces, and other community settings rather than through private physicians; requiring window guards in all high-rise apartments rather than advising parents to watch their children carefully; thoroughly inspecting meat rather than advising consumers to wash cutting boards and cook meat thoroughly; requiring landlords to keep homes free of lead paint hazards rather than warning parents to protect their toddlers from chipped paint. In each example, the former solution does not give an advantage to those with greater resources, because individual resources are unrelated and irrelevant to benefiting from the intervention.

Attend to the Characteristics of the Interventions Adopted. Even if we become far more creative in developing contextually based interventions that blanket an entire population with a health benefit, addressing many health problems will still require individual resources and action. In these cases, resource-rich persons are likely to fare better. Even in these cases, however, we can influence the trajectory of inequalities by attending to the attributes of the interventions we adopt. When we create interventions that are expensive, complicated, time-consuming to carry out, and difficult to distribute broadly, we are likely to create health disparities (Chang & Lauderdale, 2009). Conversely, to the extent that we develop interventions that are relatively affordable and easy to disseminate, we should be able to reduce the degree to which new interventions give an advantage to high SES persons. For example, Goldman and Lakdawalla (2005) analyzed two case studies supporting the idea that the introduction of difficult-to-implement treatments (in their analysis, HAART treatment for HIV/AIDS) lead to increased SES inequalities in health outcomes, whereas treatments that are simpler and require less effort (in their analysis, beta-blockers to reduce hypertension) reduce such inequalities. As Chang and Lauderdale (2009) suggest, this principle should also apply to cost: New interventions that are less expensive should result in smaller SES-based health inequalities than those that are more expensive.

Conclusion

We have sought to explicate the theory of fundamental social causes of health inequalities as it has developed since it was first published in 1995. Since that time, the theory has been extended to incorporate racism and stigmatization as fundamental causes, and multiple strategies for testing the theory have been developed. The evidence suggests substantial support for the theory, and its usefulness has been underscored, for example, by its capacity to help understand the unequal consequences of the COVID-19 pandemic. At the current time, we see FCT as a theory of the middle range that helps us understand the social pattern of disease and death from a distinctly sociological vantage point.

References

Amdam, R. (2025). *New perspectives in health promotion: Health in all policies*. Routledge.

Antonovsky, A. (1967). Social class, life expectancy, and overall mortality. *Milbank Memorial Quarterly, 45*, 31–73.

Asare, M., Owusu-Sekyere, E., Elizondo, A., & Benavidez, G. A. (2024). Exploring cervical cancer screening uptake among women in the United States: Impact of social determinants of health and psychosocial determinants. *Behavioral Sciences, 14*(9), 811.

Assari, S. (2018). Unequal gain of equal resources across racial groups. *International Journal of Health Policy and Management, 7*, 1–9.

Assari, S., & Lankarani, M. M. (2016). Race and urbanity alter the protective effect of education but not income on mortality. *Frontiers in Public Health, 4*, 100.

Bauldry, S., Thomas, P. A., Sauerteig-Rolston, M. R., & Ferraro, K. F. (2023). Racial–ethnic disparities in dual-function life expectancy. *The Journals of Gerontology: Series A, 78*(7), 1269–1275.

Bird, C. E., & Rieker, P. P. (2008). *Gender and health: The effects of constrained choices and social policies*. Cambridge Univ. Press.

Bourdieu, P. (1984). *Distinction: A social critique of the judgment of taste*. Harvard University Press.

Caraballo, C., Massey, D. S., Ndumele, C. D., et al. (2023). Excess mortality and years of potential life lost among the Black population in the US, 1999–2020. *JAMA, 329*(19), 1662–1670. https://doi.org/10.1001/jama.2023.7022

Chang, V. W., & Lauderdale, D. S. (2009). Fundamental cause theory, technological innovation, and health disparities: The case of cholesterol in the era of statins. *Journal of Health and Social Behavior, 50*, 245–260.

Clouston, S. A., & Link, B. G. (2021). A retrospective on fundamental cause theory: State of the literature and goals for the future. *Annual Review of Sociology, 47*(1), 131–156.

Clouston, S. A. P., Rubin, M. S., Phelan, J. C., & Link, B. G. (2016). A social history of disease: Contextualizing the rise and fall of social inequalities in cause-specific mortality. *Demography, 53*(5), 1631–1656.

Clouston, S. A. P., Acker, J., Rubin, M. S., Chae, D. H., & Link, B. G. (2020). Fundamental social causes of inequalities in colorectal cancer mortality: A study of behavioral and medical mechanisms. *Heliyon, 6*, e03484.

Clouston, S. A., Natale, G., & Link, B. G. (2021). Socioeconomic inequalities in the spread of coronavirus-19 in the United States: An examination of the emergence of social inequalities. *Social Science & Medicine, 268*, 113554. https://doi.org/10.1016/j.socscimed.2020.113554

Cockerham, W. (2005). Health lifestyle theory and the convergence of agency and structure. *Journal of Health & Social Behavior, 46*, 51–67.

Colen, C. G., Krueger, P. M., & Boettner, B. L. (2018). Do rising tides lift all boats? Racial disparities in health across the lifecourse among middle-class African-Americans and Whites. *SSM-Population Health, 6*, 125–135.

Courtenay, W. H. (2000). Constructions of masculinity and their influence on men's well-being: A theory of gender and health. *Social Science & Medicine, 50*, 1385–1401.

Erikson, K. T. (1966). *Wayward puritans: A study in the sociology of deviance*. Wiley.

Feagin, J. (2010). *Racist America: Roots, current realities, and future reparations*. Routledge.

Fernandez, L., Ennis, S., Porter, S. R., & Carson, E. (2022). *Mortality in a multi-state cohort of former state prisoners, 2010–2015*. US Census Bureau, Center for Economic Studies.

Freese, J., & Lutfey, K. (2011). Fundamental causality: Challenges of an animating concept for medical sociology. In B. A. Pescosolido, J. K. Martin, J. D. McLeod, & A. Rogers (Eds.), *Handbook of the sociology of health, illness, and healing: A blueprint for the 21st century* (pp. 67–81). Springer.

Glasser, M. A. (1958). Attitudes and reactions of the public to health programs: I. A study of the public's acceptance of the Salk Vaccine Program. *American Journal of Public Health and the Nation's Health, 48*(2), 141–146.

Goffman, E. (1963). *Stigma: Notes on the management of spoiled identity*. Prentice-Hall.

Goldman, D. P., & Lakdawalla, D. N. (2005). A theory of health disparities and medical technology. *Contributions to Economic Analysis and Policy, 4*, 1–30.

Hatzenbuehler, M. L., Phelan, J. C., & Link, B. G. (2013). Stigma as a fundamental cause of population health inequalities. *American Journal of Public Health, 103*(5), 813–821.

Hatzenbuehler, M. L., Rutherford, C., McKetta, S., Prins, S. J., & Keyes, K. M. (2020). Structural stigma and all-cause mortality among sexual minorities: Differences by sexual behavior? *Social Science & Medicine, 244*, 112463.

Hatzenbuehler, M. L., Lattanner, M. R., McKetta, S., & Pachankis, J. E. (2024). Structural stigma and LGBTQ+ health: A narrative review of quantitative studies. *The Lancet Public Health, 9*(2), e109–e127.

House, J. S., Kessler, R. C., Herzog, A. R., Mero, R. P., Kinney, A. M., & Breslow, M. J. (1990). Age, socioeconomic status, and health. *The Milbank Quarterly, 68*, 383–411.

House, J. S., Lepkowski, J. M., Kinney, A. M., Mero, R. P., Kessler, R. C., & Herzog, A. R. (1994). The social stratification of aging and health. *Journal of Health and Social Behavior, 35*, 213–234.

Hummer, R. A., & Hamilton, E. R. (2019). Population health in America. University of California Press.

Landes, S. D. (2024). Disability mortality disparity: Risk of mortality for disabled adults nearly twice that for nondisabled adults, 2008–19. *Health Affairs, 43*(8), 1128–1136.
Lieberson, S. (1985). *Making it count: The improvement of social research and theory*. University of California Press.
Link, B. G., & Hatzenbuehler, M. L. (2016). Stigma as an unrecognized determinant of population health: Research and policy implications. *Journal of Health Politics, Policy and Law, 41*(4), 653–673.
Link, B. G., & Phelan, J. C. (1995). Social conditions as fundamental causes of disease. *Journal of Health and Social Behavior, 35*(Extra Issue), 80–94.
Link BG, Phelan J. 2010. Social Conditions as Fundamental Causes of Health Inequalities. In Handbook of Medical Sociology, ed. CE Bird, P Conrad, AM Fremont, S Timmermans, pp. 3–17. Nashville, TN: Vanderbilt University Press.
Link, B. G., & Phelan, J. (2014). Stigma power. *Social Science & Medicine, 103*, 24–32.
Link, B. G., Northridge, M. E., Phelan, J. C., & Ganz, M. L. (1998). Social epidemiology and the fundamental cause concept: On the structuring of effective cancer screens by socioeconomic status. *Milbank Quarterly, 76*(3), 375–402.
Lutfey, K., & Freese, J. (2005). Toward some fundamentals of fundamental causality: Socioeconomic status and health in the routine clinic visit for diabetes. *American Journal of Sociology, 110*, 1326–1372.
Mackenbach, J. P., Kulhánová, I., Bopp, M., Deboosere, P., Eikemo, T. A., Hoffmann, R., Kulik, M. C., et al. (2015). Variations in the relation between education and cause-specific mortality in 19 European populations: A test of the "fundamental causes" theory of social inequalities in health. *Social Science & Medicine, 127*, 51–62.
Mackenbach, J. P., Looman, C. W. N., Artnik, B., Bopp, M., Deboosere, P., Dibben, C., et al. (2017). Fundamental causes of inequalities in mortality: An empirical test of the theory in 20 European populations. *Sociology of Health & Illness, 39*(7), 1117–1133.
Markides, K. S., & Coreil, J. (1986). The health of Hispanics in the southwestern United States: An epidemiologic paradox. *Public Health Reports, 101*(3), 253–265.
Merton RK. 1949. On sociological theories of the middle range. In Social Theory and Social Structure, ed. RK Merton. New York: Simon & Schuster, The Free Press.
Montez, J. K., Zajacova, A., Hayward, M. D., Woolf, S. H., Chapman, D., & Beckfield, J. (2019). Educational disparities in adult mortality across US states: How do they differ, and have they changed since the mid-1980s? *Demography, 56*, 621–644.
Phelan, J. C., & Link, B. G. (2015). Is racism a fundamental cause of inequalities in health? *Annual Review of Sociology, 41*(1), 311–330.
Phelan, J. C., Link, B. G., Diez-Roux, A., Kawachi, I., & Levin, B. (2004). "Fundamental causes" of social inequalities in mortality: A test of the theory. *Journal of Health and Social Behavior, 45*(3), 265–285.
Phelan, J. C., Link, B. G., & Dovidio, J. F. (2008). Stigma and prejudice: One animal or two? *Social Science & Medicine, 67*(3), 358–367.
Phelan, J. C., Link, B. G., & Tehranifar, P. (2010). Social conditions as fundamental causes of health inequalities: Theory, evidence, and policy implications. *Journal of Health and Social Behavior, 51*(1_suppl), S28–S40.
Sasson, I., & Hayward, M. D. (2019). Association between educational attainment and causes of death among White and Black US adults, 2010–2017. *JAMA, 322*(8), 756–763.
Schmitz, A., Lazarevič, P., & Luy, M. (2024). No socioeconomic inequalities in mortality among Catholic monks: A quasi-experiment providing evidence for the fundamental cause theory. *Journal of Health and Social Behavior.* https://doi.org/10.1177/00221465241291847
Walker, E. R., McGee, R. E., & Druss, B. G. (2015). Mortality in mental disorders and global disease burden implications: A systematic review and meta-analysis. *JAMA Psychiatry, 72*(4), 334–341.
Zapata-Moya, Á. R., Willems, B., & Bracke, P. (2019). The (re)production of health inequalities through preventive innovations. *Health Sociology Review, 28*, 177–193.

Chapter 5
Gender Theory and Health

Ellen Annandale

Theory and research have a reciprocal relationship. Prevailing theoretical approaches gradually fall out of fit as societies change and fresh approaches are called for. The theoretical sureties that once drove gender and health research, such as the existence of fixed, binary physical and social divides between two groups of men and women, progressively have come under question, necessitating a re-theorization of gender as more complex and pliable than hitherto recognized (Annandale, 2023). However, since gender binarism remains a very powerful force within academic, healthcare, and popular thinking, it needs to be retained within the theoretical toolkit (Lorber, 2022). Consequently, this chapter will make the case that we need to explore gender binarism and gender multiplicity as co-constitutive of health status and healthcare practices. This requires theoretical tools which reach beyond gender as a standalone concept, but simultaneously embrace its relevance for the analysis of health. It will be argued that an intersectional approach can help to accomplish this, but only if analysis retains a critical edge by taking intersections between power structures and systems of oppression as the referent rather than multiplying identity categories at the individual level (Guidroz & Berger, 2009; Hill Collins, 2019). More broadly, it will be proposed that "gender" should be regarded as a relational concept which significantly influences the health and healthcare of various genders through intersecting power structures, such as patriarchy and racism, in variable and multifaceted ways.

The chapter begins with a synopsis of the feminist origins of gender and health research, the theoretical approaches employed, a critique of them and a discussion of subsequent critical transformations. It then considers the development of new directions in research on gender and health as gender binary and cisgendered approaches came under question and researchers sought to capture the increasingly

E. Annandale (✉)
University of York, York, UK
e-mail: ellen.annandale@york.ac.uk

W. C. Cockerham (ed.), *Medical Sociology on the Move*,
https://doi.org/10.1007/978-3-031-92456-9_5

complex realities of gender in empirical research on various health issues. The final part of the chapter develops a critical analysis of the use of intersectional approaches to gender and health, taking detailed illustrations from several research studies.

Sex and Gender: Feminist Beginnings

The theoretical origins of research on gender and health lie in critical feminist analysis of the health of women and girls. Feminists' use of what came to be known by the 1970s as the sex (biology)/gender (social) distinction goes back to at least the eighteenth century (even though these terms were not used) when, through a focus on health and the body, women writers began to criticize the conventional mind-body dualism which sustained women's oppression. Though they were set apart by time and place, influential writers such as Mary Wollstonecraft (1759–1797), Harriet Martineau (1802–1876), and Charlotte Perkins Gilman (1860–1935) had a common objective of showing that women's ill-health is socially caused, rather than given by their supposedly defective biology (Gilman, [1892] 1973, 1915; Martineau, [1844] 2003; Wollstonecraft, [1792] 1992).

One of the finest illustrations of this is sociologist Perkins Gilman's semi-autobiographical novella, *The Yellow Wallpaper* ([1892] 1973) which recounts the experience of a young woman who, following a nervous breakdown, is taken to rest in an isolated, broken-down mansion under the 'loving care' of her physician husband. She becomes preoccupied by the form of a woman trapped and trying to escape from within the sprawling pattern of the yellow wallpaper decorating her bedroom. She struggles and tries to break free, but the wallpaper strangles and tortures her. Gilman herself suffered, but eventually recovered from, a period of mental illness following her marriage and the subsequent birth of her daughter. She went on to chronicle the associations between women's poor health and their situation in life, which she blamed upon the 'excessive sex distinction' created by men which had swept across every act of life in her early twentieth-century America. As she explained:

> When we say *men, man, manly, manhood* and all the other masculine derivatives, we have in the background of our minds a huge vague crowded picture of the world and its activities…And when we say women, we think *female*—the sex. (Gilman 1915, pp. 116–117, emphasis original).

While women were (and still are) reduced by others to, and confined by, their biology, men were identified as being so much more. In Gilman's estimation, we should hardly be surprised that this customary attitude brings mental illness in its wake. As she put it to women: "we have so far lived and suffered and died in a man-made world."[1]

---

[1]Gilman's 'Our Androcentric Culture' was serialised in the Forerunner, a commercial journal funded by advertisements and subscriptions which Gilman edited between 1901 and 1916. It featured only her own writing and responses to readers' letters. The first 18 parts, published between 1901 and 1910, can be found at http://www.gutenberg.org/ebooks/3017 (accessed 2 January 2025).

The solution for Gilman, and many late eighteenth and early-twentieth century contemporaries was, first, to establish that women are no more determined by their biology than are men and, second, to make clear that the patriarchal representation of women's minds and bodies as unruly and unreliable is grossly misconstrued. This fledgling embodied health feminism was still finding its theoretical wings during this time. By the final quarter of the twentieth-century, it was soaring, borne high on the sweeping winds of change brought about by what often is referred to as "second wave" feminism (generally characterized as between the 1960s and 1980s), and its employment of the powerful conceptual distinction between biological sex and social gender. This had wide appeal, but the sex/gender distinction was, and remains, a broad canvas that scholars have used in distinctive and politically inflected ways within the domain of health (Annandale, 2009). For brevity, differences between "equality feminism" and "difference feminism," within the "second wave," throw this into relief and are a useful initial illustration of the contentions that have surrounded the sex/gender concept through time.

Although "equality feminists" recognize biological specificities, the contention is that they should not be allowed to make a difference to life experiences. The biological body is muted, reflecting the supposition that men and women have "an analogous biological or natural potential that is unequally developed because the social roles imposed on the two sexes are not equivalent" (Grosz, 1995, p. 51). Consequently, the social becomes at least as important—probably more important—than the biological in accounting for the differences in the health status of women and men. For example, considering women's longer average life expectancy across most of the world, Verbrugge (1985, p. 173) placed biology fourth in rank behind "risk acquired from roles, stress, lifestyles, and long-term preventative practices, psychosocial factors, and prior healthcare."

As a visible, present-day face of equality feminism, gender mainstreaming seeks to achieve gender justice by integrating a gender perspective into institutional policies and practices (Payne & Doyal, 2012). Endorsed by the 1995 Beijing Declaration and Platform for Action of the United Nation's Fourth World Conference on Women, gender mainstreaming is espoused by supranational agencies like the WHO, national governments and institutions. For those supportive of its principles, successful mainstreaming shows that feminism "is no longer an outsider protest movement but is embedded in institutions of civil society and the state" (Walby, 2011, p. 24). Framed as women's access to the highly valued, traditionally male-defined, public sphere, gender equality is found to be associated with women's health improvement. This has stimulated an enduring stream of research on relationships between women's domestic work, paid employment and health. An extensive body of research exists, for example, on the health consequences of dual responsibility for paid work and work in the home in the global context (Ervin et al., 2022). Echoing the proposition that it is an optimum balance between social roles that promotes positive health for men and women alike, or what is considered to be "work-life balance," research has identified positive effects of "multiple roles" upon health, at least as far as time pressures do not tip this over into "role overload" (Bird & Rieker, 2008). Positive associations also have been drawn between macro national and community level measures of gender equality and the health of men and women, such as at state level, using indicators such as gender wage gaps, and the underrepresentation of women in political office (see, for example, Månsdotter et al., 2006; Mensah & Kofi Adjei, 2020).

Notwithstanding the merits of this approach, by the mid-1990s feminists and others were arguing with increasing force that characterizing the relationship between biological sex and social gender as more or less arbitrary is an unsatisfactory basis for the analysis of health and illness. This is not to say that bodies are biologically fixed through reproductive organs, genes, hormones, gonads, chromosomes, secondary sex characteristics, for example, but that these features are invested with cultural and political meaning, making biology itself, to a certain extent, a social construct (Åsberg & Birke, 2010). Social gender, by turn, acquires meaning though embodied actions. This suggests that rather than forfending biology, researchers need to ensure that it is integral to the theoretical repertoire.

From the "second wave," "difference feminists" have taken women's biological capacity as the fundamental basis of physical and mental wellbeing and a primary site of their oppression. For example, in the widely read book, *For Her Own Good,* since published in a second edition, Ehrenreich and English (2005) expose the fallacies that women have been expected to accept over the centuries in the name of science. For example, nineteenth-century doctors found uterine and ovarian 'disorders' behind every possible female complaint, from headaches to sore throats to indigestion. So weak was women's biological constitution considered to be that any deviation from the purportedly natural path of marriage, childrearing, and homemaking was judged unhealthy. In the twenty-first century, medical arguments seem to take the malice out of the oppression of women: what doctors and other healthcare practitioners propose is only "for their own good" (Ehrenreich & English, 2005). Consequently, "difference feminists" have tended to envision the route to better health and experience of healthcare for women as lying outside the mainstream, such as women-controlled, de-medicalized approaches to childbirth and, more generally, in the valuing of women's positive biological differences from men. However, as now extensively rehearsed, this risks both an essentialized account of the biological body and the establishment of two—and only two—bodies, one pregiven at birth as male, and one as female, which correspond with male or female gender identity (Annandale & Clark, 1996; Annandale, 2023).

Thus, notwithstanding their significant differences, most research on women's health stemming from "equality" and "difference" feminism has envisaged health and illness through the lens of categorical biological and/or social *difference* between men and women, taking women as the point of reference (even where comparisons are drawn to men). If privilege is invisible to those who possess it (Kimmel, 2017), then patriarchal social structures and practices not only fashion and conceal women's oppression that needs to be brought to light, but also disregard men's experience *qua* men. "Men's health" developed as a topic in its own right as recently as the mid-1990s amid budding interest in men and masculinities within academia, politics, and in policy circles. Over the ensuing period, the conceptual lens has been the conventional one of binary difference (Schofield et al., 2000), with research pointing, for example, to men's shorter average life-expectancy compared to women globally and a relative lack of attention in health policy and resource allocation to issues of men's health, with the purpose of highlighting men's disadvantage. As White et al. (2023) relate, this has lent a backlash character to men's health research with a focus on marginal statistical differences between men and women, when, the authors argue, attention should instead be on identifying the challenges that men face *qua* men. So, in brief, up until around the mid-1990s, most research supposed two gender-based health constituencies of "women's health" and "men's health" based on a robust binarism between the bodies and experiences of men and women.

New Directions, New Challenges

The assumption that "gender" refers to two distinct binary groups of men and women whose present gender expression matches their (binary) sex assigned at birth has subsequently come under significant question, particularly since the turn of the present century. During the 1990s, feminists were emphasizing that binary oppositions are inherently patriarchal since their "very structure is privileged by the male/non-male (i.e. female) distinction" (Grosz, 1990, p. 101). Consequently, to position women and men as opposites is to contribute to the oppression of women since, under patriarchy, their opposite position will always be defined negatively. Gendered differences support other oppositions in a magnet-like effect—for example, men are rational, women are irrational, women are caring, men are uncaring, and so on. It is by this process that the positively valued "healthy body" attaches to men and the negatively valued "sick body" to women (Annandale & Clark, 1996). A proposed way forward has been to deconstruct male/female, man/woman and sex/gender binaries to show that binary thinking has inured us to difference and blinded us to the heterogeneity and plurality that characterizes social life. From this perspective, elevating the suppressed term—female/woman and all that goes with it—is deficient. Closure needs to be resisted by destabilizing the hierarchical division itself so that commonalities become as important as differences such that men no longer can easily be associated with all that is valued and women with all that is not (Barrett & Phillips, 1992).

More broadly, a body of research has also drawn attention to the "fluidity and multiplicity" of men's experience (Broom & Tovey, 2009, p. 4), which points to a level of shared concern with feminist thinking on women's health to deconstruct essentialist ways of thinking about sex and gender in the health domain. As Breu puts it, "if masculinity is no longer tied to sex or straightforwardly evocative of a binarized hierarchy of gendered power, then the subject of the field itself is open to radical reconceptualization" (2022, p. 586). Thus, we have witnessed increased questioning of automatic assumptions that gender identity and experience are consequent upon biological sex assigned at birth and based on binary biological and social difference (Annandale, 2009), a process characterized as cisgenderism.

However, this does not mean that cisgender assumptions no longer predominate. They remain fundamental to the experience of social life and are embedded in institutional policies and practices. The different meanings given to gender and to the gender-health relationship reflect the ways in which various interests have brought their claims forward (Schofield, 2002). The stakes were high in the past and remain so today as various political interests jostle for primacy within academia and more widely. "'Gender' is a stretchy category that serves as a screen for collective fears about change, loss of national identity, excessive influence of the West and its cultural hegemony" (Graff & Korolczuk, 2022, p. 15). There has been a recent global surge in anti-gender politics that seek to preserve cisgender ideologies, leverage discriminatory laws that limit the bodily autonomy of women and gender diverse people, such as reproductive rights (including opposition to abortion, invitro fertilisation and surrogacy), and to disrupt policies and programmes that promote gender justice in areas such as healthcare, education and legal rights, all with detrimental consequences for health and wellbeing (Gideon & Hawkes, 2024). This often works glove in hand with anti-transgender and anti-LGBTQI politics, such as state policies which avow the traditional heterosexual family and oppose same sex marriage (Corrêa et al., 2018). As Perez-Brummer et al. (2024) relate, this is 'part of broader landscapes of intersecting forms of power and discrimination, deeply embedded with racist and heteronormative relations of power'. In parts of the global north, white men in particular have voiced an 'aggrieved entitlement' as the benefits they expected to be theirs are perceived as having been snatched away (Kimmel, 2017). The rise of hyper-masculine backlash actions through which men seek to restore loss of 'hegemonic male supremacy' in a world which now seems to favour women, is a gendered feeling (Kaiser, 2022, p. 220). A remarkable example of this was the assault on the US Capitol building in early 2021, when right-wing extremist organizations, including the Proud Boys, sought to keep Donald Trump in power following his defeat in the 2020 Presidential election. Motivated by loss of pride which they adjudged feminists had stripped away, the Proud Boys have enacted 'a gendered and racialized notion of Americanness where European men and their blood descendants are the sole creators and proprietors of the American nation' (Travis, 2023, p. 592).

Categories of social groups, such as genders, are always 'relationally co-defined' (Krieger, 2024). This means that attributions of non-binary or gender fluid identities similarly are categories interpretable only by reference to the normative gender binary and other expectations. As stated earlier, this is why we should explore gender binarism and gender multiplicity as co-constitutive of health status, the experience of illness and of healthcare practices. Binary gender exerts authority throughout social life while, simultaneously, it is being fragmented as the meaning of gender is refined to reflect a more complex variety of genders, although, obviously, the magnitude of this varies quite significantly geographically. Lorber has characterized this as the 'new gender paradox', where multiplicity is 'undermined by a continuing bi-gendered social structure that supports continued inequality' (2022, p. ix). This draws a direct association between gender binarism and inequality and gender multiplicity and equality. The corollary is that fragmenting the gender binary and related cisgenderism is an imperative for medical sociologists. However, it also signals that, since binarism and cisgenderism continue to wield substantial power, they must also be retained as part of the theoretical repertoire.

Thinking Through Gender Categories

It is hard to move away from a categorical approach to gender, even when seeking to transcend the cisgender binary. As already reflected upon, gender is relationality formed (Krieger, 2024) and this means that comparative thinking is at the heart of identifying health privileges and health disadvantages. On the one hand, it can be shown that the gender binary is 'fuzzier' than commonly depicted, since more people (especially of younger ages) identify beyond the binary, for example, as genderfluid, gender non-binary, and as two-spirit.

Alongside this, the current gender identity of transgender persons neither needs to map neatly onto sex assigned at birth (by reference, for example, to reproductive organs, genes, hormones, gonads, chromosomes, secondary sex characteristics) nor onto the gender binary (they may also identify as gender non-binary, for example). Arguably, then, there are reasons to conceptualize gender as far more fluid, emergent or interactional than it traditionally has been conceived and not necessarily to assume that medical and surgical intervention is needed to align genders and physical bodies (Johnson, 2015; Missé, 2022). But, on other hand, analysis inevitably requires the naming of gender and the construction of categories, even when this extends beyond the cisbinary. This is most marked within, but not restricted to, quantitative research. It is only very recently that surveys have been designed to take account of both sex as 'assigned at birth' and 'current gender', with options such as female, male, transman, transwoman, two-spirit, non-binary, and 'other', using fixed choice and open questions for respondents. From this foundation it is possible to enumerate categories such as cismen, ciswomen, transmen, transwomen, and people who identify outside of the binary, and to map associations with health which avoid conflating sex and gender (Kattari et al., 2020). Based on their review of gender surveys using SurveyMonkey (the leading online survey platform globally), Padgett et al., (2024) report the percentage of surveys in each country reviewed that used a 2- or 3-step gender question. Though the number of surveys conducted and the percentage using this approach, rather than asking only about sex registered at birth, varied by country, some substantial increases were identified over time. For instance, in Canada, 21% of surveys used a 2- or 3-step approach in 2021, which rose to 30% in 2015 and to 80% in 2022. For Argentina, the equivalents were 7%, 12% and 48%. Although this is a positive development, there are pragmatic reasons why it habitually fails to capture the complexity of gender. Thus, for reasons of small numbers, which make comparative analyses difficult, gender non-normative/non-cisgender categories routinely get combined for statistical analysis even though they are likely to denote very different expressions of gender identity and experience (Padgett et al., 2024). For example, trans people may identify as gender-binary, but also as gender non-binary, or as gender fluid. Consequently, while new ways of enumerating gender seem to enable hitherto invisiblized genders to be seen and to count, they still have the capacity to obscure (Singer, 2015).

It is important to get concepts and categories right (or as right as we can make them) because research consistently points to various kinds of health disadvantage for gender non-normative people. For example, Jackson et al. (2023) compared all-cause and cause-specific mortality for England using general practice databases. Their comparisons, which are limited in the ways just referred to, enumerate 'transmasculine' and 'transfeminine' people (referred to as people whose gender identities are different to those assigned at birth) and cisgender women and men. To simplify a complex analysis, the results show elevated mortality rates for transpersons compared to cispersons, especially for deaths from 'external causes'; that is, deaths due to accidents and violence, poisoning, and other adverse effects. For all-cause mortality, rates were the lowest (i.e. better) for cisgender women, followed by cisgender men, and then by transmasculine persons, with transfeminine persons having the highest (worst) rates. The authors' explanation for this is that non-cisgender persons' repeated exposure to violence, discrimination, and economic and social marginalization results in greater vulnerability to poor health outcomes and higher mortality (Jackson et al., 2023). Broadly speaking, this pattern and interpretation is supported by research more widely. For example, drawing on US national data on self-reported health status, Stacey et al. (2025) point to 'the skyrocketing increase in anti-transgender state legislation and anti-transgender violence' in the country. Their data show that 'fair or poor' self-reported health (as compared to 'very good or good' health) was highest (worse) for those who defined as 'gender nonconforming' (28.70%), followed by transwomen (26.69%), transmen (20.16%), cisgender women (16.00%) and, finally, cisgender men (15.72%).

Thinking 'Upstream'

Research of the kind just described is effective in pointing to the stark realities of health disadvantage related to gender discrimination. As feminists have long recognized, it points to gender as fundamentally a power relation through which some genders are positively valued and others negatively valued (Gideon & Hawkes, 2024). But as Connell (2021) advises, there is a risk that gender relations get sidelined when gender is approached as a personal identity and where trans and other identities are contrasted to the dominant cisgender binary. From this standpoint analytic terms like 'patriarchy' can tend to go missing (Connell, 2021). In keeping with this point, Homan (2024) explains that although self-reports of discrimination are useful, they depend on sexism (and we might add, cisgenderism) being directly visible to respondents and recognized as such in order to be measured. Moreover, research tends to focus on proximate determinants of health, typically measured at the individual level, overlooking the ultimate, upstream, multifaceted, drivers of structural gender oppression (Brown & Homan, 2023). Brown and Homan's (2023) wider call for the use of theories which focus on structural oppression as a multilevel phenomenon (macro, meso, and micro), which is systemic and intersectional in nature and operates across multiple institutions and societal domains, is a useful call to theoretical arms for research on gender and health. To this we must add a concern for location and context. As Krieger (2024) foregrounds in her 'ecosocial' framework, we need to avoid individualized and decontextualized approaches, where 'fixed binary properties of individuals are the focus'. Instead, we should be concerned with how humans embody their social and ecological contexts on a routine basis. Thus, as Krieger advises, sexism, racism, heterosexism and gender binarism together 'comprise intimately harmful, distinct, and entangled societal systems of self-serving discrimination and privilege that structure the embodiment of health inequalities' (Kreiger, 2020: 37).

The call to explore the embodiment of environments suffused by sexism, gender binarism and racism in which people live out their lives draws attention to the potential malleability (rather than givenness) of the physical body. The nexus between gender and the body is complex. The direction of research interest to date has been very much on the 'gender-shaping of biology', with far less attention given to how the biological body may, by its turn, 'express and contribute to social gender dynamics in a nexus with health'; that is, the 'biologic-shaping of gender' in a complex interactive process (Annandale et al., 2018, p. 87). This does not mean to say that biology has a determining role, but rather that 'matter and biology are active in their own right' (Frost 2011, p. 4). Bodies are responsive to their environments and 'always active in their own remaking' (Guthman & Mansfield, 2012, p. 499). Annandale et al. (2018) take female genital mutilation/cutting and its health consequences as an example of a wide-spread practice that is not only shaped by patriarchal gender relations, but also has a role itself in shaping the gender-related social experiences of girls and women. For instance, Einstein (2008, 2012), a biologist with a doctorate in neuroanatomy, explores the neurobiological repercussions of female genital mutilation/cutting (FGM/C) type 3 (infibulation with excision of the external genitalia) from a feminist perspective. Einstein argues that cutting the nerve circuits carried in the prudential, pelvic and hypogastric regions of the body may affect the rest of the body via the central nervous system, which is depicted by Einstein (and others) as 'sensitive and malleable' (2012, p. 171). Thus, the effects of FGM/C are not limited to one part of the body, but rather 'owned by the entire body, or embodied through the interconnections of all body systems and the environment' (Einstein, 2012, p. 158). Consequently, it is reasonable to suppose that the central nervous system 'plays a role in the embodiment of culture' (Einstein, 2012, p. 58, p. 155). FGM/C, then, 'configures the ways in which a woman carries herself, walks, and experiences the world' (Einstein, 2012, p. 94) and how she relates to and deals with physical and mental pain. The body becomes other than what it once was and plays an active role in shaping the social and gender-related experiences of girls and women (Annandale et al., 2018). This points not only to the active role of biological body in experience, but also to its conceivable plasticity as it responds to the social and political environment.

It is, then, important to appreciate that the bodily experience is significantly shaped by social and political contexts. Gender is fundamentally a relation of power and subjugation. In a different context, Mbembe coined the term 'necropolitics' to refer to 'the subjugation of life to the power of death' (2003, p. 39; see also, 2019). Global politics, he argues, is the work of death and the creation of the living dead. As Selin Islekel (2022) explains, necropolitics operate at the level of 'multitudes' rather than the individual body, as certain population groups are positioned as 'die-able' such that 'the actual death of and killing would not be anything out of the ordinary.' Thus, necropolitics positions deaths within the ordinary, rather than the extraordinary (Selin Islekel, 2022). The body of Mbembe's (2003, 2019) necropolitics tends to be a generic one and, as Threadcraft (2017) discusses, he remains silent on how necropolitics interests with male and female bodies. But the concept is nonetheless useful for the exploration of global health issues and, therefore, in theorising the gender and health relationship. Research by Padilla and Rodríquez-Madera (2021) on necropolitics and gender transitioning amongst transwomen in Puerto Rica provides an insightful illustration of this. They relate that 'the transgender body is systematically excluded and "designed to die"' through social exclusion and transphobic violence (2021, p. S26), in a context where medical transition is not available in the formal healthcare system. They point to literal scars on trans bodies as embodied health risks taken as they endeavor to pass as cisgender women by, for example, using injectable silicone obtained from street markets and administered extra-legally by inyeccionistas. Padilla and Rodríquez-Madera (2021) conceptualize the elevated risks of illness and death amongst transwomen as 'manifestations of necropolitical abandonment' and the scars and ailments that result as manifestations of structural and gender violence that hastens them toward death (2021, p. S27).

So far, it has been proposed that gender is relational and works through processes of power, privilege and subjugation which play out in a range of ways in different global contexts. While cisgender binarism once held sway, it is now more fitting, in some contexts, to conceptualize gender binarism and gender multiplicity as co-existing and co-constitutive of health status and healthcare practices. As expressed in the introduction to the chapter, this calls for theoretical tools which reach beyond gender as a standalone concept, but which simultaneously embrace its relevance for the analysis of health. An intersectional approach can help to realise this. However, as will now be discussed, this is achievable only if analysis retains a critical edge by taking intersections between power structures and systems of oppression as the principal object.

Intersectionality

Intersectionality was introduced in the late 1980s as a heuristic term to draw attention to the limitations of single axis thinking (Cho et al., 2013; McCall, 2005). Developed within critical race studies, the initial intent was to throw more effective light on Black women's experiences in a context where claims of 'sisterhood' were inappropriately premised on the conception of a generic white, middle-class woman (Hill Collins, 1990). Inaugurating the concept, Crenshaw (1989, p. 140) argued:

> Because the intersectional experience is greater than the sum of racism and sexism, any analysis that does not take intersectionality into account cannot sufficiently address the particular manner in which Black women are subordinated.

The speed with which intersectionality has been taken up and developed within research on gender and beyond has brought definitional dilemmas (Hill Collins, 2019). It is important that we avoid seeing gender and race just as categories to make research current and user-friendly, but rather conceptualise them as related to significant 'resistant knowledge traditions amongst subordinated peoples' (Hill Collins, 2019, p. 10). As coined by civil rights advocate and critical race scholar, Kimberlé Crenshaw (1989), intersectionality had its origins in political activism. Revisiting this in conversation with Guidroz and Berger (2009), Crenshaw points out that her use of the term was 'just a metaphor. I'm amazed at how it gets over- and under-used, sometimes I can't even recognize it in the literature anymore' (Guidroz & Berger, 2009, p. 65). The vital objective was to identify how systems of oppression overlap. Yet, as Crenshaw explains, 'a lot of people read intersectionality as just multiplying identity categories rather than constituting a structural analysis or political critique' (Guidroz & Berger, 2009, p. 70). This is troubling because intersectionality then can become 'just a listing of people and a description and no analysis of how their particular conditions are related to power structures' (Guidroz & Berger, 2009, p. 70). Although a central purpose was to break down mono-categorical thinking (for example, all women as the same), for Crenshaw, as it has developed over time, intersectionality has risked becoming just another form of identity politics. Writing with Cho, and McCall, Crenshaw expresses curiosity that intersectionality has been recast as a theory 'primarily fascinated with the infinite combinations and implications of overlapping identities' (Cho et al., 2013, p. 797), when its original analytic was structures of power and exclusion in the lives of women. Health research has been particularly liable to taking intersectionality to refer to the intersection of gender with other identity characteristics of individuals such as ethnicity, age or sexuality, rather than exploring (or also exploring) the intersection of sexism, heterosexism, racism and agism as forming peoples' health status and experiences of care (Smith et al., 2015). For Connell (2012), intersectionality effectively becomes a more sophisticated cross classification of categories (e.g., age, gender, health status, and so on), which does little to help us understand the dynamics of gender and health; that is, the 'way gender orders are created and gender inequalities are created and challenged' (Connell, 2012, p. 1676). As highlighted by Choo and Marx Ferree (2010), there is also a tendency for intersectionality to take researchers down the inadvertent path of studying the multiply marginalized, as the identification of various intersections brings to light new groups previously unmarked as suffering from inequality in significant and unique ways. The result can be what they dub 'context specialization'. Intersections become like street corners where any street (for example, gender, age, race) crosses any other without being transformed. In other words, contributions to political praxis get overlooked.

Leading intersectional theorist and black feminist, Patricia Hill Collins (1990, 2019) emphasizes that intersectionality needs to be approached as a *critical* social theory and that its critical edge needs to be sharpened. As it stands, the very open way in which it has been used over the years—which, since it can contribute to conceptual advancement, can be a strength—risks intersectionality becoming 'trapped in its own crossroads, pulled in multiple directions and drowning in ideas' (2019, p. 4). Of critical importance is the emphasis placed by Hill Collins and others on *relationality*. As she puts it, 'there would be no intersectionality without relationality', because analyzing relationships between intersectional entities is intersectionality's defining feature (Hill Collins, 2019, p. 15). Therefore, what matters is not simply devising a research sample to explore a health issue that consists of women of different ethnicities thought of as intersectional identities, for example, but addressing how their health, relations of sexism and racism intersect to construct their identities and experiences.

Consequently, for Hill Collins (2019) what is important here is the relational nature of power. She explains that relational logic operates in several ways. One of these is 'additively'; that is, by adding intersectionality theory to a research question. For example, adding race to an existing interest in gender and health. As already explained, this can be limited. But, for Hill Collins, it is nonetheless an important analytic step because it helps to disrupt the way an issue traditionally has been conceived. A further, more advanced, relational logic is 'articulation'. Here Hill Collins draws on Stuart Hall's (see Morely & Chen, 2006) concept of articulation to express how, as categories articulate with each other, they create new structures, processes and experiences. This articulation is fluid rather than fixed and occurs in different ways in different contexts. So, in healthcare contexts sexism, cisgenderism and racism may articulate to produce advantages for some people and disadvantages for others. The complexity of this may not be visible if, for example, sexism and racism are approached individually. As we will see when we look at research examples, below, health and healthcare are good illustrations of what Hill Collins refers to as a 'saturated site of power relations' (2019, p. 238).

So, two points are critical for analysis. First, intersections are not additive, but interactive. They do not simply accumulate, layered on top of each other; rather, one category (such as gender) takes its meaning from another category (such as race) and a 'uniquely hybrid creation' emerges at the intersection (Shields, 2008, p. 305). This intersection is an important object of analysis. Second, and as part of this, while the experiences of people belonging to certain categories is self-evidently important, we need to pay analytic attention to the relational logic that structures those experiences. As in other domains, the analytic currency of intersectionality has grown exponentially over the years in research in the field of gender and health. Although it is not always used exactly in the ways that its' originators intended, it has helped to enlighten our understanding of a wide range of issues. It is useful to look at some examples. In each case, the research not only draws on intersectionality but also understands gender as relational and finds explanatory power in structures and systems of oppression. The research examples have been chosen to reflect experiences in different global contexts.

Shatema Threadcraft (2016, 2017) employs necropolitics (Mbembe, 2003, 2019) to research *#blacklivesmatter* and femicide in the US. The body politic, she relates, produces the dead. She explains that, in racial politics, 'the body around which blacks can most easily rally members of the cause of racial justice…is the dead one.' (2017, p. 553). But this has the effect of cultivating a focus on some bodies and not others; specifically, on 'the slain body, which 'privileges how cismen die, how young men die, how able-bodied blacks die, over all other black deaths' (2017, p. 354). Without doubt this focus is important, but it can fail black women by making them invisible. To rectify this, Threadcraft proposed an analysis which is 'properly intersectional'. She shows that this requires a focus beyond slain bodies to also consider pathologic conditions of life, such as life in residential neighborhoods and in relation to systemic racism. Black women, she points out, experience disproportionate sexual assault, community violence, and sexual aggression resulting in a 'racialized feminine embodiment' and an 'assaulted and terrorized body'. But this is less likely to produce a *dead* body (2017, p. 555). Bringing this to the fore shows that power intersects in different ways in relation to the health of male and female black bodies and works against the likelihood that women's deaths will be counted; that is, matter. So, although it is important to research the slain body, as has been to the fore in *#backlivesmatter*, in order to appreciate how state power intersects with the female body, we also need to recognize the routinised consequences of sexism. Public spectacle is less relevant to femicide than to the broader homicide, since femicide happens more often in private than in public spaces, making it harder to rally around politically. And so, as Threadcraft (2016) explains,

> Intersectional complexity means that if those concerned with how power acts on the black female body want to keep the focus on the state and state violence in a way that is gender inclusive, they cannot focus exclusively on death and the production of the dead body. (2017, p. 569)

Although, as far as I am aware, Crenshaw does not refer to necropolitics, Threadcraft's (2016, 2017) analysis illustrates her argument that 'the intersection of racism and sexism factors into Black women's lives in ways that cannot be captured wholly by looking at the race or gender dimensions of those experiences separately' (1991, p. 1244). Continuing the theme of gendered violence, Laurel Westbrook's (2023) research in the US, injects a more nuanced approach to gender into the analytic mix. Westbrook employs the concept of a 'matrix of violence' to depict how systems of stratification (such as gender, race and sexuality) and institutions (for example, the economy, politics, law, education, media, and healthcare), interact in ways that shape patterns of fatal and nonfatal violence. As she relates, differences in the extent of identified violence amongst cisgender people, where men are more likely to be impacted than women, are well-documented. But when it comes to transgender people, attention has been upon inequalities between cisgender and transgender people as two groups (Westbrook, 2023). As she puts it, this implies that all transgender people have an equal risk of experiencing violence. Based on an original database of all known murders of transgender people, and drawing on data from the Centers for Disease Control and Prevention's National Vital Statistics

System, she analyses murders over the 30-year period 1990–2019. Among cisgender people, 20.6% (n = 111,688) of murders were of women and 79.4% (n = 431,662) of men. By contrast, among transgender people, 97.2% (n = 494) were of women and only 2.8% of men (n = 14). Thus, cismen were on average four times more likely to be murdered than cisgender women. But the disparity is reversed for transpeople, and significantly exceeds the difference between cisgender people, with transgender women more than 35 times more likely to be murdered than transgender men. Moreover, transgender women of colour were murdered with greater frequently than white transgender women. For Westbrook (2023), these disparities are explicable within a necropolitical system where social systems 'define who matters and who does not, who is *disposable* and who is not' (Mbembe, 2003, p. 27) within the 'matrix of violence', where systems of stratification and social institutions protect some people from violence while enabling violence against others.

Debadrita Chakraborty (2021) draws on necropolitics and intersectionality to explore the violence and subjugation of women in India amid social, economic, and political insecurity during and after the covid-19 pandemic. She shows how, during the pandemic, right wing state mechanisms of power pushed marginalised women into precarity, 'conferring on them the status of the living dead' (2021, p. 331). This highlights the intersection of socio-economic status and precarity and gender-based violence. Her research shows that, despite their privileged position, urban upper and middle class women found themselves vulnerable due to patriarchal conventions. Away from paid work and without former paid household help, they experienced increases in household work and childcare responsibilities as well as mental and physical abuse at the hands of their husbands. These women's homes were transformed into what Chakraborty describes as 'zones of chaos, overwork, and constant fatigue' (2021, p. 333). Lower class, lower caste and religious minority women were also subjected to mental and physical abuse, though this was far less visible in public discourse, where the plight of the upper and middle classes was to the fore. As work in the informal economy was stopped, migrant workers in the cities, such as those who worked in the homes of upper and middle class women, were forced to travel back to their homelands where state authorities took it upon themselves to sanitise their bodies, such as by making them squat on the ground while they were chemically coated with disinfectants. Chakraborty (2021, p. 337) depicts daily women workers as driven to the edge of life and 'subalternized, invisibilized, and subjected to necropolitical praxes' on the basis of gender and caste during the pandemic.

An analytic theme running though Threadcraft (2016) and Westbrook's (2023) work on murder and Chakraborty's (2021) work on Covid-19 is the 'making visible' through intersectional analysis of the disparate health-related experiences of different genders which have either been in the shadows or invisibilised in conventional single-axis analyses. Clare Wenham (2021) also brings this theme to the fore in her exploration of health security during the Zika virus outbreak in Latin America between 2015 and 2017. Wenham highlights the disconnect between global health polices which, typically, are 'gender blind' and the local realties in women in Brazil (the epicentre of the disease outbreak). As she puts it, 'health emergencies are framed as global problems, assuming mutual vulnerabilities and homogenous effects of pathogenesis across societies' (Wenham, 2021, p. 8). This leads to the invisibilization of women's experiences and of the health consequences of their experience. Zika is transmitted primarily by Aedes Mosquitoes, which mainly bite during the daytime. Zika infection is often asymptomatic, making it hard to detect and diagnose. When symptoms do appear they include rash, fever, conjunctivitis, muscle and joint pain. The incidence of Zika virus was higher amongst women than amongst men in Brazil, although, as Wenham explains, it is not clear whether this is biological or gender-role related. The gendered aspects of life could certainly make women more vulnerable as they are more likely than men to be engaged in household work during the day with closer proximity to stored and standing water (which is also more common in poorer areas), which are a breeding ground for mosquitoes, as well as being more prone to work in care roles with infected people.

Of consequence, infection during pregnancy can cause microcephaly and other malformations in babies. This was what made infection in women such a major concern during the outbreak. Resultingly, not all women—only women of reproductive age—were the focus of public health messaging. Wenham (2021) argues that women were instrumentalised as they were reduced to the biological functioning of their bodies and their reproductive capacities by global and national public health security measures, which ignored the social and political realities of their everyday lives. As she puts, it, through an 'explicit degradation of women to their reproductive functions' (2021, p. 83), women were seen as at fault for having a baby affected by Congenital Zika Syndrome (CZS). The two-fold public health message of clean your house and don't get pregnant targeted individual behaviour change among women with little or no regard for the gendered realities of their lives. It was assumed, for example, that women had self-determination over sexual activity and access to contraceptives, something which is particularly important in the context of high levels of gender-based violence, including sexual violence, in Brazil (World Bank, 2023) and that they could easily avoid use of stored and standing water.

Wenham's (2021) intersectional analysis hinges on the concept of 'in/visibility'. She asks who was visible, who was made visible, and in what ways and with what consequences in health security activities? And, relatedly, who was invisible, invisibilized (and silenced or absolved)? She shows, crucially, that women were made visible in public health messaging as they were blamed for having a baby with Zika at the same time as highly gendered dimensions of their experience were invisibilized, along with their own needs for care as women. As a corollary, despite Zika infection also being present in men, and their role in reproduction, there was a relinquishing of any responsibilities on their part. There was also little regard for differential experiences among women. As Wenham puts it, 'considering women as a homogenous group produces practices that render invisible many of the insecurities in women's daily lives' (2021, p. 93). An intersectional approach is important in this context because it brings the interactions of multiple factors in the production of vulnerability to light. In actuality, the focus of national concern was on wealthy Western women, particularly because of the upcoming summer 2016 Olympics in Rio de Janeiro which would attract from female competitors and global audiences.

The majority of women affected with Zika in Latin America were, however, black, mixed race, or of indigenous heritage, with Wenham (2021) citing data showing that 83% of women who had a child with CZS were non-white. Moreover, most of those affected in Brazil lived in the North East, the poorest part of the country.

Conclusion

It has been argued that we need to reflect critically on the binary, cisgendered approaches to gender and health that have characterized research since the inception of the field. A dual-pronged approach is called for that both acknowledges that gender binarism remains a very powerful force within societies worldwide and, therefore, exerts a considerable influence on people's experiences, but also that gender is increasingly multifaceted and complex. Consequently, a theoretical construction has been proposed whereby we take gender binarism and gender multiplicity as *co-constitutive* of health and health practices. This means conceptualizing gender as intrinsically *relational* and as finding expression in structures, processes, practices and experiences that promote advantage for some and disadvantage for others, health and wellbeing for some and affliction for others. To comprehensively address this, we need to make use of theoretical tools which reach beyond gender as a stand-alone concept by taking an intersectional approach. However, it has been argued that we need to direct analysis 'upstream' by addressing the health consequences of intersections between power structures and systems of oppression for different genders, rather than taking a limited focus on intersections between identity categories at the level of individual characteristics.

References

Annandale, E. (2009). *Women's health and social change*. Routledge.

Annandale, E. (2023). Sociologies of health and gender. In A. Petersen (Ed.), *Handbook on the sociology of health and medicine* (pp. 76–90). Edward Elgar.

Annandale, E., & Clark, J. (1996). What is gender? Feminist theory and the sociology of human reproduction. *Sociology of Health & Illness, 18*, 17–44.

Annandale, E., Wiklund, M., & Hammarström, A. (2018). Theorising women's health and health inequalities: Shaping processes of the 'gender-biology nexus'. *Global Health Action, 11*, 87–96.

Åsberg, C., & Birke, L. (2010). Biology is a feminist issue: Interview with Lynda Birke. *European Journal of Women's Studies, 17*, 413–423.

Barrett, M., & Phillips, P. (1992). Words and things: Materialism and method in contemporary feminist analysis. In M. Barrett & A. Phillips (Eds.), *Destabilising theory* (pp. 201–219). Polity.

Bird, C., & Rieker, P. (2008). *Gender and health: The effects of constrained choices and social policies*. Cambridge University Press.

Breu, C. (2022). Rethinking masculinities studies. *American Literary History, 34*(2), 586–595.

Broom, A., & Tovey, P. (2009). Introduction: Men's health in context. In A. Broom & P. Tovey (Eds.), *Men's health: Body, identity and social context* (pp. 1–8). Wiley-Blackwell.

Brown, T. H., & Homan, P. (2023). The future of social determinants of health: Looking upstream to structural drivers. *Milbank Quarterly, 101*(S1), 36–60.
Chakraborty, D. (2021). The 'living dead' within 'death-worlds': Gender crisis and covid-19 in India. *Gender, Work and Organisation, 28*(S2), 330–339.
Cho, S., Williams Crenshaw, K., & McCall, L. (2013). Toward a field of intersectionality studies: Theory, applications, and praxis. *Signs, 38*(4), 785–810.
Choo, H., & Marx Ferree, M. (2010). Practicing intersectionality in sociological research: A critical analysis of inclusions, interactions, and institutions in the study of inequalities. *Sociological Theory, 28*(2), 129–149.
Connell, R. (2012). Gender, health and theory: Conceptualising the issue, in local and world perspective. *Social Science & Medicine, 74*, 1675–1683.
Connell, R. (2021). Transgender health: On a world scale. *Health Sociology Review, 30*(1), 87–94.
Corrêa, S., Paternotte, D., & Kuhar, R. (2018). *The globalisation of anti-gender campaigns. Democracy and Society.* https://www.ips-journal.eu/topics/democracy-and-society/the-globalisation-of-anti-gender-campaigns-2761/
Crenshaw, K. (1989). Demarginalising the intersection of race and sex: A black feminist critique of antidiscrimination doctrine, feminist theory and antiracist policies. *University of Chicago Legal Forum, 139*, 139–167.
Crenshaw, K. (1991). Mapping the margins: Intersectionality, identity politics, and violence against women of color. *Stanford Law Review, 43*, 1241–1299.
Ehrenreich, B., & English, D. (2005). *For her own good: Two centuries of the experts' advice to women* (2nd ed.). Anchor Books.
Einstein, G. (2008). From body to brain: Considering the neurobiological effects of female genital cutting. *Perspectives in Biology and Medicine, 51*, 84–97.
Einstein, G. (2012). Situated neuroscience: Exploring biologies of diversity. In R. Bluhm, A. J. Jacobson, & H. L. Mailborn (Eds.), *Neurofeminism: Issues at the intersection of feminist theory and cognitive science* (pp. 145–174). Palgrave.
Ervin, J., Taouk, Y., Fleitas Alfonzo, L., Hewitt, B., & King, T. (2022). Gender differences in the association between unpaid labour and mental health in employed adults: A systematic review. *The Lancet Public Health, 7*, e775–e786.
Frost, S. (2011). The implications of the new materialisms for feminist epistemology. In H. E. Grasswick (Ed.), *Feminist epistemology and philosophy of science: Power in knowledge* (pp. 69–83). Springer.
Gideon, J., & Hawkes, S. (2024). Introduction: Gender and health-a future research agenda. In J. Gideon & S. Hawkes (Eds.), *A research agenda for gender and health* (pp. 1–20). Edward Elgar.
Gilman, C. P. (1892/1973). *The yellow wallpaper*. The Feminist Press.
Gilman, C. P. (1915). *Herland (unabridged)*. Dover.
Graff, A., & Korolczuk, E. (2022). *Anti-gender politics in the populist movement*. Routledge.
Grosz, E. (1990). Contemporary theories of power and subjectivity. In S. Gunew (Ed.), *Feminist knowledge. Critique and construct* (pp. 59–20). Routledge.
Grosz, E. (1995). *Space, time, and perversion*. Routledge.
Guidroz, M., & Berger, T. M. (2009). A conversation with founding scholars of intersectionality: Kimberlé Crenshaw, Nira Yuval-Davis and Michelle Fine. In M. T. Berger & K. Guidroz (Eds.), *The intersectional approach: Transforming the academy through race, class, and gender* (pp. 61–78). University of North Carolina Press.
Guthman, J., & Mansfield, B. (2012). The implications of environmental epigenetics: A new direction for geographic inquiry on health, space, and nature-society relations. *Progress in Human Geography, 37*, 486–504.
Hill, S. E. (2015). Axes of health inequalities and intersectionality. In S. E. Smith, C. Bambra, & S. E. Hill (Eds.), *Health inequalities: Critical perspectives (pp. 95-108)*. Oxford University Press.
Hill Collins, P. (1990). *Black feminist thought*. HarperCollins Academic.

Hill Collins, P. (2019). *Intersectionality as critical theory*. Duke University Press.

Homan, P. (2024). Health consequences of structural sexism: Conceptual foundations, empirical evidence and priorities for future research. *Social Science & Medicine, 351*, 116379.

Jackson, S. S., Brown, J., Pfeiffer, R. M., et al. (2023). Analysis of mortality among transgender and gender diverse adults in England. *JAMA Network Open, 6*(1), e2253687.

Johnson, A. (2015). Normative accountability: How the medical model influences transgender identities and experiences. *Sociology Compass, 9*(9), 803–813.

Kaiser, S. (2022). *Political masculinity: How incels, fundamentalists and authoritarians mobilise for patriarchy*. Polity.

Kattari, S., Brittain, D. R., Rossier Markus, A., & Hall, K. C. (2020). Expanding women's health practitioners and researchers' understanding of transgender/nonbinary health issues. *Women's Health Issues, 30*(1), 3–6.

Kimmel, M. (2017). *Angry white men*. Bold Type Books.

Kreiger, N. (2020). Measures of racism, sexism, heterosexism, and gender binarism for health equity research: From structural injustice to embodied harm-an ecosocial analysis. *Annual Review of Public Health, 41*, 37–62.

Krieger, N. (2024). Advancing gender transformative intersectional science for health justice: An ecosocial analysis. *Social Science & Medicine, 351*(Supplement), 1.

Lorber, J. (2022). *The new gender paradox*. Polity.

Månsdotter, A., Lindholm, L., Lundberg, M., Winkvist, A., & Őhman, A. (2006). Parental share in public and domestic spheres: A population study on gender equality, death, and sickness. *Journal of Epidemiology and Public Health, 60*, 616–620.

Martineau, H. (2003 [1844]). *Life in the sick-room* (M. Frawley, Ed.). Broadview Press.

Mbembe, A. (2003). *Necropolitics* (L. Meintjes, Trans.). *Public Culture, 15*(1), 11–40.

Mbembe, A. (2019). *Necropolitics*. Duke University Press.

McCall, L. (2005). The complexity of intersectionality. *Signs, 30*, 1771–1800.

Mensah, A., & Kofi Adjei, N. (2020). Work-life balance and self-reported health among working adults in Europe: A gender and welfare state regime comparative analysis. *BMC Public Health, 20*, 1052. https://doi.org/10.1186/s12889-020-09139-w

Missé, M. (2022). *The myth of the wrong body*. Polity.

Morely, D., & Chen, K.-H. (2006). *Stuart Hall: dialogues in cultural studies*. Routledge.

Padgett, Z., Gutierrez, S., Wronski, L., & Barari, S. (2024). Measuring the growth of gender-inclusive surveys around the world. *Survey Practice, 17*(January). https://doi.org/10.29115/SP-2023-0019

Padilla, M., & Rodríquez-Madera, S. (2021). Embodiment, gender transitioning, and necropolitics among transwomen in Puerto Rico. *Current Anthropology, 62*(Supplement 23), S26–S37.

Payne, S., & Doyal, L. (2012). Re-visiting gender justice in health and healthcare. In E. Kuhlmann & E. Annandale (Eds.), *The Palgrave handbook of gender and healthcare* (pp. 21–35). Palgrave.

Perez-Brummer, A., Valdez, N., & Scheim, A. (2024). The anti-gender threat: An ethical, democratic, and scientific imperative for NIH research/ers. *Social Science & Medicine, 351*(Supplement), 1.

Schofield, T. (2002). What does gender and health mean? *Health Sociology Review, 11*(1&2), 29–38.

Schofield, T., Connell, R. W., Walker, L., Wood, J., & Butland, D. (2000). Understanding men's health and illness: A gender-relations approach to policy, research, and practice. *Journal of American College of Health, 48*, 247–256.

Selin Islekel, E. (2022). Gender in necropolitics: Race, sexuality, and gendered death. *Philosophy Compass, 17*, e12827.

Shields, S. (2008). Gender: An intersectionality approach. *Sex Roles, 59*, 301–311.

Singer, B. T. (2015). The profusion of things. The 'transgender' matrix and demographic imaginaries in US public health. *Transgender Studies Quarterly, 2*(1), 58–76.

Stacey, L., Wisler, W., & Reczek, R. (2025). The medical institution and transgender health: The role of healthcare barriers and negative healthcare experiences. *Social Science & Medicine, 365*. https://www.sciencedirect.com/science/article/pii/S0277953624009791

Threadcraft, S. (2016). *Intimate justice: The black female body and the body politic*. Oxford University Press.
Threadcraft, S. (2017). North American necropolitics and gender: On #BlackLivesMatter and black femicide. *South Atlantic Quarterly, 116*(3), 553–579.
Travis, C. (2023). Nostalgia, hypermasculinity, and the American far right: What ever happened to being proud of your boy? *New Political Science, 45*(6), 591–612.
Verbrugge, L. (1985). Gender and health: An update on hypotheses and evidence. *Journal of Health and Social Behavior, 24*, 6–30.
Walby, S. (2011). *The future of feminism*. Polity.
Wenham, C. (2021). *Feminist global health security*. Oxford University Press.
Westbrook, L. (2023). The matrix of violence: Intersectionality and necropolitics in the murder of transgender people in the United States, 1990–2019. *Gender and Society, 37*(3), 413–446.
White, A., Connell, R., Griffith, D. M., & Baker, P. (2023). Defining 'men's health': Towards a more inclusive definition. *International Journal of Men's Community Health, 6*(1), e1–e9.
Wollstonecraft, M. (1992/1792). *A vindication of the rights of woman*. Penguin Books.
World Bank. (2023). *Gender-based violence country profile: Brazil*. https://documents.worldbank.org/en/publication/documents-reports/documentdetail/09907172316. Accessed 02 Jan 2024.

Chapter 6
Bourdieu and an Update of Health Lifestyle Theory

William C. Cockerham

The purpose of this chapter is to update health lifestyle theory and in the process illustrate the importance of Pierre Bourdieu's contributions to sociological research on this topic. Bourdieu never published work on health or medical sociology, yet many of his ideas, especially his concepts of habitus and various forms of capital (e.g., social, cultural), are increasingly utilized to provide theoretical models in health-related research (see, for example, Abel & Frohlich, 2011; Carpiano, 2006; Christensen, 2011; Cockerham, 2005, 2018, 2021a, b, 2025). The merit of his perspective is that it fully (perhaps overly in some instances) acknowledges the important role of structure in shaping and often determining human social behavior, including lifestyles. This return to a more structurally-aware approach comes decades after the demise of structural-functionalism and the ascendancy of agency-oriented theories in medical sociology and sociology generally (Cockerham, 2021a, b, 2025; Mouzelis, 2008; Smelser, 1997).

Health Lifestyles: The Agency-Structure Debate

I found the agency-structure debate to be of major importance in developing a theory of health lifestyles (Cockerham, 2005). This is because the relative contributions of agency and structure in influencing social behavior have been *the* central sociological question since the beginning of the discipline. The task of understanding the linkage between the two phenomena will always retain this centrality because it is the basis upon which society and social interaction is constructed

W. C. Cockerham (✉)
University of Alabama at Birmingham, Birmingham, AL, USA

University of Maryland, College Park, MD, USA
e-mail: wcocker@uab.edu

W. C. Cockerham (ed.), *Medical Sociology on the Move*,
https://doi.org/10.1007/978-3-031-92456-9_6

(Archer, 1995, p. 1). Although medical sociologists paid little attention to the agency-structure debate in the past, it was clearly relevant to discussions on a number of health-related topics (Pescosolido et al., 2000; Williams, 1995). Today, several studies in medical sociology address the agency-structure interface (e.g., Burdette et al., 2017; Cockerham, 2005, 2021a; Katainen & Gronow, 2024; Hammarström et al., 2015; Mollborn et al., 2021a, 2025; Øversveen, 2021; Reynolds, 2021). The agency-structure debate is particularly germane for the following question: Are the decisions people make with respect to food, exercise, smoking, and the like largely a matter of individual choice or are they principally shaped by structural variables such as social class position and gender?

One might think that lifestyle practices are a matter of individual choice. That is, a person either chooses to do healthy things as a lifestyle or not, and this is basically the whole story. On the surface, such a decision appears to be largely a matter of free will. But is this really the case? Are health and other lifestyles constructed by individuals without any specific reference to the social structures in their lives? If this is true, then why do lifestyles tend to cluster in particular patterns reflecting distinct differences between people on the basis of class, age, gender and other structural variables? It may be that health lifestyles are shaped from the top down by structural influences that people come to adopt as their own because they fit the context of how they live their life. In this scenario, structure channels health and other lifestyle practices down particular pathways instead of others that could be chosen. People still have the option to choose, but generally do so along class lines and in accordance with other structural influences that might be relevant to them. Social structures have a significant role in the selection of any lifestyle.

Consequently, in formulating a sociological theory of health lifestyles, a theorist needs to contend with the issues surrounding the relative contributions of agency and structure. Agency can be defined as the process by which individuals recall their past, imagine their future actions, critically evaluate their present circumstances, and choose their behavior based upon their assessment of a situation (Emirbayer & Mische, 1998). Theories that favor agency depict individuals as having the capacity to ultimately choose or self-direct their course of action regardless of structural constraints and influences. This capacity for self-direction underlies the operation of all forms of agency and demonstrates a fundamental freedom that people have to choose their actions (Hitlin & Elder, 2007). Symbolic interaction theory describes this very process when it discusses people constructing their social behavior on the basis of their definitions and interpretations of the situations they find themselves in (Blumer, 1969).

Structure, on the other hand, is defined by Sewell (1992, p. 19) as sets of mutually sustaining rules and procedures to the enactment of social life, along with resources, that empower or constrain social action and tend to be reproduced by that action when it occurs. Resources are of two types, either human (e.g., physical strength, dexterity, knowledge) or nonhuman (naturally occurring or manufactured) that can be used to enhance or maintain power. Sewell equates resources with the power to influence action positively or negatively as suggested by Giddens' (1984) notion of the duality of structure as both constraining and enabling. The enabling function suggests resources increase the range and style of options from which the actor can choose, but constraint means that resources also invariably limit choices to what is possible.

Following the downfall of structural-functionalism in the 1960s, agency-oriented theories moved over time to take a leading role in theorizing in sociology in the United States and United Kingdom. The theoretical tilt toward agency was in the direction of what Archer (1995) refers to as "upwards conflation." Conflation is a term in social theory that represents one-dimensional theorizing. Upwards conflation describes theories depicting individuals interacting with one another and in doing so creating social structures in a one-way, upwards path, leaving those structures incapable of acting back on individuals. Causal power in this context thus resides in the individual acting in concert with similar others to create society and the structures within it. Carried to its extreme, agency theorizing reduces social phenomena to the level of the individual (Hitlin & Elder, 2007).

This is not to say that agency-oriented theories omit considerations of structure as symbolic interaction has its notion of the "generalized other," social constructionism contains elements of Foucault's post-structuralism, Giddens' structuration theory recognizes the "duality of structure" as both constraining and enabling, and Archer's critical realism considers the effects of structural conditioning. Nevertheless, they all share the premise that agency ultimately determines social behavior. While no contemporary theory denies that either agency or structure is unimportant, theoretical debate about their differences center on the extent to which one or the other is dominant. Archer (2003) argues for example, that the capability of structure to constrain or enable individuals is contingent upon individuals exercising agency by choosing the situations in which they have an impact. Therefore, agency, in her view, is more decisive in determining behavior than structure.

While agency theorists maintain that agency will never be completely determined by structure, it is likewise clear that "there is no hypothetical moment in which agency actually gets 'free' of structure; it is not, in other words, some pure Kantian transcendental free will" (Emirbayer & Mische, 1998, p. 1004). As Scambler (2018, p. 95) accurately notes, there is no such thing as a non-structured social world. Structure is therefore present in every social context in which agency is exercised. Bauman (1999) adds to our understanding by observing that individual choices in *all* circumstances are confined by two sets of constraints: (1) choosing from among what is available and (2) social roles or codes telling the individual the rank order and appropriateness of preferences. Consequently, as Hitlin and Elder (2007, p. 177) point out, while humans may be able to control their actions, this capacity gets socially channeled in particular directions. People do have the capability to act independently of the social structures in their lives, but the occasions on which they actually do so may be rare.

For example, structural influences on health lifestyles are seen in past studies in Canada on alcohol use by married women and university students in which social situations determined how much people drank (Demers et al., 1999; Demers et al., 2002). Individuals were not autonomous actors making self-governing decisions; rather, the drinking situation itself influenced levels of consumption (Demers et al.,

2002, p. 422). Drinking with parents was constrained by their presence, for instance, while drinking with close friends in a relaxed setting was enabled. In the US, banning smoking in public places was a more effective approach to smoking cessation than individuals being targeted through educational programs (Sweat & Denison, 1995). The ban had the effect of labeling smokers as social outcasts, deviants, and threats to the health of others in their vicinity. Anti-smoking laws, social isolation, and stigma significantly decreased smoking "far beyond the results of purely individualistic approaches" (Sweat & Denison, 1995, p. S252). More recent research in the US by Mollborn and Modile (2022) likewise illustrate the effects of structure on health lifestyles. They found that the family-based socialization of socioeconomically privileged young adults produced a sense of moral worth and discipline with respect to diet and exercise that was missing in the cultural capital of the less privileged.

In England, Stead and her colleagues (2011) found that the social and symbolic meanings associated with certain foods prevented young teenagers from eating healthy lunches at school. High status ("cool") teens ate quality chocolate bars and crisps (potato chips) for lunch and drank Coca Cola or Pepsi. Teens that ate healthy or inexpensive foods were ridiculed and categorized as "nerds" or "uncool". Bananas and yoghurt were especially taboo. Thus, social status dictated lunchtime food choices for teens who wanted to be popular and accepted by their peers. Healthy eating symbolized something undesirable and exposed them to social risks. While this may seem irrational to public health experts, Stead and her associates argue that unhealthy eating can be viewed by the teenagers as profoundly rational since it avoided the risk of an impaired social identity and rejection by peers. In this circumstance, eating unhealthily could actually be positive for a teen's social and emotional well-being, even though nutritionally harmful.

Whereas these studies show structural influences have a significant effect on health lifestyles, I also found an example where structure can be so overwhelming that agency is literally rendered inert. This is seen in research by Gareth Williams (2003) reporting on high mortality among a group of Welsh coal miners in the 1930s whose work was punishing and diets meager. However, the incessant toll of childbirth and domestic labor impaired the health and shortened the lives of the women as much or more than that of the men. The structural conditions under which they lived their daily lives were so heavy that individual capabilities and capacities were ineffective. This situation, comments Williams (2003, p. 146), "provides a salutary reminder of the way in which the balance between agency, context, and structure is itself highly determined by structural forces."

Although this account might be dismissed as outdated and one would hope it no longer exists, Williams (2003) nevertheless noted that the influence of structure on agency in relation to health lifestyles can still be heavy-handed while also investigating contemporary social conditions in a working-class neighborhood in a British city. He finds that assuming people have the freedom to make healthy choices is not consistent with what many of them experience as real possibilities in their everyday lives. They understood the behavioral risk factors that made poor health more likely and for which they could be personally responsible, but they were also aware that the health risks they faced were part of social conditions that they could do little to change.

Therefore, while agency is important, it seems social structural conditions can act back on individuals and configure their lifestyle patterns in particular ways. Agency allows them to reject or modify these patterns, but structure limits the options that are available. This is not to say that considerations of agency should be minimized, but agency is not the whole story. In many situations it is not dominant but constrained. Structure invariably has a role in lifestyle decisions and I argue that it is the interaction between agency and structure that is decisive (Cockerham, 2005, 2021a, b, 2025). That is, I see health lifestyles resulting from a dialectic exchange between agency and structure in which structure's constraints and enablements operate in tandem with agency to determine practices.

Health Lifestyles: The Need for a Theory

Early medical sociology tended to focus on social and social psychological factors having a role in illness and medical care; the health-oriented behavior of people who were not sick were not a topic of investigation. However, the study of health lifestyles has become important in its own right and before proceeding to a discussion of health lifestyle theory, we should first consider the need for such a theory. Social factors not only cause disease, but they also cause health and the primary mechanism by which health is socially manufactured or undermined is through lifestyles (Cockerham, 2005, 2021a, b, 2023, 2025). Everyone has a lifestyle that is practiced on a daily basis and to ignore such a fundamental form of behavior undercuts our ability to fully account for social conduct (Giddens, 1991). Although medical sociology neglected the study of lifestyle constellations that were relevant for health for many years, this situation has changed with the realization that such lifestyles are indeed a regular part of everyday living and have a major role in health outcomes. In past periods of history, when life expectancy was shorter, a person's health was more or less taken for granted; that is, an individual was either naturally healthy or unhealthy and that was simply the way life had turned out for the person.

This situation is now different with a majority of people expecting to live to advanced ages and in the process becoming more susceptible to chronic diseases associated with lifestyles. Chronic diseases—such as heart disease, cancer, stroke, and diabetes—cannot be cured by medical treatment and certain lifestyle practices, such as smoking, alcohol and drug abuse, eating high fat foods, and unprotected sex in the case of sexually-transmitted diseases, cause these afflictions and end life prematurely. Modernity now brings the requirement to actively work to stay healthy in order to avoid these problems and prolong life spans. However, while some people are protective of their physical well-being, others, either in ignorance or purposively, practice bad health habits that are self-destructive. Why? Katainen and Gronow (2024, p. 36) suggest that unhealthy habits are "creative solutions to problems confronted in everyday life and reflect individuals' relationships to the material and social world around them." Drinking alcohol, smoking, overeating, and the like, can be a means of stress reduction, self-fulfillment, enjoyment, relaxation, or mode of socializing with friends.

Nonetheless, health today has become viewed as an achievement—something that people are supposed to work at to enhance their quality of life or risk illness and premature death if they do not (Clarke et al., 2003; Martschukat, 2021). As Giddens (1991) and Turner (1992) concluded long ago, lifestyle options have become integrated with bodily regimens or routines aimed at physical maintenance. People in advanced societies are normatively assigned personal responsibility for their health and even the design of their own bodies along socially acceptable lines (Turner, 1992; VanHeuvelen & VanHeuvelen, 2021). This is seen in the recent analysis of contemporary social life by Martschukat (2021, p. 136), a social historian, who determined that people in advanced societies are currently living in an "Age of Fitness" in which "the active pursuit of fitness pushed its way to the center of social organization and individual existence."

The epidemiological transition in the twentieth century from acute to chronic illnesses was not the only development promoting the role of health lifestyles in daily life and the need for a theory. Another reason is the late modern decline in the status and professional authority of physicians through lessened control over the medical marketplace, health care decisions requiring the permission of insurers, and greater movement toward the mutual participation model of the physician-patient relationship in which the patient shares in decision-making about his or her medical care. This circumstance has accelerated with the advent of Internet medicine and the wide diffusion of medical knowledge in the public domain (Drentea & Moren-Cross, 2005; Fox et al., 2005). Adopting a healthy lifestyle accords people some personal control over their health as a preventive measure.

Additionally, as Giddens (1991) points out, lifestyles not only fulfill practical ends, but also express a person's self-identity. Giddens therefore defines a lifestyle as a more or less integrated set of practices which an individual embraces, not only because such practices satisfy utilitarian needs, but because they give material form to a particular narrative of self-identity (Frie & Janssen, 2009; Jaye et al., 2018; Mollborn & Lawrence, 2018; Mollborn et al., 2021a; Mollborn & Modile, 2022). What people consume in their lifestyle practices reflects their social status as different groups have different patterns of consumption (Atkinson, 2024; Bourdieu, 1984; Carpiano et al., 2008; Stead et al., 2011). Knowing a person's lifestyle explains a great deal about the person, including their social status.

Health Lifestyles: The Foundation

As noted, sociologists have been slow to recognize the effects of lifestyles on behavior and ultimately on health. One reason may have been the influence of Thorstein Veblen's ([1899] 1994) classic, the *Theory of the Leisure Class*, that affixed the term "lifestyle" to modes of leisure adopted by the upper class. The term "lifestyle" became synonymous with upper class styles of living and what many considered trivial forms of consumerism by the affluent. Only the wealthy had the time and the money to have a "style" to their lives. As we now know, it was a mistake to suppose that lifestyles are confined to those in more privileged material circumstances. Everybody has a lifestyle, even the poorest of the poor (Giddens, 1991).

Weber

Max Weber ([1922] 1978) provides the deepest insight into the lifestyle concept among the classical theorists and, in doing so, made three lasting contributions. First, he associated lifestyles with status groups, noting that people in such groups shared a similar lifestyle distinct from other groups. To be a member of a group and share its status, a person was expected to adopt its style of life. Even though an individual may have a "lifestyle," lifestyles themselves are a collective phenomenon, reflecting patterns of living characteristic of particular groups and especially social classes. Although Weber's methodologies often reflected an individualist and agency-oriented "bottom-up" approach to the study of social structure, he did not view patterns of social action as the uncoordinated practices of disconnected individuals (Kalberg, 1994). Instead, he saw such action in terms of regularities and uniformities repeated by numerous actors over time that formed general patterns of behavior. His focus was on the way in which people act in concert, not individually.

The bridge from agency to structure for Weber was his use of "ideal types," consisting of structural entities like his concept of bureaucracy or macro-level processes like the spread of formal rationality in Western society whose construction allowed him to make general statements about collective forms of social behavior (Kalberg, 1994). For example, in *The Protestant Ethic and the Spirit of Capitalism* (1958), Weber emphasized structure in an essentially "top-down" fashion by showing how social institutions (Calvinist religion) and widespread belief systems (the spirit of capitalism) were powerful forces in shaping the thoughts and behavior of individuals (Sibeon, 2004). In order for a manner of life to emerge that could adapt to the peculiarities of capitalism and come to dominate others, Weber (1958, p. 55) finds "that it had to originate somewhere, and not in isolated individuals alone, but as a way of life common to whole groups of men [people]."

Second, Weber pointed out that lifestyles were based not on what people produced, but what they consumed. Consumption is not independent of production. As Ritzer (Ritzer & Yagatich, 2012), argues, the distinction between production and consumption is false in that all acts invariably involve both processes. In order to consume something, it has to be first produced, and the process of production often requires the consumption of something. In the case of health lifestyles, consumption seems to hold sway over production. Even though it can argued that positive health lifestyles are intended to produce good health, that production consumes goods, services, and time, and ultimately the health produced is used or consumed over time. Therefore, lifestyle differences between groups are primarily based on their relationship to the means of consumption in a society. Moreover, while economic modes of production set the parameters within which styles of consumption occur, it does not determine specific forms of it. This is because the consumption of goods and services conveys a *social* meaning that displays the status and social identity of the consumer. Consumption can therefore be regarded as a set of social and cultural practices that *establish* differences between groups, not merely a means of expressing differences that are in place because of economic factors (Bocock, 1993; Bourdieu, 1984).

And third, Weber's most important contribution to conceptualizing lifestyles in sociological terms is to impose a dialectical capstone over the interplay of choices and chances (Cockerham et al., 1997). What Weber calls "life chances" is defined by Dahrendorf (1979. p. 73) as the "crystallized probability of finding satisfaction for interests, wants and needs, thus the probability of the occurrence of events which bring about such satisfaction." The probability of finding satisfaction is anchored in structural conditions. Life chances are therefore a proxy for structure and life choices represent agency. Choices and chances work off each other to determine a lifestyle. People have needs, wants, and social identities that they match up with their chances in life and select a lifestyle supported by and realistic for their social position. Despite the powerful influence of structure, Weber accords choice the greater role.

What Weber provides us that is central to formulating a contemporary theory of health lifestyles is that: (1) such lifestyles are collective, health-related practices characteristic of particular groups and classes; (2) while they produce health, the aim of this activity is ultimately one of consumption as people use their health for some end, such as work, a longer life, increased vitality, enhanced enjoyment of their physical body, or a good physical appearance; and (3) that the interplay of agency and structure establish and shape the practices that comprise their expression and form.

Giddens

Another contribution to health lifestyle theory comes from Anthony Giddens (1991) who describes how late modernity influences contemporary lifestyles by undercutting traditional practices and promoting a diversity of choices. Global transformations of our sense of time, space, and distance, combined with certain disembedding factors (like increasingly sophisticated and abstract monetary systems, the widespread availability of rapid digital communications, and the penetration of technical knowledge throughout society), advance constant change. In these circumstances, people are likely to be pushed by social situations into choosing a particular lifestyle that connects their options to a more or less stable pattern that provides consistency for their self-identity in a time of ongoing change.

Giddens also maintains that even persons in the lowest social classes have some choice because no culture, in his view, eliminates choice altogether in day-to-day affairs and the poor have distinctive cultural styles and activities that require choices, such as trying to survive conditions of poverty. While he does not overlook the influence of external sources on the lifestyles of individuals generally, he favors agency over structure in lifestyle selection because of the role of choice in the construction of self- identity. Nevertheless, Giddens (1984) importantly contributes to our understanding of structure with his notion of the duality of structure, namely that structures are both constraining and enabling at the same time. That is, structures set limits on what people can choose, but they also provide resources (e.g., status, class position, finances) that can help them realize their choices. This constraining and enabling function guides people into lifestyles that are realistic for them.

What we primarily gain from Giddens in developing a theory of health lifestyles is recognition of (1) late modernity's role in fostering a diversity of lifestyle choices, (2) the necessity of having to choose (3) the tendency of choices to cluster in particular patterns (4) the role of lifestyles in reflecting the self-identity of the individual, and (5) the dual function of structure as a constraint or enabler of choices.

Bourdieu

Unlike Weber and Giddens, Bourdieu shows a clear preference for structure over agency as seen in his strong emphasis upon the effects of class hierarchies on behavior. The seminal study detailing class as the most decisive variable in the determination of health lifestyles is Bourdieu's book *Distinction* (1984). Based on a survey of French professionals (upper-middle class) and working class respondents that included sports preferences and eating habits, Bourdieu found the working class to be more attentive to maintaining the strength of the male body than its shape, and to favor food that is cheap, nutritious, and abundant. In contrast, the professional class prefers food that is tasty, healthy, light, and low in calories. As for leisure sports such as sailing, skiing, golf, tennis, and horseback riding, he found a stratified system and noted that the working class not only faces economic barriers, but also social barriers in the form of hidden entry requirements of family tradition, obligatory dress and behavior, and early socialization. Additionally, these sports were usually practiced in exclusive locations with chosen partners and required investments of money, time, and training that the working class lacks. The working class, in contrast, opts for sports that are popular with the general public and accessible to all classes. These are sports like soccer, wrestling, and boxing that feature strength, endurance, and violence.

Consequently, Bourdieu formulated the notion of "distance from necessity" that emerges as a key explanation of class differences in lifestyles. He points out that the more distant a person is from having to acquire economic necessity, the greater the freedom and time that person has to develop and refine personal tastes in line with a more privileged class status. Lower social strata, in turn, tend to adopt the tastes consistent with their class position, in which obtaining items of necessity (such as inexpensive foods and housing) is paramount. For example, Bourdieu (1984, p. 177) observes that as one rises in class position, the proportion of income spent on food diminishes, and that within the food budget, the proportion spent on heavy, fattening foods, which are also cheap—pasta, potatoes, bacon, and pork—declines, whereas an increasing proportion is spent on leaner, lighter, non-fattening foods and especially fresh fruits and vegetables.

Bourdieu finds that social classes not dominated by the ordinary interests and urgencies of making a daily living claim superiority in social and cultural tastes over those who have only fundamental levels of material well-being. Cultivating a taste in good wines typically signifies higher status, or, if beer is the preferred drink, then foreign or craft-brewed beers are likely to be favored over cheap domestic brands. "As the objective distance from necessity grows," states Bourdieu (1984, p. 55), "life-style increasingly becomes the product of what Weber calls a 'stylization of life', a systematic commitment which orients and organizes the most diverse practices—the choice of a vintage or a cheese or the decoration of a holiday home in the country." The greater the social distance from struggling to obtain necessity, the greater the refinement of lifestyle practices. The relevance of the distance from necessity concept is seen in health lifestyles where classes higher on the social scale have the time and resources to adopt the healthiest practices.

The most important of Bourdieu's theorizing with respect to lifestyles is his use of habitus. Although the concept of a habitus can be traced back to the Greek scholar Aristotle around 350 BCE (Hinote, 2014; Wacquant, 2016), the contemporary notion of habitus originates with Edmund Husserl ([1952] 1989, pp. 266–93) who used the term in 1913 to describe *habitual action* that is intuitively followed and practically performed. The concept was expanded by Bourdieu (1977, pp. 72–95) to serve as his core explanation for the agency-structure relationship in lifestyle dispositions (Bourdieu, 1984, pp. 169–225). Bourdieu (1990, p. 53) defines habitus as "systems of durable, transposable dispositions, structured structures predisposed to operate as structuring structures, that is, as principles which generate and organize practices and representations that can be objectively adapted to their outcomes without presupposing a conscious aiming at ends or an express mastery of the operations necessary in order to attain them." Put another way, the habitus serves as a cognitive map or set of perceptions that routinely guides and evaluates a person's choices and options. It provides enduring dispositions toward acting deemed appropriate by a person in particular social situations and settings. Included are dispositions that can be carried out even without giving them a great deal of thought in advance. They are simply habitual ways of acting when performing routine tasks.

The influence of exterior social structures and conditions are incorporated into the habitus, as well as the individual's own inclinations, preferences, and interpretations. The dispositions that result not only reflect established normative patterns of social behavior, but they also encompass action that is habitual and even intuitive. Through selective perception the habitus molds aspirations and expectations into what Bourdieu calls "categories of the probable" that impose perceptual boundaries on dispositions and the potential for action. "As an acquired system of generative schemes," observes Bourdieu (1990, p. 55), "the *habitus* makes possible the free production of all the thoughts, perceptions, actions, inherent in the particular conditions of its production—and only those." Thus the habitus has perceptual boundaries. One can only know what one knows and act accordingly.

When Bourdieu speaks of the internalization of class conditions and their transformation into personal dispositions toward action, he is describing conditions similar to Weber's concept of life chances that determine materially, socially, and culturally what is probable, possible, or impossible for a member of a particular social class or group (Swartz, 1997, p. 104). Individuals who internalize similar life chances share the same habitus because, as Bourdieu (1977, p. 85) explains, they are more likely to have similar shared experiences: "Though it is impossible for *all* members of the same class (or even two of them) to have the same experiences, in the same order, it is certain that each member of the same class is more likely than any member of another class to have been confronted with the situations most frequent for members of that class." As a result, there is a high degree of affinity in lifestyle choices among members of the same class. Bourdieu maintains that while they may depart from class standards, personal styles are never more than a deviation from a style of a class that relates back to the common style by its difference.

Even though Bourdieu allows agency some autonomy (e.g., agents are determined only to the extent they determine themselves), his emphasis on structure with respect to routine operations of the habitus clearly delineates a far lesser role for agency than the individualist approach to health lifestyles advocating a free range of choices. Consequently, some have argued that Bourdieu strips agency of much of its critical reflexive character and is, in fact, a determinist perspective even though he denies it (Bohman, 1999). Turner and Wainwright (2003, p. 273), however, disagree and find that Bourdieu gives "full recognition" to "agency through his notions of strategy and practices," while illustrating the powerful role of institutions and resources "in shaping, constraining, and producing human agency." Simon Williams (1995) also defends Bourdieu by pointing out that the habitus is not a barrier to choice and his perspective accounts for the relative durability of differences in lifestyles between social classes.

I would argue that the *process* of experience rescues Bourdieu's concept of habitus from the charge of "downward conflation." According to Archer, downward conflation refers to theorizing in which structures unilaterally mold the social practices of individuals and have a complete monopoly over causation, thereby shaping behavior from above in a one-way downward direction. However, through experience, agency acquires new information and rationales for prompting creativity and change by way of the habitus. As Bourdieu (Bourdieu & Wacquant, 1992, p. 133), explains, even though experiences confirm habitus, since there is a high probability that most people encounter circumstances that are consistent with those that originally fashioned it, the habitus nevertheless "is an *open system of dispositions* that is constantly subjected to experiences, and therefore constantly affected by them in a way that reinforces or modifies its structures." Thus the habitus can be creative and initiate changes in dispositions, although this potential is not stressed in Bourdieu's earlier work.

Silva (2016), however, finds that Bourdieu's depiction of habitus is more elastic in his later work. Bourdieu's (2000, pp. 160–61) later perspective is that the habitus changes when confronted with new conditions and its degrees of integration with the perceptions of the individual can vary. Moreover, the dispositions generated by the habitus can not only be changed, but rejected, weakened through nonuse, subjected to tension, or out of line with the parameters of a particular field.

While dispositions toward practices originate in the habitus, the practices themselves are carried out in social contexts that Bourdieu conceptualizes as "fields." Fields are networks or configurations of objective relations (domination, subordination, etc.) between social positions (Bourdieu & Wacquant, 1992). Fields thus contain people who dominate and others who are dominated (Bourdieu, 1998a, p. 40). A field therefore constitutes a structured social space or what Bourdieu describes as an "arena" in which people and institutions use their capital—economic, cultural, and social—to maneuver for advantage in a hierarchical structure of relationships. Amounts and types of capital determine positions in the hierarchy relative to others in the field. Some positions are clearly more powerful and so the power relations of a field typically shape the interaction that takes place within it. Korp (2008) maintains that healthy lifestyles can be viewed as the habitual practices of groups that dominate social fields where healthy living is considered important. The opposite could be the case in fields with different power dynamics. The exercise of agency is therefore influenced from outside the individual by fields and capital, while habitus shapes it from the inside.

Bourdieu calls for the rejection of theories that either explicitly or implicitly claim that the weight of structure on individuals takes away their behavioral options. This assertion shows him opposing determinism, although he also maintains that the rejection of mechanistic theories of behavior does not imply that we should bestow on some creative free will the exclusive power to generally constitute the meanings of situations and determine the intentions of others. The dispositions generated by the habitus tend to be compatible, in his view, with the behavioral parameters set by the wider society; therefore, usual and practical modes of behaving—not unpredictable novelty—typically prevail. Consequently, Bourdieu emphasizes structure more than agency even though he accords agency the capacity to direct behavior when motivated; otherwise, his perspective largely accounts for routine behaviors that people enact without having to analyze or even think much about unless deeper attention is required.

Bourdieu's major contributions to our understanding of health lifestyles therefore fall into three major areas: (1) his concept of the "distance from necessity" as the origin of class differences in lifestyle practices (2) identifying the role of habitus in creating and reproducing lifestyles, and (3) emphasizing this role to show how structure, or in Weberian terms, life chances determine lifestyle choices. He is at his best in analyzing how lifestyles produce distinctions between social classes.

The merit of Bourdieu's (1984) approach is that he maintains there is a structural dimension to lifestyle practices rather than individuals making random or uncoordinated choices on their own. What he accomplishes is to bring structure back into forefront of contemporary theoretical discourse by emphasizing the power of invisible objective structures that nonetheless shape practices. These structures, especially class position, actively influence and potentially determine behavioral outcomes through a person's subjective interpretation of their circumstances (Monnier, 2007; Swartz, 1997). Bourdieu advances a structural theory of social practices that connects individual action to culture, structure, and power relationships with his notions of capital and field that influence the individual externally and habitus that internalizes the influence of external structures within the individual's own behavioral repertoire. From my perspective, Bourdieu's notion of habitus is central to a theory of health lifestyles as it provides the individual with the social parameters or boundaries for his or her choices that channel a person down a particular pathway as opposed to others that might be chosen.

As I have said elsewhere (Cockerham, 2005, p. 53), sociological concepts reflecting literally all theories of social life attest to the fact that *something* (namely structure) exists beyond the individual to give rise to customary patterns of behavior. These concepts range from Durkheim's ([1895] 1950, p. 13) notion of social facts as "every way of acting, fixed or not, capable of exercising on the individual an external constraint" to Mead's (1934, p. 155) view of the "generalized other" as the organized attitudes of the whole community and the social process through which "the community exercises control over the conduct of its individual members." To assign individuals complete freedom in their lifestyle choices overlooks the pervasive boundaries placed on those choices by the social structures in their lives.

Health Lifestyles: A Theory

Before presenting an updated theory of health lifestyles, it is logical to first define the subject being theorized. My definition (Cockerham, 2000, 2005; Cockerham et al., 1997) is as follows: health lifestyles are collective patterns of health-related behavior based on choices from options available to people according to their life chances. This view incorporates the dialectical relationship between life choices and life chances proposed by Weber ([1922, pp. 531–9] 1978, pp. 926–39) and the duality of structure suggested by Giddens (1987, pp. 60–61). While health and other lifestyle choices are voluntary, life chances—which represent structure, especially class position—either empower or constrain choices as choices and chances work off each other to determine behavioral outcomes. That is, the person has the capability of choosing his or her lifestyle, but the choices are limited by what is possible and strongly influenced by the style common to one's class position, age, gender, and the like. The theory is therefore based on the premise that health lifestyles are not the uncoordinated behaviors of disconnected individuals, but rather are personal routines that merge into an aggregate form that are characteristic of specific groups and classes. This paradigm is presented in Fig. 6.1. The arrows between boxes indicate hypothesized causal relationships.

Beginning with Box 1, in the top box in Fig. 6.1, four categories of structural variables are listed that have the capacity to shape health lifestyles: (1) class

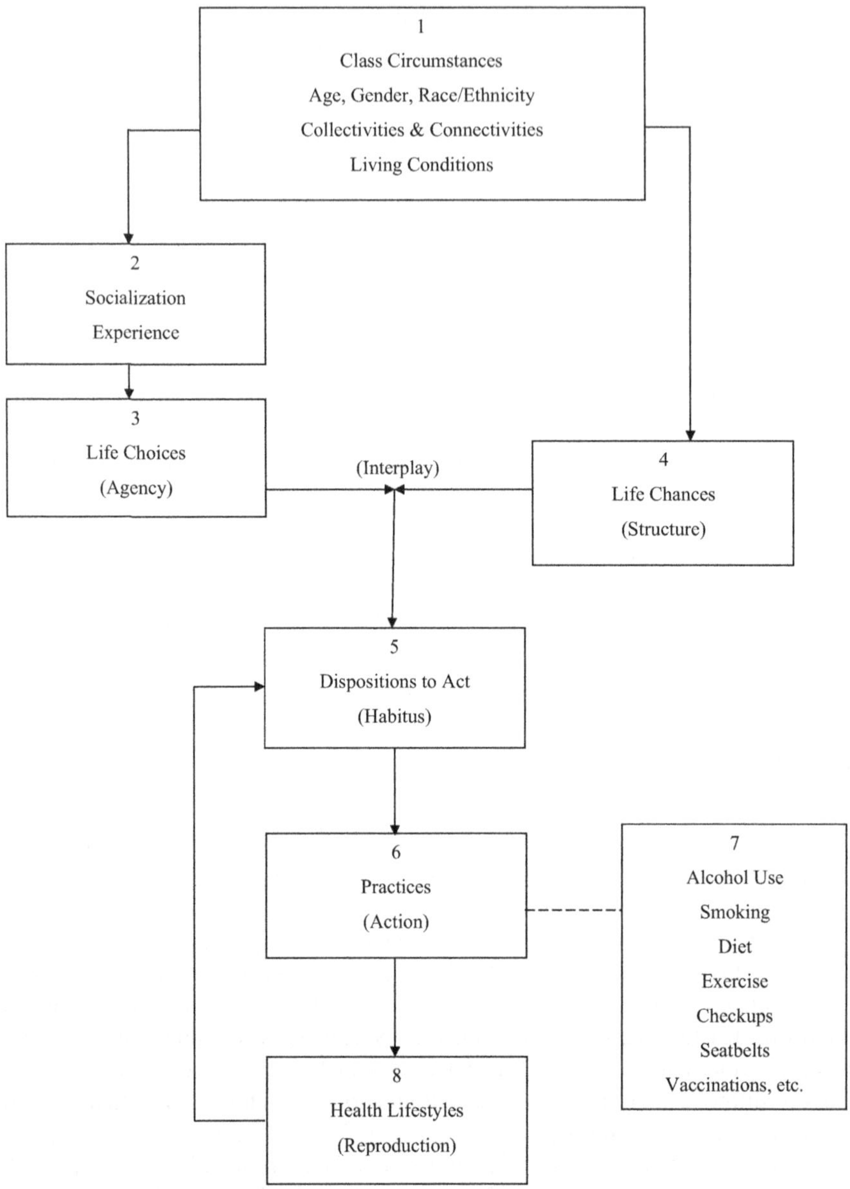

Fig. 6.1 Health lifestyles paradigm

circumstances (2) age, gender, and race/ethnicity (3) collectivities and connectivities, and (4) living conditions. What is meant "by capacity to shape" is that each of these categories can affect the lifestyle choices made by individuals. They do so in ways suggested by Bauman (1999, p. 72) in that they provide an *agenda of choices* (a set of available choices, but the composition of the set itself is seldom for the chooser to decide) and the *code of choosing* (social rules that tell the chooser what is appropriate or inappropriate). In the first instance, structural conditions, not the individual, establish the range of choices available for the person to choose from; in the second situation, structural conditions provide the rank order of preferences for the individual. For example, an individual's class circumstances determine what is available to choose from and what *should* be chosen. This starting point suggests that the model is one of downward conflation; however, this is not the case, since as will be discussed, agency enters the model in Box 3.

Class Circumstances

The first category of structural variables in Box 1 is class circumstances that, from all accounts, is the most powerful influence on lifestyle forms. Not only is this claimed by a host of sociological theorists ranging from Veblen to Bourdieu, but also it is supported by the research literature. Virtually every study confirms that the lifestyles of the upper and upper-middle classes are the healthiest of any socioeconomic strata in Western society and progressively worsen the lower one descends the social ladder. More affluent classes have the highest participation in leisure-time sports and exercise, healthier diets, moderate drinking, little or no smoking, more physical checkups by physicians, and greater opportunities for rest, relaxation, and coping successfully with stress (Andrews et al., 2017; Burdette et al., 2017; Carpiano et al., 2008; Christensen & Carpiano, 2014; Eriksen et al., 2024; Lawrence et al., 2020; McCoy et al., 2024; van den Broek, 2021). The upper and upper-middle classes are also the first to have knowledge of new health risks and, because of their greater resources, are most able to adopt new health strategies and practices (Link & Phelan, 2000; Missinne et al., 2015). The advantaged classes are able to move in a more fluid fashion to embrace new health behaviors, such as adopting low cholesterol and low carbohydrate diets. They were able to reduce their risk of heart disease in the United States (which at one time was high relative to the lower class) so that lower class individuals are now at greater risk.

A decisive component of class standing in the social gradient of health is education (Andersson et al., 2022; Mirowsky & Ross, 2003). Better educated people are typically healthier because they have the knowledge to help them lead healthier lives with respect to their lifestyles and seek preventive and curative forms of medical care when they need it. While education is obviously a critical factor for one's health, it is nevertheless part of a broader dimension of class membership that enables people in higher social strata to be healthier over the life course. The other factors are income that provides them with the financial resources to live a healthy life and occupational status that provides them with self-esteem and a sense of responsibility. Although it is clear that education plays an especially powerful role in the selection of health lifestyle practices, income and occupational status join education as the major components of social class or socioeconomic status (SES).

According to Adler and her associates (1994), the three SES variables—education, income, and occupation—are interrelated but not identical nor fully overlapping. Since associations between SES and health are found with each of these variables, Adler et al. (1994, p. 15) suggest that a boarder underlying dimension of social stratification or social ordering exists that exerts a potent influence on health-related behavior. That is, education is not just a characteristic of individuals, but it can also be viewed in combination with the other components of class to constitute a broad structural variable that produces top-down distinctions in the quality and form of health lifestyles. Moreover, it determines the social context for the practice of such lifestyles. So while education, income, and occupational status are separate individual qualities, collectively they constitute a structural variable whose influence is evident when people express the tastes, distinctions, outlooks, behaviors, and lifestyles common to their class as a whole.

Furthermore, Weber (1946) not only found that lifestyles expressed distinct differences between status groups and their adoption was a necessary feature of upward social mobility, but he also observed that powerful social strata were "social carriers" of lifestyles. These carrier strata were important causal forces in their own right as they transmitted class-specific norms, values, religious ethics, and ways of life across generations (Kalberg, 1994). As Bourdieu (1984) observes, patterns of lifestyles in one generation are reproduced over the time in the next generations that appear and the powerful influence of class on health lifestyles continues. The upper middle class typically serves as a social carrier of positive health lifestyles because its "distance from necessity"—to use Bourdieu's (1984) terminology—allows them the leisure time, access to sources of authoritative knowledge, and resources to learn about appropriate health behavior and adopt such behavior as a public model for other classes.

Age, Gender, and Race/Ethnicity

Stratification variables such as age, gender, and race/ethnicity were not considered by Weber, but contemporary empirical studies show that these variables also influence health lifestyles. Age affects health lifestyles in many ways. As I (Cockerham, 2023, p. 445) have previously stated: "As people age, they carry their health lifestyle along with them as part of an age-specific cohort into the next stage of their life course, modifying or keeping the lifestyle as is while adjusting to an older and physically different body." Exercise, for example, is one major health lifestyle activity that declines and is often lost with advancing age (Rees Jones et al., 2011). Age groups have distinctive lifestyle practices, including young children who are not passive in expressing their preferences to their caretakers (Mollborn et al., 2014, 2021b, 2025; Mollborn & Lawrence, 2018) and adolescents who are prone to experiment at their time of life (adams et al., 2022).

Yet we additionally know that class can intersect with age to produce further differences in lifestyle practices within age groups, as seen in teenage smoking that appears significantly more among the lower strata than the middle and upper classes (Andersson et al., 2022) and in the socialization of children from higher SES families who are taught to be healthy (Mollborn et al., 2014; Mollborn et al., 2021b, 2025). Rees Jones and his colleagues (2011) found that class becomes less important as men age for exercise, but other practices like smoking and alcohol use retain a strong class patterning. Rees Jones et al. conclude that these health lifestyles become fixed or "locked in" and remain socially structured even in later life. The concept of a selective lifestyle "lock-in" along class lines illustrates the durability of class influences on health lifestyles over the life course.

As for gender, it is clearly a significant variable in that women eat more healthy foods, drink less alcohol, smoke less, visit doctors more often for preventive care, wear seatbelts more frequently when they drive, and, with the exception of exercise, have healthier lifestyles overall than men (Annandale, 2021; Cockerham, 2005, 2018;). Furthermore, in adolescence, males tend to adopt the health lifestyles of their fathers and females those of their mothers, thereby setting the parameters for the transmission of gender-specific health practices into adulthood (Mollborn et al., 2020). But whereas gender is a strong predictor of health lifestyle practices, its effects can also be moderated by class distinctions, as people higher on the social scale, regardless of gender, eat healthier diets, smoke less, and participate more in leisure-time exercise (Cockerham, 2021a).

Race and ethnicity are presumed to be important, but there is a paucity of research directly comparing the health lifestyles of different racial and ethnic groups, especially for Asians and Hispanics. Black-White comparisons in the United States show that Whites often drink alcohol, smoke, exercise, and practice weight control more than Blacks (Cockerham et al., 2017, 2022; Hattery & Smith, 2011; Pampel, 2008; Saint Onge & Krueger, 2011), but more research is needed.

An effort to rectify this situation with respect to nutrition in the Black population is found in the work of Hattery and Smith (2011). They link poor diets to diabetes, colon cancer, infant mortality, and premature deaths. Being disproportionally more likely to be poor, Blacks were less likely to eat healthily and exercise. "And, just as the poor in other parts of the world are more vulnerable to diseases like malaria and cholera," states Hattery and Smith (2011, p. 55), "the poor, and increasingly African Americans, are more vulnerable to the diseases associated with an unhealthy lifestyle." Another study of health lifestyles and cardiovascular disease found that Blacks had a higher probability of excessive caloric intake than Whites that was indicative of a greater potential for obesity (Cockerham et al., 2017). There is also evidence that exercise declines more steeply for Blacks than Whites across the course of adulthood, yet this pattern may be caused by Blacks having more functional health problems and living in less safe neighborhoods (Saint Onge & Krueger, 2017). The risk of victimization in an unsafe neighborhood can significantly undermine the motivation to engage in outdoor exercise. Other research by Saint Onge and Krueger (2011) finds that non-Hispanic Whites and more educated individuals exercise more than non-Hispanic Blacks, Hispanics, and less educated persons. Non-Hispanic Whites and the educated also disproportionately participate in facility-based exercise (swimming, tennis, golf), while non-Hispanic Blacks favor team sports (basketball) and fitness activities (running, walking) and Hispanics gravitate toward team sports (soccer). Recreational facilities are often absent in low-income areas and the ability to participate in team sports declines much earlier in life than facility-based exercise. This gives non-Hispanic Whites and better educated persons an advantage in exercising longer as they age. Saint Onge and Krueger observe that the type and extent of leisure-time physical activity is shaped by the cultural identities and social circumstances of the participants.

Most studies on health and race, however, address levels of morbidity and mortality rather than specific health practices. These studies often suggest that racial disparities in health are largely but not exclusively determined by class position, with disadvantaged socioeconomic circumstances and the adverse life experiences associated with them promoting poor health (Angel & Angel, 2021; Erving & Satcher, 2021; Bradby & Nazroo, 2021). Clearly, more research is needed to determine the extent of racial differences in health lifestyle practices and the extent to which such lifestyles are affected by racial discrimination (Phelan & Link, 2015).

Research on the relationship between health lifestyles and different ethnic groups is also lacking, including how to best conceptualize and measure ethnicity. Existing studies of ethnicity, like those of race, have focused more on the overall health profiles of ethnic groups than on health lifestyles. Nevertheless, Karlsen and Nazroo (2002) found that the structural influences seen in ethnic-oriented patterns of discrimination and harassment, along with lower class social status, had greater effects on health than personal identities. Such identities were considered products of agency in that they were self-constructed and internally defined by the individual. That is, how the individual defined him or herself in relation to their ethnicity was not as important for their health as structural conditions beyond the individual, namely discrimination.

Collectivities and Connectivities

Collectivities are collections of actors linked together through specific social relationships and networks, such as the workplace, kinship, religion, and politics. The shared norms, values, ideals, and social perspectives of such collectivities has been held to constitute inter-subjective "thought communities" beyond individual subjectivity that reflect a particular collective world view (Zerubavel, 1997). The notion of thought communities is akin to Mead's (1934) concept of the generalized other in that both are abstractions of the perspectives of social collectivities or groups that enter into the thinking of the individual. While people may accept, reject, or ignore the normative guidance rendered by such groups, group views are nonetheless likely to be taken into account when choosing a course of action (Berger & Luckmann, 1967). Weber ([1922] 1978) notes that concepts of collective entities have meaning in the minds of individuals, partly as something actually existing and partly as something with normative authority. "Actors," states Weber ([1922] 1978, p. 14), "thus in part orient their action to them, and in this role such ideas have a powerful, often a decisive, causal influence on the course of action of real individuals."

Religion and political ideology are examples of collective perspectives that have implications for health lifestyles. This is seen in the usual preference of religious persons and groups for positive health lifestyles since their beliefs invariably promote healthy living in the form of good nutrition, exercise, and personal hygiene, while discouraging alcohol use and smoking cigarettes (Hill et al., 2007; Idler, 2021). However, the full extent of the relationship between religiosity and health lifestyles is not known because of a lack of relevant studies. This is an important area that needs further research.

Little is also known about ideology and health lifestyles. Research on the effects of the socialist heritage in Russia after the fall of the Soviet Union in 1989 show that pro-socialists (those who are in favor of a return to state socialism as it was under communism) had less healthy lifestyles than anti-socialists, even though neither group demonstrated exceptionally positive health practices (Cockerham et al., 2002). Pro-socialists had a particularly passive approach to health lifestyles that seemed left over from Soviet times. The choices of individuals in Soviet society were confined to a single social and political ideology (communism) and expected to conform to it. When a person got sick, the state was responsible for taking care of that person as a benefit of state socialism. Individual incentives in health matters were not encouraged. Thus it could be argued that communism was bad for one's health as it failed to promote healthy lifestyle practices and improve the general health of those subject to it. A leftover from Soviet times is one of the largest gender gaps in life expectancy in world, with Russian women outliving their male counterparts 9.8 years on average as recently as 2023.

A more recent study in the US on a COVID-19 pandemic-related lifestyle (e.g., social distancing, mask usage, hand sanitizing, and vaccinations) found that political conservatism was associated with risker pandemic lifestyle practices (Hill et al., 2022). Conservatives exhibited less empathy for the welfare of others, a more authoritarian outlook, and less likelihood of perceiving the pandemic as a threat to themselves and the broader society. Although vaccination had the greatest capability of ending the pandemic, it became a divisive lifestyle practice in the US because of the fear of harm from vaccines and a political issue as an infringement on individual rights. However, the extent to which ideology affects health lifestyles beyond these two examples remains unknown.

In the past, there was also little research on family and kinship group influences concerning health lifestyles, but this changed with the research of Mollborn and her colleagues that finds such influence can be strong, primarily in socioeconomically advantaged families (Mollborn & Lawrence, 2018; Mollborn & Modile, 2022; Mollborn et al., 2021b, 2025). Most individuals are born into a family of significant others—significant because they provide the child with a specific social identity and sense of self. This identity includes not only an appraisal of physical and intellectual characteristics, but knowledge about the family's social and medical history. In addition to learning the family's social status, perspective, and cultural orientation, the child learns about the health threats most common for the family and the measures needed to cope with them. As the child becomes older and takes as his or her own the values and attitudes of the immediate family, community, and wider society as presented through the mediating influence of the family, the child is considered properly socialized in that he or she behaves in accordance with group-approved rules.

Children can either accept or reject the social perspective of their family as representative of their own social reality. Yet the reality presented to them in the process of primary socialization is set by adults who determine what information is provided and assessments of the validity of opposing viewpoints. Although children are not necessarily passive in the socialization experience, what is important is that they have no choice in the selection of their significant others so that identification with them is quasi-automatic (Berger & Luckmann, 1967). This further means that children's internalization of their family's interpretation of social reality is quasi-inevitable and Bourdieu (1990) finds is instrumental in forming the habitus. Although the initial social world presented to children by their significant others may be weakened by later social relationships and views, it can nonetheless be a lasting influence. Parental influence, for example, has been found in the Mollborn studies to be an important and persistent influence on the preventive health beliefs of their children and significant in shaping their health lifestyles.

Whereas collectives are social networks of people who serve as a normative authority for health lifestyles, connectivities are electronic social networks which operate as computational authority on lifestyle practices (Airoldi, 2022, p. 145). These electronic networks center on an individual's biodata instead of group norms and represent another form of health lifestyle participation. Connectivities function as a reference metric for electronically measuring and determining the effectiveness of various lifestyle practices on the body. They are also a major source of health information, as well as a means to interact with health care providers electronically. This is made possible by widespread use of digital technologies, such as smartwatches, Fitbit health and fitness trackers, patient-centered apps, health care provider apps, and electronic links to websites for webinars, exercise and yoga services, virtual classes, social media groups, streaming video sites, blogs, podcasts, and the like for participating in and managing health lifestyles. Connectivities are a major feature of modern health lifestyle practices and a new addition to health lifestyle theory that needs to be included in future studies (Cockerham, 2023).

Living Conditions

Living conditions are a category of structural variables pertaining to differences in the quality of housing and access to basic utilities (e.g., electricity, gas, heating, sewers, indoor plumbing, safe piped water, hot water), neighborhood facilities (e.g., grocery stores, parks, recreation), and personal safety. Such conditions may also apply to other sites where people spend their lives, such as their place of work or employment. To date there has been little research linking living conditions to health lifestyles, but the connection is important. Blaxter (1990) found in a nationwide British survey that still has relevance for today when she determined that the environment within which a person lives strongly affects health-related behavior. Health lifestyles were most effective in positive living situations and least effective in unhealthy conditions, such as substandard housing, pollution, lack of public services and medical facilities, poor quality food, sewage and drainage problems, exposure to insects and rodents, and high levels of neighborhood unemployment, crime, alcoholism, and drug abuse.

Blaxter concluded that socioeconomic circumstances and the living environment determined the extent to which health lifestyles can be practiced effectively. This is an important finding in that it shows the structural conditions of people's lives makes it probable or improbable they can actually achieve a positive health lifestyle. Blaxter (1990, p. 216) finds that if living conditions are good, healthy behavior appears to have a strong influence on health, but if they are bad, then behavior makes little difference and is often unhealthy. Consequently, living a healthy lifestyle was not simply a matter of individual choice, but to a large extent depended upon a person's social and material environment for its success.

In the United States, for instance, living in disadvantaged neighborhoods has been associated with poor health (Arcaya et al., 2016) and growing up in affluent neighborhoods has been found to have positive long-term health effects (Vartanian & Houser, 2010). Living in poor neighborhoods significantly contributes to low participation in vigorous outdoor exercise and obtaining healthy foods. Therefore, living conditions can constrain or enhance health lifestyles.

Socialization and Experience

Class circumstances and the other variables shown in Box 1 in Fig. 6.1 provide the social context for socialization and experience as depicted by the arrow leading to Box 2. This is consistent with Bourdieu's (1977) view that dispositions to act in particular ways are constructed through socialization and experience, with class position providing the social context for this process. The present model, however, adds the additional structural categories—age, gender, race/ethnicity, collectivities and connectivities, and living conditions—depicted in Box 1, since they also comprise part of the social environment within which socialization and experience occur.

Whereas primary socialization represents the imposition of society's norms and values on the individual by significant others and secondary socialization results from later institutional training, experience is the learned outcome of day-to-day activities that comes about through social interaction and the practical exercise of agency. It is through both socialization and experience that the person or actor acquires reflexive awareness and the capacity to perform agency, but experience—with respect to life choices—provides the essential basis for agency's practical and evaluative dimensions to evolve over time. This is especially the case as people confront new social situations and conditions.

Life Choices (Agency)

Figure 6.1 shows that socialization and experience (Box 2) provides the capacity for life choices (agency) depicted in Box 3. As previously noted, the term "life choices" was introduced by Weber as one of the two major components of lifestyles (the other is life chances) and refers to the self-direction of one's behavior. It is an English language translation of *Lebensführung*, which in German literally means conducting or managing one's life. Life choices are a process of agency by which individuals critically evaluate and choose their course of action. Weber's notion of life choices accounts for the interpretive process whereby the potential outcomes of choices are imagined, evaluated, and reconstructed in the mind and then selected and acted upon to achieve desired goals (Emirbayer & Mische, 1998). Weber (1949) maintained that individuals have the capacity to interpret their situation, make deliberate choices, and attach subjective meaning to their actions. All social action in his view takes place in contexts that imply both constraints and opportunities, with the actor's interpretive understanding (*Verstehen*) of the situation guiding behavioral choices (Kalberg, 1994).

Life Chances (Structure)

Class circumstances and to a lesser degree the other variables in Box 1 constitute life chances (structure) shown in Box 4. Life chances are the other major component of lifestyles in Weber's model. Weber was ambiguous about what he meant by life chances, but the term is usually associated with the advantages and disadvantages of relative class situations. Consequently, the higher a person's position in a class hierarchy, the better the person's life chances or probabilities for finding satisfaction and vice versa. Dahrendorf (1979, p. 65) adds the following clarification; "for Weber, the probability of sequences of action postulated in the concept of chance is not merely an observed and thus calculable probability, but is a probability which is invariably anchored in structural conditions." Thus a person's probabilities for satisfaction that comprise his or her life chances are based on the structural conditions in their life, especially their class position. Weber's thesis is that chance is socially determined and social structure is an arrangement of chances. Therefore, life chances represent the influence of structure in Weber's *oeuvre* and this paradigm.

Choice and Chance Interplay

The arrows in Fig. 6.1 indicate the dialectical interplay between life choices (Box 3) and life chances (Box 4). This interaction is clearly Weber's most important contribution to conceptualizing lifestyle construction (Cockerham et al., 1993, 1997).

Choices and chances operate in tandem to determine a distinctive lifestyle for individuals, groups, and classes. Life chances (structure) either constrain or enable choices (agency); agency is not passive in this process, however. As Archer (2003) explains, whether or not constraints and enablements are exercised as causal powers is based on agency choosing the practices to be activated. "Constraints," says Archer (2003, p. 4), "require something to constrain, and enablements something to enable." Consequently, people have to consider a course of action if their actions are to be either constrained or enabled. People therefore align their goals, needs, and desires with their probabilities for realizing them and choose a lifestyle according to their assessments of their resources and class circumstances. Unrealistic choices are not likely to succeed or be selected, while realistic choices are based upon what is structurally possible.

In this context, choices and chances are not only connected dialectically, but are analytically distinct. As Archer (1998, p. 369) points out: "Because the emergent properties of structures and the actual experiences of agents are not synchronized (due to the very nature of society as an open system), then there will always be the inescapable need for a two-part account." Weber provides such a framework. He conceptualizes choice and chance as separate components in the activation and conduct of a lifestyle and merges the different functions of agency and structure without either losing their distinctiveness.

Up to this point, the health lifestyles paradigm has indeed been an example of Archer's (1998) notion of downward conflation in which individual behavior is molded by structure in the form of class circumstances, gender, collectivities, etc. However, even though structure is dominant in the beginning because people are socialized and have experiences within the context of the pre-existing social structures that comprise their world, agency enters the model at the mid-point where choices and chances interact and outcomes are chosen from what is available. In this way, the one-dimensional theorizing that the term "conflation" represents in Archer's critique of the macro–micro debate in sociology is hopefully avoided. The health lifestyle model presented here, seeks to blend agency and structure and be neither fully upward nor downward in its approach. As Hammarström et al. (2015, p. 14) recognize, health lifestyle theory is an "agency within structure model," which is correct. A basic premise of the theory is that people choose their lifestyle but their choices are constrained or enabled by what is structurally possible and influenced by the style common to their position in society. Nevertheless, I recognize that there is an imbalance favoring structure since structure proceeds individuals and subjects them to molding through socialization, even though they are nonetheless able to think for themselves, choose, and be creative in their behavior if they feel it is appropriate. However, behavior in familiar settings or day-to-day fields is typically routine, and the reality of this situation is that the habitus seems especially powerful in shaping behavioral practices largely along structural lines.

Dispositions to Act (Habitus)

Figure 6.1 shows that the interaction of life choices and life chances produce individual dispositions to action (Box 5). These dispositions constitute a habitus that, as noted, is a cognitive map or set of perceptions routinely guiding and evaluating a person's choices and options. It is a process of thinking in which social norms and cultural conventions are internalized in the mind, along with the individual's own inclinations, preferences, and interpretations. The habitus produces enduring dispositions toward acting that are not only normative, but habitual and even intuitive. One of its principal functions is that of providing a unity of style linking the practices of a single agent to a class of agents that brings together agents or individuals who are very similar to each other and different from members of other classes (Bourdieu, 1998b). Therefore, Bourdieu finds that the habitus retranslates the relational characteristics of a social position into a lifestyle reflecting a unitary set of choices of practices that differentiates itself from the choices of persons in other classes.

As for health lifestyles, the dispositions that are generated are either focused directly on health maintenance or include considerations of health in their adoption, or, conversely, give little or no thought to health outcomes and may even disregard such outcomes even though implications for health nonetheless exist. Consequently, health lifestyles are binary. That is, they usually fall into one or the other of two categories: good or bad. This binary characteristic means that the outcome generated from the interplay of choices and chances have either positive or negative effects on health. Positive health lifestyles are intended to avoid risk and are oriented toward achieving or maintaining one's overall health and fitness. Negative health lifestyles put one at risk for illness and earlier mortality. Yet the health lifestyles of many, perhaps most people, are likely to be neither uniformly positive nor all negative (concordant) but a combination of both healthy and unhealthy (discordant) practices. At least this appears to be the norm (Saint Onge & Krueger, 2017), especially in adolescence and young adulthood when these age groups experiment with unhealthy behaviors (adams et al., 2022; Lawrence et al., 2020; Mollborn et al., 2021a).

Completing the Model

Figure 6.1 shows that dispositions (Box 5) produce practices (action) that are represented in Box 6. The practices that result from the habitus can be based on deliberate calculations, or as noted, habits and intuition. Bourdieu (1984) helps us to realize that practices linked to health lifestyles can be so integrated into routine behavioral repertories that they can be acted out more or less unthinkingly once established in the habitus. He observes that people tend to adopt generalized strategies (a sense of the game) oriented toward practical ends in routine situations that they can habitually follow without having always to stop to analyze them. As a routinized feature of everyday life, it is therefore appropriate to view health lifestyles as guided more by a practical than abstract logic (Williams, 1995).

The four most common practices measured in studies of health lifestyles are alcohol use, smoking, diet, and exercise. These are shown in Box 7 along with other practices such as vaccinations and mask wearing that comprise other typical forms of action taken or not taken. The practices themselves may be positive or negative, but they nonetheless comprise a person's overall pattern of health lifestyles as represented in Box 8. It is important to note that these practices sometimes have a complexity of their own. Smoking tobacco in any form is negative, but moderate alcohol use (preferably red wine) was once thought to reduce the risk of heart disease, is now considered harmful. Eating fresh fruits and vegetables is positive, but consuming meat can be either positive or negative depending on how it is cooked, its fat content, and how often it is consumed. Relatively vigorous leisure-time exercise has more health benefits than physical activity at work because the latter is subject to stress from job demands and time schedules, while walking and other everyday forms of exercise have some value. However, measures of leisure-time exercise may not fully represent the physical activities of women who take care of children and do housework. It is therefore necessary that researchers take the multi-faceted features of health lifestyle practices into account when analyzing them.

Action (or inaction) with respect to a particular health practice leads to its reproduction, modification, or nullification by the habitus through a feedback process. This is seen in Fig. 6.1 by the arrow showing movement from Box 8 back to Box 5. This is consistent with Bourdieu's (1977, 1984) assertion that when dispositions are acted upon they tend to produce or modify the habitus from which they are derived. As conceptualized by Bourdieu, the habitus is the centerpiece of the health lifestyle model.

Conclusion

A central theme of this chapter is that any individualistic paradigm of health lifestyles is too narrow and unrealistic because it fails to consider structural influences on health lifestyle choices. In order to correct this approach and formulate a theory where none previously existed, an updated health lifestyle model is presented here that accords structure a role consistent with its influence in the empirical world. There are times when structure outweighs but does not negate agency and other times when structure may overwhelm agency, and these situations need to be included in concepts explaining health lifestyle practices. A structural orientation does not mean that action is structurally predetermined; rather, it recognizes that social structures strongly influence the thoughts, decisions, and actions of individuals (Sibeon, 2004). After all, isn't this what sociology is really about—namely, the systematic study of society?

Furthermore, it seems very rare that agency ever truly frees itself from structure. At least this is the position taken by Emirbayer and Mische (1998) whose seminal paper defines what agency actually is and I would agree. The only possible exception would seem to be that of experiencing intense emotion in which rational thought is suspended by the contingencies of the moment. Yet when the moment passes, the constraints and enablements of structure reassert themselves as rationality returns and the individual takes control over his or her emotions.

The theoretical model presented here does favor structure and is obviously strongly influenced by Weber and Bourdieu. Although Bourdieu, in particular, has his critics, his notion of habitus nevertheless represents a novel and logical conceptualization of the internalization of external structures in the mind and perceptual processes of the individual. The result is a registry of dispositions to act in ways that are practical and usually consistent with the socially approved behavioral pathways of the larger social order or some class or group therein. Deviant behavior, of course, is an exception and in this situation, the behavioral pathways chosen are a rejection of society's norms and values. Otherwise, most social behavior is consistent with the norms and outcomes deemed appropriate by society for the situation.

This model of health lifestyles states that four categories of (1) structural variables, namely (a) class circumstances (b) age, gender, and race/ethnicity (c) collectivities, and (d) living conditions, provide the social context for (2) socialization and experience that influence (3) life choices (agency). These structural variables also collectively constitute (4) life chances (structure). Choices and chances interact and commission the formation of (5) dispositions to act (habitus), leading to (6) practices (action), involving (7) alcohol use, smoking, diets and other health-related actions. Health practices constitute patterns of (8) health lifestyles whose reenactment results in their reproduction (or modification) through feedback to the habitus.

The theory is an initial representation of the health lifestyle phenomenon and is subject to verification, change, or rejection through future empirical application. It is an update of an initial theoretical formulation concerning a major aspect of day-to-day social behavior for which no other theory now exists. Moreover, it moves beyond current theoretical trends reflecting an emphasis upon individualism to bring considerations of structure consistent with the reality of everyday life back into the conceptual focus of theory in medical sociology.

References

Abel, T., & Frohlich, K. L. (2011). Capitals and capabilities: Linking structure and agency to reduce health inequalities. *Social Science and Medicine, 74*, 236–244.

Adams, J., Lawrence, E. M., Goode, J. A., Schaefer, D. R., & Mollborn, S. (2022). Peer network processes in adolescents' health lifestyles. *Journal of Health and Social Behavior, 63*, 125–141.

Adler, N. E., Boyce, T., Chesney, M. A., Cohen, S., Folkman, S., Kahn, R. L., et al. (1994). Socioeconomic status and health: The challenge of the gradient. *American Psychologist, 10*, 15–24.

Airoldi, M. (2022). *Machine habitus*. Polity.

Andersson, M., Maralani, V., & Wilkinson, R. (2022). Origins and destinations, but how much and when? Educational disparities in smoking and drinking across adolescence and Young adulthood. *Population Research and Policy Review, 41*, 521–558.
Andrews, H., Hill, T., & Cockerham, W. C. (2017). Educational attainment and dietary lifestyles. *Advances in Medical Sociology, 18*, 101–120.
Angel, R. J., & Angel, J. L. (2021). Latinos and equity in health care access in the U.S. In W. Cockerham (Ed.), *The Wiley Blackwell companion to medical sociology* (pp. 303–321). Wiley Blackwell.
Annandale, E. (2021). Health and gender. In W. Cockerham (Ed.), *The Wiley Blackwell companion to medical sociology* (pp. 237–257). WileyBlackwell.
Arcaya, M. C., Tucker-Seeley, R. D., Kim, R., Schnake-Mahl, A., So, M., & Subramanian, S. V. (2016). Research on neighborhood effects on health in the United States: A systematic review of study characteristics. *Social Science & Medicine, 168*, 16–29.
Archer, M. S. (1995). *Realist social theory: The morphogenetic approach*. Cambridge University Press.
Archer, M. S. (1998). Realism and morphogenesis. In M. Archer, R. Bhaskar, A. Collier, T. Lawson, & A. Norrie (Eds.), *Critical Realism* (pp. 356–381). Routledge.
Archer, M. S. (2003). *Structure, agency, and the internal conversation*. Cambridge University Press.
Atkinson, W. (2024). *Class* (2nd ed.). Polity.
Bauman, Z. (1999). *In search of politics*. Stanford University Press.
Berger, P. L., & Luckmann, T. (1967). *The social construction of reality*. Anchor.
Blaxter, M. (1990). *Health lifestyles*. Routledge.
Blumer, H. (1969). *Symbolic interaction*. Prentice-Hall.
Bocock, R. (1993). *Consumption*. Routledge.
Bohman, J. (1999). Practical reason and cultural constraint: Agency in Bourdieu's theory of practice. In R. Schusterman (Ed.), *Bourdieu: A critical reader* (pp. 129–152). Blackwell.
Bourdieu, P. (1977). *Outline of a theory of practice*. Polity.
Bourdieu, P. (1984). *Distinction*. Harvard University Press.
Bourdieu, P. (1990). *The logic of practice*. Stanford University Press.
Bourdieu, P. (1998a). *On television*. New Press.
Bourdieu, P. (1998b). *Practical reason: On the theory of action*. Stanford University Press.
Bourdieu, P. (2000). *Pascalian meditations*. Stanford University Press.
Bourdieu, P., & Wacquant, L. J. D. (1992). *An invitation to reflexive modernity*. University of Chicago Press.
Bradby, H., & Nazroo, J. Y. (2021). Health, ethnicity, and race. In W. Cockerham (Ed.), *The Wiley Blackwell companion to medical sociology* (pp. 258–278). Wiley Blackwell.
Burdette, A. M., Needham, B. L., Taylor, M. G., & Hill, T. D. (2017). Health lifestyles in adolescence and self-rated health into adulthood. *Journal of Health and Social Behavior, 58*, 520–536.
Carpiano, R. M. (2006). Toward a neighborhood resource-based theory of social capital for health: Can Bourdieu and sociology help? *Social Science and Medicine, 62*, 165–175.
Carpiano, R. M., Link, B. G., & Phelan, J. C. (2008). Social inequality and health: Future directions for the fundamental cause explanation. In A. Lareau & D. Conley (Eds.), *Social class* (pp. 232–263). Russell Sage.
Christensen, V. T. (2011). Does parental capital influence the prevalence of child overweight and parental perceptions of child weight-level. *Social Science and Medicine, 79*, 469–477.
Christensen, V. T., & Carpiano, R. M. (2014). Social Class differences in BMI among Danish women: Applying Cockerham's health lifestyle approach and Bourdieu's theory of lifestyle. *Social Science & Medicine, 112*, 12–21.
Clarke, A. E., Shim, J. K., Mamo, L., Fosket, J. R., & Fishman, J. R. (2003). Biomedicalization: Technoscientific transformations of health, illness, and U.S. Biomedicine. *American Sociological Review, 68*, 161–194.
Cockerham, W. C. (2005). Health lifestyle theory and the convergence of agency and structure. *Journal of Health and Social Behavior, 46*, 51–67.

Cockerham, W. C. (2018). Health lifestyles and the search for a concept of a gender-specific habitus. *Social Theory & Health, 16*, 142–155.

Cockerham, W. C. (2000). The sociology of health behavior and health lifestyles." In C. E. Bird, P. Conrad, and A. M. Fremont (Eds.), *Handbook of medical sociology*, 5th Edition (pp. 159–172). Prentice-Hall.

Cockerham, W. C. (2021a). *Sociological theories of health and illness*. Routledge.

Cockerham, W. C. (2021b). Health lifestyles: Bringing structure Back. In W. Cockerham (Ed.), *The new Blackwell companion to medical sociology* (pp. 159–183). Wiley-Blackwell UK.

Cockerham, W. C. (2023). Health lifestyle theory in a changing society: The rise of infectious diseases and digitalization. *Journal of Health and Social Behavior, 64*, 437–451.

Cockerham, W. C. (2025). *Social causes of health and disease* (4th ed.). Polity.

Cockerham, W. C., Abel, T., & Lüschen, G. (1993). Max Weber, formal rationality, and health lifestyles. *Sociological Quarterly, 34*, 413–435.

Cockerham, W. C., Rütten, A., & Abel, T. (1997). Conceptualizing contemporary health lifestyles: Moving beyond Weber. *Sociological Quarterly, 38*, 321–342.

Cockerham, W. C., Christine Snead, M., & DeWaal, D. F. (2002). Health lifestyles in Russia and the socialist heritage. *Journal of Health and Social Behavior, 43*, 42–55.

Cockerham, W. C., Bauldry, S., Hamby, B. W., Shikany, J. M., & Bae, S. (2017). A comparison of black and white racial differences in health lifestyles and cardiovascular disease. *American Journal of Preventive Disease, 52*, S56–S62.

Cockerham, W. C., Bauldry, S., & Sims, M. (2022). Obesity-related health lifestyles of late middle-age African Americans: The Jackson heart study. *American Journal of Preventive Medicine, 63*, S47–S55.

Dahrendorf, R. (1979). *Life chances*. University of Chicago Press.

Demers, A., Bisson, J., & Palluy, J. (1999). Wives' convergence with their husbands' alcohol use: Social conditions as mediators. *Journal of Studies of Alcohol, 60*, 368–377.

Demers, A., Kairouz, S., Adlaf, E. M., Glickman, L., Newton-Taylor, B., & Marchand, A. (2002). Multilevel analysis of situational drinking among Canadian undergraduates. *Social Science and Medicine, 55*, 415–424.

Drentea, P., & Moren-Cross, J. L. (2005). Social capital and social support on the web: The case of an internet mother site. *Sociology of Health & Illness, 27*, 920–943.

Durkheim, E. ([1895] 1950). *The rules of sociological method*. Free Press.

Emirbayer, M., & Mische, A. (1998). What is agency? *American Journal of Sociology, 103*, 962–1023.

Eriksen, I. M., Kari, S., Langnes, T. F., & Walseth, K. (2024). The formation of classed health lifestyles during youth. *Sociology of Health & Illness, 46*, 137–152.

Erving, C. L., & Satcher, L. A. (2021). In W. Cockerham (Ed.), *The Wiley Blackwell companion to medical sociology* (pp. 279–302). Wiley Blackwell.

Fox, N., Ward, K., & O'Rourke, A. (2005). Pro-anorexia, weight-loss drugs, and the internet: An 'anti-recovery' exploratory model of anorexia. *Sociology of Health & Illness, 27*, 944–972.

Frie, K., & Janssen, C. (2009). Social inequality, lifestyle and health—A non-linear canonical correlation analysis based on the approach of Pierre Bourdieu. *International Journal of Public Health, 54*, 213–222.

Giddens, A. (1984). *The constitution of society: Outline of a theory of structuration*. Polity.

Giddens, A. (1987). *Social theory and modern sociology*. Stanford University Press.

Giddens, A. (1991). *Modernity and self-identity*. Stanford University Press.

Hammarström, A., Lundman, B., Ahlgren, C., & Wiklund, M. (2015). Health and masculinities shaped by agency within structures among young unemployed men in a northern Swedish context. *PLOS ONE, 10*, 1–18. https://doi.org/10.1371/journal.pone.0124785

Hattery, A., & Smith, E. (2011). Health, nutrition, access to healthy food and well-being among African Americans. In A. Lemelle, W. Reed, & S. Taylor (Eds.), *Handbook of African American health* (pp. 47–59). Springer.

Hill, T. D., Ellison, C. G., Burdette, A. M., & Musick, M. A. (2007). Religious involvement and healthy lifestyles: Evidence from a survey of Texas adults. *Annals of Behavioral Medicine, 34*, 217–222.

Hill, T. D., Garcia-Alexander, G., Davis, A. P., Bjorklund, E. T., Vila-Henninger, L. A., & Cockerham, W. C. (2022). Political ideology and pandemic lifestyles: The indirect effects of empathy, authoritarianism, and threat. *Discover Social Science and Health, 2*, 14. https://doi.org/10.1007/s44155-022-00014-0

Hinote, B. P. (2014). Habitus, Class, and health. In W. Cockerham, R. Dingwall, & S. Quah (Eds.), *The Wiley Blackwell encyclopedia of health, illness, behavior, & society* (pp. 741–747). Wiley Blackwell.

Hitlin, S., & Elder, G. H., Jr. (2007). Time, self, and the curiously abstract concept of agency. *Sociological Theory, 25*, 170–191.

Husserl, E. ([1952] 1989). Ideas pertaining to a pure phenomenology and to a phenomenological philosophy. Kluwer Academic.

Idler, E. L. (2021). Health and religion. In W. Cockerham (Ed.), *The new Blackwell companion to medical sociology* (pp. 370–388). Wiley Blackwell.

Jaye, C., Young, J., Egan, R., Llewellyn, R., Cunningham, W., & Radue, P. (2018). The health lifestyle in longevity narratives. *Social Theory & Health, 16*, 361–378.

Jones, R., Ian, P., Olia, W., Peter, H., Goya Wannamethee, S., & Morris, R. W. (2011). Class and lifestyle 'lock-in' among middle-aged and older men: A multiple correspondence analysis of the British Regional Heart Study. *Sociology of Health & Illness, 33*, 399–419.

Kalberg, S. (1994). *Max Weber's comparative historical sociology*. University of Chicago Press.

Karlsen, S., & Nazroo, J. Y. (2002). Agency and structure: The impact of ethnic identity and racism on the health of ethnic minority people. *Sociology of Health & Illness, 22*, 36–52.

Katainen, A., & Gronow, A. (2024). Habits and the socioeconomic patterning of health-related behaviour: A pragmatist perspective. *Social Theory and Health, 22*, 36–52.

Korp, P. (2008). The symbolic power of 'healthy lifestyles'. *Health Sociology Review, 17*, 18–26.

Lawrence, E., Mollborn, S., Goode, J., & Pampel, F. (2020). Health lifestyles and the transition to adulthood. *Socius, 6*. https://doi.org/10.1177/2378023l0942070

Link, B. G., & Phelan, J. (2000). Evaluating the fundamental cause explanation for social disparities in health. In C. Bird, P. Conrad, & A. Fremont (Eds.), *The handbook of medical sociology* (5th ed., pp. 33–46). Prentice Hall.

Martschukat, J. (2021). *The age of fitness*. Polity.

McCoy, C. A., Johnston, E., & Hogan, C. (2024). The impact of socioeconomic status on health practices via health lifestyles: Results of qualitative interviews with Americans from diverse socioeconomic backgrounds. *Social Science & Medicine, 344*, 116618.

Mead, G. H. (1934). *Mind, self, and society*. University of Chicago Press.

Mirowsky, J., & Ross, C. E. (2003). *Education, social status, and health*. Aldine de Gruyter.

Missinne, S., Daenekindt, S., & Bracke, P. (2015). The social gradient in preventive healthcare use: What we can learn from socially mobile individuals? *Sociology of Health & Illness, 37*, 823–838.

Mollborn, S., & Lawrence, E. (2018). Family, peer, and school influences on children's developing health lifestyles. *Journal of Health and Social Behavior, 59*, 133–150.

Mollborn, S., & Modile, A. (2022). 'Dedicated to being healthy': Young adults' deployments of health-focused cultural capital. *Social Science and Medicine, 293*, 114648.

Mollborn, S., James-Hawkins, L., Lawrence, E., & Fomby, P. (2014). Health lifestyles in early childhood. *Journal of Health and Social Behavior, 55*, 386–402.

Mollborn, S., Lawrence, E. A., & Hummer, R. A. (2020). A gender framework for understanding health lifestyles. *Social Science & Medicine, 265*, 113182.

Mollborn, S., Lawrence, E. M., & Saint Onge, J. (2021a). Contributions and challenges in health lifestyle research. *Journal of Health and Social Behavior, 62*, 388–403.

Mollborn, S., Rigles, B., & Pace, J. (2021b). "Healthier than just healthy": Families transmitting health as cultural capital. *Social Problems, 68*, 574–590.

Mollborn, S., Pace, J. A., & Rigles, B. (2025). Children's health lifestyles and the perpetuation of inequalities. *Journal of Health and Social Behavior., 66*, 2–17. https://doi.org/10.1177/00221465241255946
Monnier, C. A. (2007). Pierre Bourdieu. In G. Ritzer (Ed.), *The Blackwell encyclopedia of sociology* (Vol. 1, pp. 347–350). Blackwell.
Mouzelis, N. P. (2008). *Modern and postmodern social theorizing*. Cambridge University Press.
Øversveen, E. (2021). Structural determination and social practice: Towards a new understanding of 'structure' in health inequality research. *Social Theory & Health, 21*, 1–16.
Pampel, F. C. (2008). Racial convergence in cigarette use from adolescence to the mid-thirties. *Journal of Health and Social Behavior, 49*, 484–498.
Pescosolido, B. A., McLeod, J., & Alegría, M. (2000). Confronting the second contract: The place of medical sociology in research and policy for the twenty-first century. In C. Bird, P. Conrad, & A. Fremont (Eds.), *Handbook of medical sociology* (5th ed., pp. 411–426). Prentice Hall.
Phelan, J. C., & Link, B. G. (2015). Is racism a fundamental cause of inequalities in health? *Annual Review of Sociology, 41*, 18.1-18.20.
Reynolds, M. M. (2021). Health power resources theory: A relational approach to the study of health inequalities. *Journal of Health and Social Behavior, 62*, 493–511.
Ritzer, G., & Yagatich, W. (2012). Contemporary theory. In G. Ritzer (Ed.), *The Wiley-Blackwell companion to sociology* (pp. 98–118). Wiley-Blackwell.
Saint Onge, J. M., & Krueger, P. M. (2011). Education and racial-ethnic differences in types of exercise in the United States. *Journal of Health and Social Behavior, 52*, 197–211.
Saint Onge, J. M., & Krueger, P. M. (2017). Health lifestyle behavior among U.S. Adults. *SSM-Population Health, 3*, 89–98.
Scambler, G. (2018). *Sociology, health and the fractured society*. Routledge.
Sewell, W. H. (1992). A theory of structure: Duality, agency, and transformation. *American Journal of Sociology, 98*, 1–29.
Sibeon, R. (2004). *Rethinking social theory*. Sage.
Silva, E. (2016). Unity and Fragmentation of the habitus. *The Sociological Review, 64*, 166–183.
Smelser, N. (1997). *Problematics of sociology*. University of California Press.
Stead, M., McDermott, L., MacKintosh, A. M., & Adamson, A. (2011). Why healthy eating is bad for young people's health: Identity, belonging and food. *Social Science and Medicine, 72*, 1121–1139.
Swartz, D. (1997). *Culture and power: The sociology of Pierre Bourdieu*. University of Chicago Press.
Sweat, M. D., & Denison, J. A. (1995). Reducing HIV incidence in developing countries with structural and environmental interventions. *AIDS, 9*, S251–S257.
Turner, B. S. (1992). *Regulating bodies: Essays in medical sociology*. Routledge.
Turner, B. S., & Wainwright, S. P. (2003). Corps de ballet: The case of the injured dancer. *Sociology of Health & Illness, 25*, 269–288.
van den Broek, T. (2021). Early-life circumstances, health behavior profiles, and later-life health in Great Britain. *Journal of Aging and Society, 33*, 317–330.
VanHeuvelen, T., & VanHeuvelen, J. S. (2021). Between-country inequalities in health lifestyles. *International Journal of Comparative Sociology, 62*, 203–223.
Vartanian, T. P., & Houser, L. (2010). The effects of childhood neighborhood conditions on self-reports of adult health. *Journal of Health and Social Behavior, 51*, 291–306.
Veblen, T. ([1899] 1994). *Theory of the leisure class*. Dover Wainright.
Wacquant, L. (2016). A concise genealogy and anatomy of habitus. *The Sociological Review, 64*, 64–72.
Weber, M. (1946). *From max Weber: Essays in sociology*. Oxford University Press.
Weber, M. (1949). *The methodology of the social sciences*. Free Press.
Weber, M. (1958). *The protestant ethic and the spirit of capitalism*. Scribners.
Weber, M. ([1922] 1978). *Economy and society* (Vol. 1). University of California Press.

Williams, S. J. (1995). Theorising class, health and lifestyles: Can Bourdieu help us? *Sociology of Health & Illness, 17*, 577–604.
Williams, G. (2003). The determinants of health: Structure, context and agency. *Sociology of Health & Illness, 25*, 131–154.
Zerubavel, E. (1997). *Social mindscapes*. Harvard University Press.

Chapter 7
The Life Course Perspective and Dynamics Around Health

Claudine Burton-Jeangros

Introduction

The health of successive generations is shaped by changing social, technological, political and economic conditions. Social norms regarding healthy lives are also dynamic, diversely shaping aspirations. In addition to these collective transformations, people experience modifications in their own social and biological circumstances over their life course, and their personal health adjusts with aging. Nevertheless, inequalities in health are constantly reproduced: individuals with more privileges are better able to avoid disease, and they live longer than those with less privileges. The observation that individual bodies are inevitably reactive to social circumstances is at the heart of health and medical sociology. The life course perspective aims to address these changes in health and in society while possibly helping to understand how inequalities endure (Burton-Jeangros, 2020; Burton-Jeangros et al., 2015).

The life course interdisciplinary framework emerged in the social sciences in the 1960s, but it initially paid limited attention to health. At the end of the twentieth century, however, developments in life course epidemiology emphasized the importance of time in individuals' health trajectories, as these are unfolding in their social context. This approach was made possible by the increasing accumulation of longitudinal data allowing the testing of associations between health and social circumstances over successive life stages and across generations.

The life course perspective has generated growing interest among scholars of various disciplines and has become part of the rich theoretical apparatus mobilized to approach health inequalities. It helps move away from risk factor epidemiology

C. Burton-Jeangros (✉)
Institute of Sociological Research & LIVES Swiss Center of Expertise for Life Course Research, University of Geneva, Geneva, Switzerland
e-mail: claudine.jeangros@unige.ch

W. C. Cockerham (ed.), *Medical Sociology on the Move*,
https://doi.org/10.1007/978-3-031-92456-9_7

focused on biological and behavioral determinants of health to encompass the complexity of social determinants over time. At the same time, it addresses the challenges of biosocial mechanisms that contribute to shaping health inequalities. Its potential is reflected in the increasing number of publications in reference journals (*Social Science and Medicine*, *Journal of Health and Social Behavior*, *Sociology of Health and Illness* notably) adopting a life course perspective. In addition, the life course perspective has pervaded policy principles at the World Health Organization and at the national level in many countries.

This chapter intends to show how the life course perspective can contribute to various domains of health and medical sociology. Population aging, a massive societal phenomenon impacting relationships across society, places at the center of attention the importance of time, as an individual and collective issue shaping the distribution of health and its multiple determinants. In addition to the introduction of a temporal perspective in health inequality scholarship, attention should also be paid to the time-related meanings that people elaborate with respect to their health or illness conditions and their impact on psychosocial processes.

After introducing the life course perspective and its diffusion in epidemiology, the second part of the chapter develops five sections covering elements relevant to approaching health dynamics in health and medical sociology. First, mechanisms related to changes in social positions throughout the life course are discussed. Second, interactions across life domains, including notably the relationships between work, family and health trajectories, are addressed. The importance for health of complex social locations and social identities according to the intersectionality perspective is then approached. Fourth, the integration of a life course perspective from the institutional perspective on health inequalities is presented. The last section tackles the importance of meanings attached to health and illness as a measure of people's agency in that respect.

The Life Course Perspective

The life course perspective emerged in the 1960s as an interdisciplinary framework addressing the complexity of human lives from a dynamic perspective, combining developments in psychology and sociology (Alwin, 2012; Shanahan et al., 2016). Interest was then growing about the life span of individuals, along a developmental approach focused on organic processes across all life stages. At the same time, increasing attention was being given to the consequences of structural change for individuals' lives in the decades following the Second World War. Comparisons of the life course of successive cohorts, i.e., groups of individuals growing and aging in different social contexts shaped by historical events, revealed the relevance of studying the development of human lives in their context. The American sociologist Glen Elder pioneered this perspective in his book *Children of the Great Depression* (Elder, 1974), with a study based on longitudinal data following over several decades the trajectories of children born between 1920 and 1930 in the United

States. It was concluded that the social origins and age of the children at the time of the economic crisis mattered in the development of their biographies.

In addition to these two disciplines, demography, anthropology, history, and economics also engaged in this perspective, leading to an ambitious interdisciplinary research agenda, which approaches the life course as "a steady flow of an individual's actions and experiences, which modify domain-specific biographical states and affect individual wellbeing over time" (Bernardi et al., 2019, p. 7). Extending the interest in the intersection of biography and history, as formulated by Mills in the sociological imagination, the life course perspective formulated theoretical propositions bringing together developmental processes at the individual level, people's life trajectories and social change (Alwin, 2012).

These propositions were formalized in five overarching principles to address these mechanisms (Elder et al., 2003). The first emphasizes the lifelong development of individuals, suggesting that early life circumstances matter, as well as later conditions, throughout life stages. The second stresses the timing of transitions, whether they are expected—i.e., getting married at the average age of one's cohort—or unexpected transitions—having cancer at an early age. A third idea relates to the central role of context and time, which intimately shape biographies and thus calls for comparisons across social groups and cohorts. A fourth element situates individuals within their social networks with the notion of linked lives, i.e., people do not go through their lives alone or detached from others, and their trajectories can be importantly affected by the persons with whom they live. The fifth principle relates to the core sociological question of structure and agency, with attention given to agency and the capacities of individuals to shape their own trajectories amidst social constraints. The conceptual map offered by these principles supported advances across disciplines.

In sociology, life course research has paid notable attention to work and family trajectories, and different concepts have been developed to account for their transformations over time (Azar, 2024). Differentiation focuses on life course variability, considering whether individuals encounter more variety over time in their life statuses as a result of changes in the labor market and family dynamics. Standardization refers to how much life transitions and their timing are normative in a specific context, i.e. whether they are aligned on a single norm such as retirement age. Finally, institutionalization is focused on the extent to which life stages are regulated through laws or organizational rules, such as marital partnerships.

To account for the perspective's sustained developments over the past decades and to integrate the numerous propositions that have emerged across disciplines, Bernardi et al. (2019) synthesized three main axes for research. The first axis refers to the importance of time—the "time-related interdependence of the life course"—and indicates that individuals' current circumstances are influenced by their past conditions, which together influence their future prospects. The second axis, "interdependence across life domains", emphasizes that resources available in specific areas (family, work and health, for example) influence opportunities and outcomes in other domains. The third axis, labeled "multilevel interdependence of the life course", considers the associations of people with others through family relations, social networks, and institutions. These axes are represented as the edges of a cube to stress how their respective mechanisms are themselves interrelated through second-order interdependencies (being diagnosed with a chronic disease affects work opportunities; hence, it influences access to economic resources over time) and third-order interdependencies (this relation could be mitigated by how social policies compensate sick workers).

These theoretical propositions will be further addressed in the coming sections, as they have been progressively introduced in the understanding of health inequality dynamics, along trajectories developing throughout individuals' life course and taking place in contrasted contexts.

Life Course Epidemiology

Initial developments in the life course perspective did not pay attention to health, possibly reflecting a division between sociological specialties and a long-standing reluctance to integrate biological elements in sociological reasoning (Landecker & Panofsky, 2013). Hence, health gained a place in the life course landscape through advances in epidemiology over the 1990s (Ben-Shlomo & Kuh, 2002). These findings were related to growing preoccupations in life sciences with population aging and the associated growth of chronic conditions in later life. The shortcomings of cross-sectional epidemiological research, which involves evaluating the associations between health conditions and risk exposures, notably behaviors or physiological factors, to explain the origins of noncommunicable diseases have become increasingly obvious. In parallel, access to a growing body of longitudinal data has offered novel opportunities to better understand the etiology of disease. The initial steps are associated with Barker's work in the United Kingdom on biological programming, with research showing relationships between mothers' situations during pregnancy, assessed by nutrition and birth weight, and their children's coronary heart diseases in adulthood (Barker, 1995). It was later extended to the Developmental Origins of Health and Disease, with birth cohorts providing rich longitudinal data over decades (Power et al., 2013).

The initiators of the field identified three phases in the development of life course epidemiology (Ben-Shlomo et al., 2016). The first involves research interested in the influence of early-life factors on clinical chronic disease endpoints. The second phase expanded through the integration of a larger range of outcomes (such as disability, oral health, and musculoskeletal disorders) and exposures related to biological, psychological and social factors. The third phase corresponds to stronger connections between life course epidemiology and the study of aging, with an interest in compensatory or mediating effects between detrimental conditions early in life and later health. These stages emphasize the strengthening of the interdisciplinary scope of life course epidemiology over time.

Life course epidemiology involves considering the interactions existing between biological states and social lives or, in terms of Fassin (2018) between biology and biography. Successive biological life phases, such as conception, prenatal, prepubertal, pubertal, maturity and senescence, are distinguished (Ben-Shlomo et al., 2016). Some research is also interested in the reproduction of health across generations and among twins (Houweling & Grünberger, 2024; Steves et al., 2012). In addition to the mounting empirical evidence assessing the dynamics of life-long circumstances and health conditions, various theoretical models have been proposed to account for the mechanisms shaping these interactions (Bartley & Kelly-Irving, 2024; Kuh et al., 2004; Wagner et al., 2024).

The critical or sensitive periods hypothesis suggests that specific stages or the timing of some transitions trigger conditions affecting health. This has been related to biological and social exposures at specific life stages, which are expected to have lasting consequences for health, such as lead exposure or poor nutrition in childhood. This model assumes that the "long arm of childhood conditions" might have direct effects on health, suggesting that some exposures would have irreversible effects (Steiber, 2019). However, such consequences often emerge decades later in the life course, with a long period of latency that makes it difficult to associate a specific cause with these effects (Hertzman & Boyce, 2010).

The pathway model is interested in the sequence of multiple exposures and their impact on health, hence considering how exposures can generate indirect health effects through shaping the life course. Here, adult socioeconomic circumstances, influenced by earlier life conditions, are considered important as they possibly mediate health in the long run. Socialization is mentioned as a second mechanism through which parenting practices influence health behaviors (related, for example, to alcohol, tobacco, and nutrition) and preferences across generations within a family (Steiber, 2019).

Another model emphasizes the accumulation of either advantages or disadvantages throughout life. Dannefer (2003, p. S327) suggested that there exists a "systemic tendency for interindividual divergence in a given characteristic (e.g., money, health, or status) with the passage of time". The proposition is associated with Matthew effects, according to which a limited initial gap grows over time through the increasing accumulation of resources by the privileged ones against the progressive depletion of the initially less resourceful people (Merton, 1968), and with Bourdieu's (1979) theory of social reproduction. It emphasizes the strength of social mechanisms that repeatedly distribute resources in an uneven manner across social groups. In life course epidemiology, this model suggests a possible synergy occurring across determinants of health over time, which is expected to generate increasingly diverging trajectories over aging.

These models are helpful for formulating hypotheses and interpreting empirical findings. However, their application is limited in different ways. First, their assumptions partly overlap, and it often remains challenging to test their respective role in the understanding of processes shaping health outcomes (Hallqvist et al., 2004). Second, chronic conditions tend to emerge rather late in the life course, with a potentially long temporal gap since exposure to adverse determinants, making it difficult to disentangle their specific influences when they are observed decades later. Third, selection effects occur since individuals in poorer health are more likely to not be represented in research samples, notably through differential attrition due to mortality in longitudinal studies. According to the age-as-leveler hypothesis (Lynch, 2003), as a consequence of selection, inequalities are likely to decrease over later life stages since only the better-off individuals remain alive.

These models, regularly discussed in life course epidemiology scholarship, have been differentiated into developmental and structural perspectives (Jones et al., 2019). The first is interested in the plasticity of the human body, considering that it is highest in critical and sensitive periods; hence, external exposures are expected to have an important impact on development and to affect health later in life. These individual-level mechanisms are typically assessed through animal studies and quasi-experimental designs. The structural perspective, on the other hand, is interested in biopsychosocial mechanisms shaping the distribution of population health and longevity. It attributes health inequalities to social exposures through contrasted life experiences and their associated stressors while also paying attention to people's agency, shaped by their social identity and socioeconomic resources.

However, a number of scholars invite us to move beyond such a distinction by embracing the relations between social and biological processes, with the concepts of biological embodiment and epigenetics. The notion of embodiment proposed by Krieger (2005) considers that bodies are "active and engaged entities". This suggests that individuals incorporate the world in which they live through an incorporation encompassing societal circumstances and ecological conditions (Kelly-Irving & Delpierre, 2021). This process is presented as possibly adaptative, allowing individuals to adjust to their changing environments owing to their body plasticity. In research on early-life development, biological embedding connects social experience with bodily transformations, offering a conceptual bridge across the social and natural sciences (Hertzman & Boyce, 2010). It highlights the processes under which experience is incorporated or gets under the skin and modifies individual biology. The complexity of these processes is elaborated at the multiple levels at which bodies can be affected, including "neurobiology, physiological pathways, genes, and gene regulation" (Hertzman & Boyce, 2010).

The concept of epigenetics refers to causal interactions between social regulation and gene regulation (Landecker & Panofsky, 2013) on the basis of their interactions. First, social structure and social regulation are related to gene structure and gene regulation, with direct and causal relationships between the former and the latter. Second, similar genetic make-up can be expressed in contrasted bodily outcomes. Social scientists have long been reticent in considering biological or genetic factors in their research; however, these new findings call for their "critical engagement" since refusing to consider these interactions is currently limiting (Harris & Schorpp, 2018). The inclusion of biomarkers in databases rich in social indicators (for example, the UK Household Longitudinal Study, the Survey of Health, Aging and Retirement in Europe (SHARE)) is offering new avenues for developing and testing hypotheses about social–biological interactions. The policy implications of such findings should also be considered since they can provide evidence on the importance of social regulation, for example, supporting the regulation of chemical exposure (Landecker & Panofsky, 2013). In addition, they can counterbalance the relevance of developments in genetic engineering as a solution to improve population health.

This section emphasizes how epidemiology helps introduce health in the life course approach while proposing new theoretical insights into the complex mechanisms connecting social and biological lives from a dynamic perspective. It still focuses mostly on how exposure, including a range of determinants at the micro, meso and macro levels, can impact health, approaching it as an outcome affected by individuals' social and economic resources. It matters for sociology since health is here considered more than a mere biological condition, only affected by physiological or genetic processes. However, taking epigenetics and embodiment mechanisms seriously implies considering not only how social life affects individual and collective health but also reverse relations. The next section presents further theoretical elaborations about these complex interactions.

The Contributions of the Life Course Perspective to Health and Medical Sociology

The second part of the chapter explores the social gradient in health from a dynamic perspective and within social interactions shaped by historical and social contexts. Along the three axes of the cube proposed by Bernardi et al. (2019), the life course perspective can contribute to health inequality research by examining in greater depth the processes shaping the distribution of health over individual and collective time. In addition, it invites to consider biosocial mechanisms across not only life domains but also across people whose lives are linked and within institutional arrangements. Finally, taking social interactions seriously implies taking into account how relationships with relatives, other social categories or health professionals contribute to shaping health and illness trajectories and their associated meanings. These aspects are addressed in the next five sections.

Health and Social Condition Dynamics

The social gradient in health is systematically observed at the population level, repeating itself across periods, contexts, indicators of health and social circumstances. It cuts across social hierarchies to shape health and disease trajectories linearly along differentiated levels of social privileges (Hertzman & Boyce, 2010). Along Durkheim, it can thus be defined as a social fact, since the distribution of population health across social categories reflects collective properties overriding individual situations (Hertzman, 2012). By considering how biological and social processes interact over individual trajectories and across historical times, the life course perspective explicitly adds a dynamic component to the social determinants of health framework (Marmot, 2015) or the fundamental cause theory (Link & Phelan, 1995).

Empirical evidence about these mechanisms has accumulated, with findings based on European data showing that early-life circumstances affect health later in life across a number of different health outcomes (Cullati et al., 2023). However, a scoping review of socioeconomic conditions and multimorbidity in old age also emphasized that adult socioeconomic circumstances can mediate the role of unfavorable early-life circumstances (Wagner et al., 2022). Such a reduction in the impact of social origin on later health calls for caution toward a possibly too deterministic stance of the developmental perspective, since compensatory mechanisms can modify the accumulation of disadvantages/advantages (Holman & Walker, 2021). At the same time, differences are regularly observed with gender stratification: adult circumstances attenuate or even erase early life circumstances for men, but this is not the case among women (Cullati et al., 2023). It is proposed that women might encounter fewer opportunities than men do to compensate for the role of early-life factors, an issue further considered below when examining work–family trajectories.

Another line of sociological research looks at the influence of social mobility on health, hence considering how health can be shaped by movements across generations. It aims to assess the specific role of mobility beyond the differences observed across individuals situated in contrasting social positions. With reference to Sorokin's early work, it is considered important to assess the disruptive impact of social mobility beyond the accumulation model (Steiber, 2019). Changing social position would be stressful since it creates distance from the class of origin while situating oneself in a new social category whose codes and norms are unfamiliar. The adaptation needed to cope with changing social circumstances might generate social isolation and anxiety. More specifically, downward social mobility, experienced as hurtful or humiliating, would be associated with poorer mental health. An empirical study on satisfaction with health performed on German household panel data confirmed the association between health satisfaction in young adulthood and the experience of social mobility. However, in later adulthood, socioeconomic position became more important than mobility, suggesting that its impact is limited in time.

A larger study based on European Social Survey data from 28 countries reported an association between social mobility and depressive symptoms among men: upward mobility protected them, whereas downward mobility was associated with greater depressive symptoms than among those who had remained immobile (Gugushvili et al., 2019). Among women, on the other hand, depressive symptoms were not affected by social mobility. These findings suggest potential for additional research examining the effects on health of time spent in specific SES positions (duration), the scope of mobility (in an adjacent social class or over several positions), the stages in the life course at which these transitions occur, and the sequence of changes in socioeconomic status (Holman & Walker, 2021).

Nevertheless, the enduring nature of the social gradient in health, repeated across studies, is puzzling in light of constant macrolevel transformations in biological and social vulnerability across generations. Wadsworth (1997) proposed a distinction between changes in biological environments, referred to as time-related biological vulnerability, and transformations in social environments, referred to as time-associated social vulnerability. In the first type of vulnerability, population health changes across time and contexts, and the main causes of mortality and morbidity in high-income countries are currently different from those that prevailed over the past centuries. Such patterns of health and disease are partly associated with transformations in medicine and health care, since new technologies and access to health care contribute to modifications of biological vulnerability. Furthermore, collective health norms and practices also change over time as a result of prevention campaigns and therapeutic advances. Hence, comparing cohorts implies considering which transformations they encounter at different life stages (for example, smoking regulation and access to antibiotics).

In the second type of vulnerability, social conditions also keep changing (Ranci, 2010), as described in the sociology of work (from manual to service employment), sociology of the family (increasing rate of divorce, family recompositions), or sociology of education (growing duration of education). In addition, social policy transformations over successive stages of the welfare system modify the opportunities and compensation offered to individuals over their life course, which likely influence their health chances or risks. It seems reasonable to expect that these multiple changes interfere with the connections between biology and biography; however, they have a limited impact on the social gradient in health.

Next to macrolevel transformations, interactions between social and health conditions can be approached at the microlevel. Pearlin et al. (2005) elaborated on how social and economic conditions, through their enduring consequences and associated stressful events, equate with exposure to serious stressors. In this paper, three processes are described to account for how hardships of different forms disrupt the continuities of life. First, the role of stressful circumstances as instigated in social status and its variations can impact health; however, this is conceptualized here in terms of indirect exposure associated with demands and hardships related to social position. Exposure to continuous ambient stressors may reduce the sense of personal safety and induce negative concepts of the self and frustrations when trying to achieve aspirations. Second, chronic or repetitive hardships generate recurrent stressors as a result of experiences of discrimination based on class, race or gender, for example: "We may speculate that people who have experienced unfair treatment because of race or other ascription fall into a state of vigilant anticipation, awaiting its next occurrence. We suggest that the psychic pain inflicted by discrimination may very well stem from the anticipation of its future occurrence as well as from its past occurrences" (Pearlin et al., 2005, p. 209). The third mechanism refers to stress proliferation, where an initial stressor (related, for example, to trauma in early life or disruption in social roles and statuses later in life) expands into additional or secondary stressors. These assumptions find some empirical support in a systematic review of lay understandings of health inequalities in the United Kingdom (Smith & Anderson, 2018). Across the reviewed studies, people were aware of the role of their changing working conditions and related housing opportunities, which, when acting jointly, exacerbated stress and anxiety, fuelled by stigma and guilt. Stress and fear were frequently mentioned as a likely psychosocial pathway between their social circumstances and their deteriorated health.

These elements suggest that the social gradient in health resists changing social and biological vulnerability and is fueled by psychosocial mechanisms relating specific social positions to a number of stress exposures embedded in social hierarchies.

Health and Resources Among Life Domains

Biological embodiment and epigenetics invite the consideration of both social causation and social selection mechanisms, along the life course principle of lifelong development. Indeed, when a dynamic approach is adopted, individual health conditions can also be considered resources for future personal achievements. Good health, which is associated with higher prospects, can act as a resource for other life domains. Moreover, owing to its interaction with living conditions, health status is a consequence or an outcome of the resources available in other domains, as described in the previous section. This interactive approach is encouraged by the proposition to examine interdependencies across life domains, as stated by Bernardi et al.(2019, p. 100258): "One can assume that actors seek constellations of activities that are reciprocally supportive across domains or for which a single resource simultaneously serves multiple life domains".

These interdependencies justify considering health selection mechanisms, which suggest that individuals in poorer health have more limited social opportunities. While caution was initially important when these were used to dismiss the existence of health inequalities, it also seems crucial to consider how health is a resource for both individuals and society. Owing to their rapid and massive consequences, the HIV epidemic and the COVID-19 pandemic have well illustrated this; however, the elevated proportion of people diagnosed with one or multiple chronic health conditions currently represents a high toll for social functioning at both the individual and collective levels. From his functionalist perspective, Parsons (1964) suggested that society needs a population in good health to perform efficiently.

With respect to interdependencies across life domains, work and family represent major social roles over adulthood to be explored in their dynamic relationships with health. These explorations must consider gender stratification since men and women remain unequal across these three domains. Research assessing the influence of family circumstances on health initially focused on women only (Annandale & Hunt, 2000), testing the impact of the accumulation of social roles, in various combinations of family and paid work, on their health. Theoretical assumptions suggest potential role conflict due to difficulties in meeting demands associated with the accumulation of roles, and role enhancement considering that endorsing work and family is beneficial in terms of psychophysiological functioning (Uccheddu et al., 2022). Given that being in a couple, having children and being employed are favorable determinants of health when considered separately, the available data now allow to build trajectories that consider the transitions, duration, and combination of these social roles and their associations with health.

In a systematic review of the literature, a number of factors related to work–family trajectories appeared to be supportive of health; these factors included longer education, continuous engagement in the labor market and later parenthood (Machů et al., 2022). In contrast, people whose trajectories were characterized by early parenthood, raising children alone and having limited employment reported poorer health. Furthermore, women's trajectories were more heterogeneous than men's trajectories were, reflecting uneven gender commitment to family roles. Indeed, women experienced more work interruptions than men who had more stable and full-time engagement in work. In various patterns across European countries in terms of the relationship between work-family trajectories and health, men's health later in life is more affected by their working conditions, whereas women's health is more affected by their family engagements (Uccheddu et al., 2022). These findings emphasize the importance of considering gendered trajectories of social roles when assessing health inequalities. Furthermore, changing patterns in labor division between men and women over recent generations confirm the relevance of endorsing a life course perspective. Nevertheless, if women engage more in the paid labor market today, the division of domestic work remains uneven. Research on its specific impact on health remains limited.

The life course perspective also involves paying attention to linked lives: notably, family interactions can offer a number of economic, social, and psychological resources that are important for health (Carr & Springer, 2010). Moreover, these interactions can represent stressors and hence threaten the health of family members (Umberson et al., 2006). Furthermore, many transitions, such as marriage, divorce, parenthood, retirement, and health events, not only have a direct effect on available resources but affect several members of a household simultaneously (Koehly & Manalel, 2023). The convoy model of social relations is focused on these interactions, notably among couples but also across generations in the context of parenting or care giving at an older age. Testing whether linked lives have positive or negative consequences for health and well-being, depending on their quality and functions, requires data collected across people, which is, for example, the case of household panel data. Despite efforts to conceptualize these mechanisms (Umberson et al., 2010), empirical evidence remains limited. As an illustration, an analysis of how couple dynamics can impact preventive care revealed an association between women's mammography screening and the regular dental check-up of their male partner when he was a child (Missinne, 2015).

When health is considered both a resource and an outcome across life domains, the importance of gender inequalities calls for a more complex analysis of health inequality dynamics while taking into account the multiple forms of stratification present in society, as suggested in the next section.

Health in Intersectional Trajectories

In the progressive complexification of theoretical and empirical developments, more factors of stratification have been integrated into life course research through the intersectionality lens (Holman & Walker, 2021). It is interested in how people's positions and resources are affected by social class, gender, age, race or ethnicity, migratory background, or sexual orientation, to name the most frequently cited ones. The intersection of these factors defines not only specific social locations but also social identities, which are shaped and reinforced by relationships with others. Indeed, interdependencies between sexism, racism, and ageism define social interactions as well as systems of privilege and oppression, which matter for life chances and for health. These systems are dynamic since "the 'matrix of domination' changes over historical time, and people therefore experience sexism, age, racism, etc., differently in different historical periods" (Holman & Walker, 2021, p. 252). Mechanisms of discrimination may change as a result of transformations in the institutional context (through anti-discrimination laws, for example); however, they are still reproduced over time despite new constraints. These complex stratification mechanisms shape intersectional trajectories resulting from synergies between the life course and the intersection of contrasted social positions. This calls for empirical research testing how these multiple patterns of inequality and discrimination at the individual and collective levels shape health outcomes.

The intersectionality lens, which sheds new light on the trajectories of unequal aging, can be connected with a number of theoretical insights. Along with processes of discrimination conceptualized as a determinant of health (Hatzenbuehler et al., 2013; Pescosolido & Martin, 2015), considering how intersectional positions impact social locations and relations with others over time seems particularly relevant. The concept of weathering, which addresses the relationship between racism and health conditions, refers to how chronic exposure to socioeconomic disadvantages accelerates biological aging (Bartley & Kelly-Irving, 2024). Intersectionality can also be associated with cumulative advantage processes, suggesting that, owing to their social positions, some individuals are constantly exposed to multiple challenges and stressors. Finally, it sheds light on the biological embodiment dynamic in which intersectionality connects various forms of social oppression with health inequalities (Kelly-Irving & Delpierre, 2021). Bringing embodiment and intersectionality together contributes to challenging genetic essentialism through "a clearer understanding of how biological and health differences observed between social groups (e.g., income, occupation, race/ethnicity) are driven by a dynamic interaction between humans and their socially stratified environments across the life course." (Kelly-Irving & Delpierre, 2021, p. 1184).

Some empirical evidence about the importance of intersectionality in health trajectories has been established in the United States. Analyses revealed that, in terms of hypertension risk trajectories, black or Hispanic women were more affected, a risk obscured in analyses looking separately at race/ethnicity and gender since among white people, hypertension was less common among women (Richardson &

Brown, 2016). This showed that the effects of race/ethnicity and gender are multiplicative and not simply additive. Race and ethnicity inequalities in health are particularly relevant for assessing the role of changing living conditions over time in their influence on health, especially when they are related to migration trajectories. Another study hence examined the intersection of racial/ethnic inequality, nativity and age with respect to chronic conditions and functional limitations (Brown, 2018). It concluded that minorities, whether US-born or foreign-born, experienced an earlier decline in their health than did US-born whites. This "premature aging", or physiological "wear and tear", was characterized by a gap of several years—6 years for chronic conditions and over 10 years for functional limitations—between the more privileged and less privileged groups in society. These inequalities were interpreted as a result of pervasive racial and ethnic stratification in the United States, exposing minorities to multiple forms of racism. These interpretations can again be related to findings from lay understandings of health inequalities, in which disadvantaged people refer to shame and stigma, feelings that are "commonly connected to concerns about feeling 'judged', 'disrespected' and labeled 'poor'" (Smith & Anderson, 2018, p. 162). They were aware of the importance of these elements in their poorer mental health and unhealthy behaviors. These results anchor psychosocial mechanisms within specific contexts of interactions on the basis of enduring social hierarchies.

The concept of intersectionality emerged in gender studies, which are more inclined to use qualitative research designs. Its integration in health research is rather recent (Hankivsky, 2012), and while its potential has been acknowledged, developments have remained slow (Harari & Lee, 2021), which is notably attributed to epistemological incompatibility between the concept and quantitative analyses. This systematic review identified some shortcomings in the integration of intersectionality, including frequent limitations to the three stratification factors of class, gender and race; a focus on marginalized groups without addressing the continuum of positions and integrating the role of privileged categories in the reproduction of inequalities; a focus on a limited number of explanatory mechanisms, notably discrimination, while not paying attention to others such as intimate partner violence; and the still rare inclusion of a life course perspective. However, new opportunities for analyses are anticipated with increasing access to survey data linked with administrative information and biobanks (Holman & Walker, 2021).

The Institutional Turn in Health Inequalities Research

The social determinants of health framework emphasize the importance of public policies for population health; however, the role of institutions has long been neglected in research (Gkiouleka et al., 2018). Social positions of privilege or disadvantage are not only individual attributes; and institutional theory is interested in how institutional arrangements contribute to shaping population health (Beckfield et al., 2015). Three institutional mechanisms were formulated relating to the extent of redistribution of resources through welfare, the compression of inequalities within set limits, and the mediation looking at relations between diverse types of resources. Indeed, formal structures affect life domains by shaping access to housing, education, employment, and family support (Holman & Walker, 2021). The fundamental cause theory suggests that health inequalities are tightly associated with social stratification, since people in higher positions have access to resources that matter for health, including knowledge, money, power and social connections, that offer them protection against poor health (Link & Phelan, 1995). Hence, it is legitimate to assess the capacity of institutions to mitigate inequalities through their politics of resource redistribution.

Variations in welfare regimes are usually operationalized through typologies differentiating liberal regimes based on market regulation and providing minimal welfare (UK, USA), conservative or Bismarckien regimes based on earnings and managed by employers, Scandinavian regimes characterized by generous and universal schemes, Latin regimes described as fragmented and relying heavily on family structures and the voluntary sector, and finally Eastern European regimes related to previous communist countries characterized by low provision of services, marketisation and decentralization (Bambra & Eikemo, 2008). Available data across European countries allow multilevel analyses to evaluate whether more or less generous welfare provisions have an impact on health trajectories. Longitudinal analyses thus examine how different arrangements mediate the effects of early disadvantage on health later in life. While differences are observed, with gender variations (Sieber et al., 2020; Uccheddu et al., 2022), the results are often difficult to interpret owing to the complexities underlying the regimes. Hence, variations across countries were tested on other indicators, such as the percentage of expenditure in social protection of the national gross domestic product. This indicator of welfare state generosity showed a positive effect on women's health trajectories but not on men's health trajectories (Sieber et al., 2021).

Considering the extent and persistence of gender dynamics in social roles, another study investigated how much defamilization policies moderate the impact of the life course on women's mental health later in life (Azar, 2024). These policies aim at supporting women's autonomy toward caregiving responsibilities to allow them to engage more fully in the paid labor force. Here, again, such policies had contrasting consequences for women's health, as their life and work trajectories differed across contexts. The notions of diversification, standardization and institutionalization introduced earlier are indicative of the complexity of trajectories across time and context.

This theoretical perspective opens promising research questions; however, it struggles to assess how welfare regimes might have impacted the health trajectories of successive generations. On the one hand, welfare state provisions continue adjusting to changing configurations of social risks (Ranci, 2010). On the other hand, their consequences might be delayed, emerging later in life. In addition, against the diversity of intersectional trajectories described in the previous section, it is difficult to test the specific influence of public policies across national contexts, especially since the life course perspective suggests that time and context matter. Studies on local policies designed for specific populations should thus be encouraged.

Temporalities of Health, Illness and Disease

This last section suggests that next to medical appreciation of what it means to be in good health or sick, people's changing understanding of their own health over time is important from a life course perspective. Notions such as illness trajectories, biographical disruption, or health memories emphasize the dynamic processes through which people interpret and act on their health. Narratives around experiences of chronic conditions and the prevention of risks can be related to the principle of agency, which involves "both actual capacities/resources and individuals' perceptions of those capacities/resources" (Hitlin & Kirkpatrick Johnson, 2015, p. 1432). These narratives also shed light on how individuals navigate their health trajectories against their actual resources across life domains and amidst structural constraints. Paying attention to people's agency takes some distance from a deterministic or top-down view according to which people necessarily endorse medical and scholarly definitions of what it means to be healthy or sick (Burton-Jeangros & Fargnoli, 2023). Health and medical sociology is indeed replete with findings addressing resistance, contradictions and conflicts between health professionals and the public (Burton-Jeangros, 2024).

Medical history typically adopts a linear appreciation of time, emphasizing the success of medicine and the continuous progress of therapeutic developments. However, professional narratives of success have been hampered by re-emergence of infectious diseases, resistance to antibiotics and vaccine hesitancy. In addition to the vocabulary of premature deaths and preoccupation with technical and medical capacities to extend human longevity, which is often oblivious to social inequalities (Gutin & Hummer, 2021), paying more attention to the social temporalities of health and illness seems relevant. Hence, this section brings together various insights related to health temporalities, as they shed further light on the biopsychosocial mechanisms contributing to health inequalities.

People develop their own interpretations of health along with the historical and contextual circumstances they have encountered, and their personal experiences, hardships and aspirations also matter (Burton-Jeangros & Fargnoli, 2023). In addition to the static WHO definition of health as "a state of complete physical, mental and social wellbeing", it has been defined as "the ability to cope with challenges of existence within a specific context; hence, it is highly contextual and circumstantial" (Amzat & Razum, 2022). The emic versus etic distinction proposed by medical anthropology is useful here to differentiate local, situated meanings of health and illness from their professional definitions. People's experiences also emphasize health multidimensionality, as formulated by the biopsychosocial model, suggesting dynamic connections between somatic and mental health over time (Engel, 1977). The concept of syndemics developed in anthropology refers to the frequent interactions of two or more diseases in association with unfavorable social conditions (Singer & Clair, 2003). Hence, in their lived experiences, people often handle ambiguity and uncertainty, and their trajectories unfold against medical scenarios, shaped by a professional division of labor separating dimensions of health between non-communicable, infectious and mental conditions (Green & Lynch, 2022).

Different concepts highlight the complexity of temporalities existing around the experiences of chronic diseases and their multiple consequences in individuals' lives beyond their medical management. From a biographical perspective, Strauss (1987) elaborated the notion of illness trajectories, differentiating them from the course of illness defining successive physiological stages of health conditions according to professional definitions. The term "illness trajectories" was coined to consider the work performed by patients to handle their condition over time, with an emphasis on two features affecting this health work. First, the contingencies in the evolution of illness itself, in professional management and its biographical implications, are important to consider. Second, people's work or patient engagement in treatment needs to be emphasized. The notion of biographical disruption was proposed by Bury (1982) to consider the impact of the diagnosis of a chronic condition on an individual's perception of the self, with serious consequences for self-identity. However, the timing of the disruption appeared important, with the disruption of a chronic disease being elevated for younger people but not for elderly individuals, integrating illness in the normal course of their aging (Jowsey, 2016).

In contrast to medical knowledge and work favoring a calendar or clock time, which is typical of modern Western contexts, chronic illness affects individuals' sense of time and expectations toward the future (Jowsey, 2016, p. 1093): "Meanings attributed to past and present experiences and practices, as well as future plans and imaginings, acquire new significance with chronic illness". Studies on subjective life expectancy have revealed how the awareness of one's own finitude can change the way people think and act about their future (Ferraro, 2016). Next to self-transformations and a new sense of time, illness affects relations with others. A study on heterosexual HIV-infected women's trajectories in Switzerland revealed how they struggled over the long run with the social and medical consequences of their condition (Fargnoli, 2021). Their lived experience did not match the narrative of success developed by medical doctors about treated patients being undetectable. Instead, these women had to handle the side effects of treatments, often dismissed by professionals, recurrent suspicions about the way they had been infected since they did not belong to mainstream categorizations of HIV-infected people, as well as stigmatizing reactions encouraging them to remain silent about their condition. These elements show the manifold implications of living with a chronic condition, which is susceptible to affecting trajectories across life domains and in relation to others.

In addition, individual and collective health memories matter; on the basis of personal past events or collective health experiences, they shape present understandings (Harrison et al., 2024). Current health conditions are not only affected but also assessed along 'shadows of the past' (Bernardi et al., 2019). People's perceptions in relation to time can be considered ‘reflexive judgments’ (Ferraro, 2016), affecting their interpretations of health amidst their social conditions. In that respect, histories of marginalization can matter for some groups who feel discriminated against or excluded from health care, experienced as “slow violence” by “chronic disease patients facing abandonment” (Green & Lynch, 2022, p. 435). When professionals and medical structures do not pay attention to health inequalities, they reinforce feelings of estrangement that can contribute to the mechanisms observed in the intersectional trajectories described above. Resistance to medical and public health prescriptions and framings can thus be preferred, as a way to resist blame, labeling or stigma (Smith & Anderson, 2018).

These elements give room to the principle of agency, situated at the other extreme of the institutional theory presented in the previous section, while they depict the importance of power dynamics in the backstage of health trajectories unfolding.

Conclusions

The integration of the life course perspective into health and medical sociology opens renewed avenues for research that benefit from the accumulation of rich longitudinal data, mostly quantitative but also qualitative. However, empirical developments supported by the multiplication of opportunities in data analysis techniques (including longitudinal qualitative analyses) need to be guided by theoretical propositions. This chapter presents the main orientations proposed from the life course perspective to address biosocial mechanisms shaping health inequalities over individual and collective time. In addition to the importance of biological and social interactions shaping individual bodies, social mechanisms across generations, within families, between people and the institutional landscape they live in appear crucial for health chances.

The social determinants of health framework suggests that health care opportunities are only one element shaping health, among a large number of factors. The life course perspective certainly confirms that multiple influences matter for health and repeatedly shape the social gradient in health beyond individual experiences. This perspective challenges, once more, medical reductionism with its emphasis on individual and behavioral risk factors. The integration of linked lives, intersectionality, and institutional arrangements emphasize the importance of social relations in health inequalities, including power dynamics between the privileged and unprivileged that keep reproducing differences in social and health stratification. The elements presented in this chapter hopefully highlight the relevance, but also challenges, of strengthening a research agenda on these issues.

This ambitious approach involves engaging with a range of disciplines, notably epidemiology and anthropology. Accordingly, the scope of methods should be expanded by mobilizing both quantitative and qualitative findings. To fully address the role of the multiple factors shaping embodiment processes, from the macrolevel of public policies to the microlevel of psychosocial mechanisms, rich data are necessary. Longitudinal comparative data encompassing biological and social indicators are increasingly available. However, some gaps persist, such as in assessing the influences taking place within couples and families or in measuring the complexity of migration or family trajectories.

The life course perspective emphasis on dynamics around health issues has clear policy implications. To address health inequalities, vulnerable populations, defined as those who accumulate exposures throughout their life course as a result of their devalued position in social hierarchies, should be targeted (Frohlich & Potvin, 2008). It has also been proposed along intersectionality analyses to favor 'proportionate universalism' on the basis of people's actual needs (Holman & Walker, 2021). The long arm of childhood conditions over health in later life calls for interventions focused on the early stages of life and investments in providing equal opportunities among children. This implies supporting their families while taking into account persisting gender stratification over adulthood and older ages. In addition, both the positive and negative resources associated with linked lives, notably within families, call for policies attentive to such dynamics beyond individual compensation schemes.

References

Alwin, D. F. (2012). Integrating varieties of life course concepts. *The Journals of Gerontology Series B: Psychological Sciences and Social Sciences, 67B*(2), 206–220. https://doi.org/10.1093/geronb/gbr146

Amzat, J., & Razum, O. (2022). *Globalization, health and the global south: A critical approach.* Routledge.

Annandale, E., & Hunt, K. (2000). *Gender inequalities in health.* Open University Press.

Azar, A. (2024). Work–family life course trajectories and women's mental health: The moderating role of defamilization policies in 15 European Territories. *Journal of Health and Social Behavior, 65*(4), 468–488. https://doi.org/10.1177/00221465241265435

Bambra, C., & Eikemo, T. A. (2008). Welfare state regimes, unemployment and health: A comparative study of the relationship between unemployment and self-reported health in 23 European countries. *Journal of Epidemiology & Community Health, 63*(2), 92–98. https://doi.org/10.1136/jech.2008.077354

Barker, D. J. P. (1995). Fetal origins of coronary heart disease. *BMJ, 311*(6998), 171–174. https://doi.org/10.1136/bmj.311.6998.171

Bartley, M., & Kelly-Irving, M. (2024). *Health inequality: An introduction to concepts, theories and methods* (3rd ed.). Polity Press.

Beckfield, J., Bambra, C., Eikemo, T. A., Huijts, T., McNamara, C., & Wendt, C. (2015). An institutional theory of welfare state effects on the distribution of population health. *Social Theory & Health, 13*(3), 227–244. https://doi.org/10.1057/sth.2015.19

Ben-Shlomo, Y., & Kuh, D. (2002). A life course approach to chronic disease epidemiology: Conceptual : Models, empirical challenges and interdisciplinary perspectives. *International Journal of Epidemiology, 31*, 285–293.

Ben-Shlomo, Y., Cooper, R., & Kuh, D. (2016). The last two decades of life course epidemiology, and its relevance for research on ageing. *International Journal of Epidemiology, 45*(4), 973–988. https://doi.org/10.1093/ije/dyw096

Bernardi, L., Huinink, J., & Settersten, R. A. (2019). The life course cube: A tool for studying lives. *Advances in Life Course Research, 41*, 100258. https://doi.org/10.1016/j.alcr.2018.11.004
Bourdieu, P. (1979). *La distinction: Critique sociale du jugement*. Éditions de Minuit.
Brown, T. H. (2018). Racial stratification, immigration, and health inequality: A life course-intersectional approach. *Social Forces, 96*(4), 1507–1540. https://doi.org/10.1093/sf/soy013
Burton-Jeangros, C. (2020). Life course approaches in global health. In I. R. Haring, I. Kickbusch, D. Ganten, & M. Moeti (Eds.), *Handbook of global health* (pp. 1–28). Springer International Publishing. https://doi.org/10.1007/978-3-030-05325-3_42-1
Burton-Jeangros, C., & Fargnoli, V. (2023). Vulnerability around health issues: Trajectories, experiences and meanings. In D. Spini & E. Widmer (Eds.), *Withstanding vulnerability throughout adult life* (pp. 189–204). Springer Nature Singapore. https://doi.org/10.1007/978-981-19-4567-0_12
Burton-Jeangros, C. (2024). Experiences of Health Risks : Prevention, Power Dynamics and Inequalities. Springer Nature Switzerland. https://doi.org/10.1007/978-3-031-65377-3
Burton-Jeangros, C., Cullati, S., Sacker, A., & Blane, D. (Eds.). (2015). *A life course perspective on health trajectories and transitions* (Vol. 4). Springer International Publishing. https://doi.org/10.1007/978-3-319-20484-0
Bury, M. R. (1982). Chronic illness as biographical disruption. *Sociology of Health and Illness, 4*(2), 167–182. papier.
Carr, D., & Springer, K. W. (2010). Advances in families and health research in the 21st century. *Journal of Marriage and the Family, 72*, 743–761. papier.
Cullati, S., Sieber, S., Van Der Linden, B. W. A., Orsholits, D., Von Arx, M., Boisgontier, M. P., & Cheval, B. (2023). Childhood socioeconomic disadvantage and health in the second half of life: The role of gender and welfare states in the life course of Europeans. In I. D. Spini & E. Widmer (Eds.), *Withstanding vulnerability throughout adult life* (pp. 217–238). Springer Nature Singapore. https://doi.org/10.1007/978-981-19-4567-0_14
Dannefer, D. (2003). Cumulative advantage/disadvantage and the life course: Cross-fertilizing age and social science theory. *Journal of Gerontology, 58B*(6), S327–S337.
Elder, G. H. (1974). *Children of the great depression: Social change in life experience*. Chicago University Press.
Elder, G. H., Johnson, M. K., & Crosnoe, R. (2003). The emergence and development of life course theory. In I. J. T. Mortimer & M. J. Shanahan (Eds.), *Handbook of the life course* (pp. 3–19). Springer US. https://doi.org/10.1007/978-0-306-48247-2_1
Engel, G. (1977). The need for a new medical model: A challenge for biomedicine. *Science, 196*(4286), 129–136. https://doi.org/10.1126/science.847460
Fargnoli, V. (2021). *InVIHsibles: Trajectoires de femmes séropositives*. Editions Antipodes.
Fassin, D. (2018). *La vie: Mode d'emploi critique*. Éditions du Seuil.
Ferraro, K. F. (2016). Life course lens on aging and health. In M. J. Shanahan, J. T. Mortimer, & M. K. Johnson (Eds.), *Handbook of the life course* (pp. 389–406). Springer International Publishing. https://doi.org/10.1007/978-3-319-20880-0_18
Frohlich, K. L., & Potvin, L. (2008). Transcending the known in public health practice. *American Journal of Public Health, 98*(2), 216–221. https://doi.org/10.2105/AJPH.2007.114777
Gkiouleka, A., Huijts, T., Beckfield, J., & Bambra, C. (2018). Understanding the micro and macro politics of health: Inequalities, intersectionality & institutions—A research agenda. *Social Science & Medicine, 200*, 92–98. https://doi.org/10.1016/j.socscimed.2018.01.025
Green, J., & Lynch, R. (2022). Rethinking chronicity: Public health and the problem of temporality. *Critical Public Health, 32*(4), 433–437. https://doi.org/10.1080/09581596.2022.2101432
Gugushvili, A., Zhao, Y., & Bukodi, E. (2019). 'Falling from grace' and 'rising from rags': Intergenerational educational mobility and depressive symptoms. *Social Science & Medicine, 222*, 294–304. https://doi.org/10.1016/j.socscimed.2018.12.027
Gutin, I., & Hummer, R. A. (2021). Social inequality and the future of US life expectancy. *Annual Review of Sociology, 47*, 501–520. Annual Reviews. https://doi.org/10.1146/annurev-soc-072320-100249

Hallqvist, J., Lynch, J., Bartley, M., Lang, T., & Blane, D. (2004). Can we disentangle life course processes of accumulation, critical period and social mobility? An analysis of disadvantaged socio-economic positions and myocardial infarction in the Stockholm Heart Epidemiology Program. *Social Science & Medicine, 58*(8), 1555–1562. https://doi.org/10.1016/S0277-9536(03)00344-7

Hankivsky, O. (2012). Women's health, men's health, and gender and health: Implications of intersectionality. *Social Science & Medicine, 74*(11), 1712–1720. https://doi.org/10.1016/j.socscimed.2011.11.029

Harari, L., & Lee, C. (2021). Intersectionality in quantitative health disparities research: A systematic review of challenges and limitations in empirical studies. *Social Science & Medicine, 277*, 113876. https://doi.org/10.1016/j.socscimed.2021.113876

Harris, K. M., & Schorpp, K. M. (2018). Integrating biomarkers in social stratification and health research. *Annual Review of Sociology, 44*(1), 361–386. https://doi.org/10.1146/annurev-soc-060116-053339

Harrison, M., Smith, A. K. J., & Adams, S. (2024). Matters of time in health and illness. *Health Sociology Review, 33*(1), 1–9. https://doi.org/10.1080/14461242.2024.2319943

Hatzenbuehler, M. L., Phelan, J. C., & Link, B. G. (2013). Stigma as a fundamental cause of population health inequalities. *American Journal of Public Health, 103*(5), 813–821.

Hertzman, C. (2012). Putting the concept of biological embedding in historical perspective. *Proceedings of the National Academy of Sciences, 109*(Supplement_2), 17160–17167. https://doi.org/10.1073/pnas.1202203109

Hertzman, C., & Boyce, T. (2010). How experience gets under the skin to create gradients in developmental health. *Annual Review of Public Health, 31*(1), 329–347. https://doi.org/10.1146/annurev.publhealth.012809.103538

Hitlin, S., & Kirkpatrick Johnson, M. (2015). Reconceptualizing agency within the life course: The power of looking ahead. *American Journal of Sociology, 120*(5), 1429–1472. JSTOR. https://doi.org/10.1086/681216

Holman, D., & Walker, A. (2021). Understanding unequal ageing: Towards a synthesis of intersectionality and life course analyses. *European Journal of Ageing, 18*(2), 239–255. https://doi.org/10.1007/s10433-020-00582-7

Houweling, T. A. J., & Grünberger, I. (2024). Intergenerational transmission of health inequalities: Towards a life course approach to socioeconomic inequalities in health—A review. *Journal of Epidemiology and Community Health, 78*(10), 641–649. https://doi.org/10.1136/jech-2022-220162

Jones, N. L., Gilman, S. E., Cheng, T. L., Drury, S. S., Hill, C. V., & Geronimus, A. T. (2019). Life course approaches to the causes of health disparities. *American Journal of Public Health, 109*(S1), S48–S55. https://doi.org/10.2105/AJPH.2018.304738

Jowsey, T. (2016). Time and chronic illness: A narrative review. *Quality of Life Research, 25*(5), 1093–1102. JSTOR.

Kelly-Irving, M., & Delpierre, C. (2021). Framework for understanding health inequalities over the life course: The embodiment dynamic and biological mechanisms of exogenous and endogenous origin. *Journal of Epidemiology and Community Health, 75*(12), 1181–1186. https://doi.org/10.1136/jech-2021-216430

Koehly, L. M., & Manalel, J. A. (2023). Interconnected social convoys: Understanding health and well-being through linked personal networks. *Advances in Life Course Research, 56*, 100541. https://doi.org/10.1016/j.alcr.2023.100541

Krieger, N. (2005). Embodiment: A conceptual glossary for epidemiology. *Journal of Epidemiology & Community Health, 59*(5), 350–355. https://doi.org/10.1136/jech.2004.024562

Kuh, D., Ben Shlomo, Y., & Ezra, S. (Eds.). (2004). *A life course approach to chronic disease epidemiology*. Oxford University Press. https://doi.org/10.1093/acprof:oso/9780198578154.001.0001

Landecker, H., & Panofsky, A. (2013). From social structure to gene regulation, and back: A critical introduction to environmental epigenetics for sociology. *Annual Review of Sociology, 39*(1), 333–357. https://doi.org/10.1146/annurev-soc-071312-145707

Link, B. G., & Phelan, J. (1995). Social conditions as fundamental causes of disease. *Journal of Health and Social Behavior, 35*, 80. https://doi.org/10.2307/2626958

Lynch, S. M. (2003). Cohort and life-course patterns in the relationship between education and health: A hierarchical approach. *Demography, 40*(2), 309–331. JSTOR. https://doi.org/10.2307/3180803

Machů, V., Arends, I., Veldman, K., & Bültmann, U. (2022). Work-family trajectories and health: A systematic review. *Advances in Life Course Research, 52*, 100466. https://doi.org/10.1016/j.alcr.2022.100466

Marmot, M. G. (2015). *The health gap: The challenge of an unequal world.* Bloomsbury.

Merton, R. K. (1968). The Matthew effect in science. *Science, 159*(3810), 56–63.

Missinne, S. (2015). Moving towards a better understanding of socioeconomic inequalities in preventive health care use: A life course perspective. In C. Burton-Jeangros, S. Cullati, A. Sacker, & D. Blane (Eds.), *A life course perspective on health trajectories and transitions* (Vol. 4, pp. 111–131). Springer International Publishing. https://doi.org/10.1007/978-3-319-20484-0_6

Parsons, T. (1964). Social structure and dynamic process: The case of modern medical practice. In T. Parsons (Ed.), *The social system*. The Free Press.

Pearlin, L. I., Schieman, S., Fazio, E. M., & Meersman, S. C. (2005). Stress, health, and the life course: Some conceptual perspectives. *Journal of Health and Social Behavior, 46*(2), 205–219. https://doi.org/10.1177/002214650504600206

Pescosolido, B. A., & Martin, J. K. (2015). The stigma complex. *Annual Review of Sociology, 41*(1), 87–116. https://doi.org/10.1146/annurev-soc-071312-145702

Power, C., Kuh, D., & Morton, S. (2013). From developmental origins of adult disease to life course research on adult disease and aging: Insights from birth cohort studies. *Annual Review of Public Health, 34*(1), 7–28. https://doi.org/10.1146/annurev-publhealth-031912-114423

Ranci, C. (2010). *Social vulnerability in Europe: The new configuration of social risks*. Palgrave Macmillan. http://public.eblib.com/choice/publicfullrecord.aspx?p=578907

Richardson, L. J., & Brown, T. H. (2016). (En)gendering racial disparities in health trajectories: A life course and intersectional analysis. *SSM - Population Health, 2*, 425–435. https://doi.org/10.1016/j.ssmph.2016.04.011

Shanahan, M. J., Mortimer, J. T., & Kirkpatrick Johnson, M. (2016). Introduction: Life course studies—Trends, challenges, and future directions. In M. J. Shanahan, J. T. Mortimer, & M. K. Johnson (Eds.), *Handbook of the life course* (pp. 1–23). Springer International Publishing. https://doi.org/10.1007/978-3-319-20880-0_1

Sieber, S., Cheval, B., Orsholits, D., van der Linden, B. W. A., Guessous, I., Gabriel, R., Kliegel, M., von Arx, M., Kelly-Irving, M., Aartsen, M. J., Boisgontier, M. P., Courvoisier, D., Burton-Jeangros, C., & Cullati, S. (2020). Do welfare regimes moderate cumulative dis/advantages over the life course? Cross-national evidence from longitudinal SHARE data. *The Journals of Gerontology: Series B, 75*(6), 1312–1325. https://doi.org/10.1093/geronb/gbaa036

Sieber, S., Orsholits, D., Cheval, B., Ihle, A., Kelly-Irving, M., Delpierre, C., Burton-Jeangros, C., & Cullati, S. (2021). Social protection expenditure on health in later life in 20 European countries: Spending more to reduce health inequalities. *Social Science & Medicine, 292*, 114569. https://doi.org/10.1016/j.socscimed.2021.114569

Singer, M., & Clair, S. (2003). Syndemics and public health: Reconceptualizing disease in bio-social context. *Medical Anthropology Quarterly, 17*(4), 423–441. https://doi.org/10.2307/3655345

Smith, K. E., & Anderson, R. (2018). Understanding lay perspectives on socioeconomic health inequalities in Britain: A meta-ethnography. *Sociology of Health & Illness, 40*(1), 146–170. https://doi.org/10.1111/1467-9566.12629

Steiber, N. (2019). Intergenerational educational mobility and health satisfaction across the life course: Does the long arm of childhood conditions only become visible later in life? *Social Science & Medicine, 242*, 112603. https://doi.org/10.1016/j.socscimed.2019.112603

Steves, C. J., Spector, T. D., & Jackson, S. H. D. (2012). Ageing, genes, environment and epigenetics: What twin studies tell us now, and in the future. *Age and Ageing, 41*(5), 581–586. https://doi.org/10.1093/ageing/afs097

Strauss, A. L. (1987). Illness trajectories. *Folia Sociologica, 13*.
Uccheddu, D., Emery, T., Gauthier, A. H., & Steverink, N. (2022). Gendered work-family life courses and late-life physical functioning: A comparative analysis from 28 European countries. *Advances in Life Course Research, 53*, 100495. https://doi.org/10.1016/j.alcr.2022.100495
Umberson, D., Williams, K., Powers, D. A., Liu, H., & Needham, B. (2006). You make me sick: Marital quality and health over the life course. *Journal of Health and Social Behavior, 47*(1), 1–16.
Umberson, D., Crosnoe, R., & Reczek, C. (2010). Social Relationships and Health Behavior Across the Life Course. *Annual Review of Sociology, 36*(1), 139–157. https://doi.org/10.1146/annurev-soc-070308-120011.
Wadsworth, M. E. J. (1997). Health inequalities in the life course perspective. *Social Science and Medicine, 44*(6), 859–869.
Wagner, C., Carmeli, C., Chiolero, A., & Cullati, S. (2022). Life course socioeconomic conditions and multimorbidity in old age—A scoping review. *Ageing Research Reviews, 78*, 101630. https://doi.org/10.1016/j.arr.2022.101630
Wagner, C., Carmeli, C., Jackisch, J., Kivimäki, M., van der Linden, B. W. A., Cullati, S., & Chiolero, A. (2024). Life course epidemiology and public health. *The Lancet Public Health, 9*(4), e261–e269. https://doi.org/10.1016/S2468-2667(24)00018-5

Chapter 8
Theories of the Rise, Fall, and Contemporary Challenges to the Profession of Medicine

Bernice Pescosolido

Introduction

Since the rise of industrialization, the modern profession of medicine has stood among the most powerful, if not the most powerful, of occupational groups in society. Medicine and its practitioners are the arbiters of life and death; of possibilities realized, possibilities dashed and possibilities reclaimed; and of evaluations of "normal" and "abnormal." The expansion of medicine's claim over more and more life spheres has been chronicled and criticized (see Olafsdottir, Conrad, both in this volume). In contemporary society, we turn to physicians to understand what we do, what we should eat, and whether we should punish or treat those who step outside society's norms. And, despite claims that the power of the medical profession may be waning, no viable alternatives have come forth to replace the allopathic system. Even "complementary alternative medicine" (both indigenous and New Age) has been absorbed, transformed, or otherwise brought under its jurisdiction (Astin et al., 1998).

In this chapter, the rise of the modern medical profession to this position of power and prominence will be traced through a recounting of sociological theories. This history can be crafted as a story that begins with the glorious and inevitable march of progress, moves to the inside of an aspiring profession, increasingly considers the other social actors, contexts, and processes that enabled the medical profession, and ends, at least to this point, with the full constellation of other institutions and organizations that have the potential to support or encroach on its boundaries. This recounting may take on the flavor of a "grand narrative" with all of its strengths and flaws (see Klein, 2004). However, as a sociology of knowledge, it reflects the dominance of the theoretical ideas of the times in which these theories were

B. Pescosolido (✉)
Indiana University, Bloomington, IN, USA
e-mail: pescosol@indiana.edu

W. C. Cockerham (ed.), *Medical Sociology on the Move*,
https://doi.org/10.1007/978-3-031-92456-9_8

fashioned. Perhaps more importantly, it reveals a story of incorporating more and more aspects of context that come together to shape the profession's fate. As Nobel Laureate and political scientist Elinor Ostrom (2009) advised us, understanding the whole of a complex phenomenon requires understanding the *interaction* of specific structures, forces, and processes. I argue that each theory set took on an explanation of critical parts of the complex interactions that constructed the privileged status that the profession of medicine holds. Together, they provide a thorough understanding of the rise to power but, as yet, an incomplete understanding of its present and future. Towards the end of this chapter, the issues that have most recently attracted sociological interest about the profession of medicine will be discussed. As has been the case since the 1980s, the subfield's attention to physicians remains "light" at best, though some exciting areas of research have emerged.

At the risk of being ethnocentric, I will focus primarily on the American case. Much of the work has been done on the U.S. This is perhaps not surprising, as the U.S. is the country where the medical profession achieved the greatest power and, despite concerns over its future, continues to have a degree of control over aspects of its work never achieved in other societies. The American case represents an integral part of how "professions" came to be defined, and its comparison with other countries allowed a separation of what is essential to professional status and what is not.

Clearly, the modern nation state exerted influence in determining the exclusive jurisdiction of allopathic medicine vis-à-vis other systems of medicine (e.g., the initial support for traditional Chinese medicine under Mao and the Communist Party in China, Unschuld 1992) and the extent to which the allopathic system was privately or publically owned and funded (e.g., as part of welfare state in the United Kingdom and the Nordic countries; Berlant, 1975; Porter, 2001). Just as critically, political power shaped the nature of colonial medicine in Africa (e.g., Lyons, 1988) and Asia (Brown, 1979), where allopathic medicine was used as a tool of colonial dominance, and in the public systems in the Soviet Union or Chile, where state socialist ideologies explicitly addressed class-based inequalities in the provision of care (Waitzkin, 2011). Thus, almost right from the beginning, Freidson (1970a) marked the critical division between the profession's power over the *content* of its work (e.g., diagnosis, treatment) in contrast to control of the *terms* of its work (i.e., the socio-cultural arrangements under which physicians provided services). Yet, in modern times, it is not clear whether that distinction has proved durable, as US insurance companies require preauthorization, set limits on care, and, essentially, reject doctors' orders. Nevertheless, an overview of the complex story of how sociological theories of the medical profession engaged and even stood at the forefront of altering larger theoretical trends and foci (e.g., the shift from concerns with the rise of professional power to debates over its decline) requires focusing the analytic lens on one country facilitates feasibility.

Sociological Theories of the Medical Profession in Historical Context

All theories—from medical science to mainstream sociology to the Marxist critique—agree on five fundamental and interrelated factors. Understanding these similarities provides an essential foundation upon which to lay out sociological theories focused on the U.S. profession of medicine. First, medicine is one of the "big three" occupations that has clearly and unambiguously staked a claim as a "profession." Despite the rather ubiquitous current use of the term to apply to any number of occupations, only medicine, law, and clergy have a special and privileged position based on unique expertise. Whether that claim was/is justified or "natural" becomes part of the theoretical history. What is also clear is that, as Freidson (1970b) noted, in contemporary society medicine appears to "trump" other professions in terms of power (e.g., determining if an individual can or cannot be tried for a crime depending on their assessment of mental status). Second, while a special role for healers has existed in every known society and while the precursor to the modern physician was established during the Middle Ages, what we now think of as a "physician" (i.e., an allopathic and science-based practitioner) only came to prominence at the beginning of the twentieth century in the U.S. and somewhat earlier in European countries (e.g., roughly the 1860s in Germany; the 1880s in Great Britain; Hollingsworth, 1986). Third, science, specifically the "Great Break" (i.e., Germ Theory + Anesthesia + Antisepsis), marked the beginning of the modern medical profession. Despite knowledge of anthrax in ancient societies, French, German, and British scientists around 1860 first documented that this disease was associated with a rod-shaped, blood born body (later called a bacillus; see Turnbull & Shadomy, 2011). This is widely considered to be the initial step in the development of the germ theory of modern medicine, the dominant paradigm separating modern physicians from all sorts of other healers. Combined with the development of anesthesia (Pernick, 1987) and the call to use antiseptics (Haller, 1981), the germ theory represented a major departure from the hot/cold, elemental theories and bloodletting practices of physicians of the day (Freidson, 1970b; Lindemann, 2010). Fourth, physicians in the late nineteenth century were not held in higher esteem in their communities than were practitioners of other healing traditions, including homeopathy, midwifery, and folk healing. With their medical bag holding mainly purgatives, opium-based medicines (e.g., laudanum), and tools for blood-letting, even the great physicians of that time (e.g., Benjamin Rush in Philadelphia) offered little that was unique. Because of the harsh and even lethal effects of existing therapies, the public held little regard for medicine and especially hospitals, considering them only as a last resort and "a place to die" (see Warner, 1986 on the "therapeutic gloom" of the period). Fifth, in the U.S., all theories point to the Flexner Report of 1910, commissioned by the Carnegie Foundation for the Advancement of Teaching, as sealing the fate of the U.S. healthcare system and the profession of medicine. Given its fundamental interest in education, the Carnegie Foundation hired Abraham Flexner to visit existing medical schools, many of which were proprietary. School administrators opened their doors, anticipating the private foundation funding that might come from their participation. However, much to their surprise and dismay, Flexner took a strong stance on the viability of and support for only the few, newly established medical schools, such as Johns Hopkins, which adopted a scientific curriculum based on the German university. He argued that all other schools should be closed, and they often were. The Flexner Report rippled through the existing landscape of medicine, and discussions of its role and stakeholder motivations are interpreted differently in theories of the rise of the profession, as we shall see below.

Phase I: The Initial Foray—Looking "Inside" to Unique Characteristics

With medicine's own histories detailing the Great Break, and the victories in World War II serving as the staging platform, sociologists and their colleagues from history, political science, anthropology, public health, and other disciplines sought to understand the modern profession of medicine. They rejected the "Great Man" theories of medicine (e.g., Walsh, 1907) in favor of looking to the characteristics of modern practice and practitioners that separated them from other occupations in the medical arena and joined it with the other great professions of law and religion. But even before American sociologists focused their analytic lens in this direction, Sir Alexander Morris Carr-Saunders and Paul A. Wilson in England wrote *The Professions* (1933). Carr-Saunders, initially trained as a natural scientist, turned his attention to many social problems, including eugenics (which he supported). In this classic treatise, the focus was squarely on the obligations of professionals and their duty to serve others, seeing this as a "higher calling." What distinguished professions from other occupations were those characteristics that are still seen as the hallmarks of the professions—a specialized body of expert and esoteric knowledge, long formalized (not apprenticeship-based) training in universities, and the establishment of a professional association that oversaw licensing criteria and the development/enforcement of a code of ethics.

In American sociology, Talcott Parsons (1951) first articulated a theory of the profession, using medicine as an exemplar in his larger theory of modern society. In *The Social System*, he saw illness as a practical problem of all societies and he put forth the basic structural functionalist argument. All societies must respond to health and disease in order to have a working society. Thus, all societies create specialized, institutionalized roles for patient and practitioner, who together, work to restore individuals back to health as productive members of society. The status of physician in modern society, based on the progress and promise of science, came with rights and obligations (see Fig. 8.1).

In a more abstract way, then, Parsons followed Carr-Saunders and Wilson in articulating those characteristics that separated the profession from other occupations. First, the profession of medicine is characterized by an *achievement*

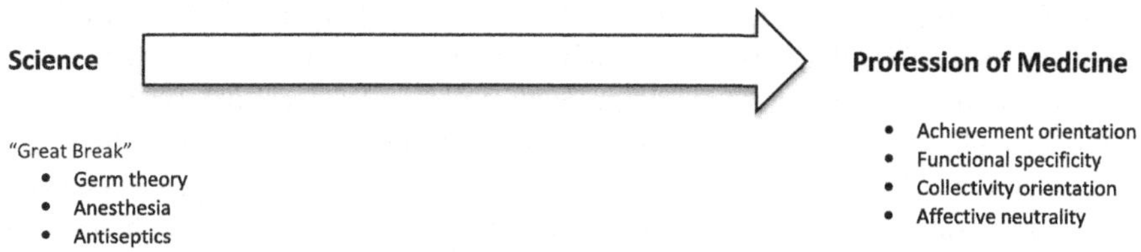

Fig. 8.1 Sociological theories of the medical profession, Phase I: Parsons' model (1951)

orientation. Entry into the role is based on technical competence acquired during a long and rigorous training period. Through formal schooling, physicians acquire the knowledge, skill, certification, and confidence to attend to illness. In essence, physician roles come not from skills handed down or inherited along family lines; rather it is a learned profession. Second, the role of the physician is *functionally specific*. Unlike the more generalized role of healers in premodern societies, physicians are to limit their profession and practice to their scientific training and expertise. They do not serve as "wise men" whose role encompasses understanding and solving all social problems. Third, physicians are expected to approach their work with *affective neutrality*. Illness is cast as an objective problem and patients must be dealt with in a professional and scientifically neutral way. Finally, the profession of medicine's role is characterized by a *collectivity orientation*. Physicians are obligated to put the welfare of patients above all else, especially personal and financial interests. Thus, the profit motive is not central to their work, and the exploitation of sickness for personal gain is strongly prohibited. Parsons specifically contrasted medical work and "commercialism," seeing the latter as the "most serious and insidious evil with which it has to contend" (1951: 435).

Phase II: The Construction of the Profession—Physicians as Self-Interested, Proactive Actors Requiring Political and Public Support

Pioneered by Eliot Freidson (Freidson, 1970a, b), this second phase is defined by the concept of professional dominance. Freidson rejected the notion that the power and prestige of the profession of medicine was somehow naturally conferred. As with his concept of the "sick role," Parsons' version of the "professional role" came to be seen as an ideal type in the Weberian sense. In contrast, Freidson and those who followed in this tradition conceptualized one brand of healers in the heterogeneous medical marketplace of the 1800s as actively and consciously working together to create a special status. Science-based medicine offered a striking departure from previous attempts at healing and promised better living by bringing medicine under the canopy of science (Rosenberg, 1987). Science was the "hook" upon which allopathic physicians seized to set themselves apart.

Along with Jeffrey Berlant (1975), Magali Sarfatti-Larson (1977) and others, Freidson made clear that this was not an inevitable march of progress nor the only path to a modern profession of medicine. Rather, physicians were determined actors who, through American Medical Association (AMA) leadership, developed a centrally defined political agenda, characterized by the "trappings" of professionalization (e.g., codes of ethics) and an organization of resources to separate themselves from other medical and folk practitioners of the time.

Freidson saw the list of unique characteristics of the professions from earlier theories as deliberately crafted by emerging allopathic physicians to lay claims to preeminence, autonomy and self-regulation. Thus, sociologists in the professional dominance tradition delineated the processes by which occupations actively struggled to become professions. To use Magali Safartti-Larson's term, the "professional project" of aspiring middle-class men was to establish a new view of the body (as machine), disease (as based on the germ theory), and appropriate in-house training of and standards for practitioners (in lab-based, university-attached medical schools; codes of ethics).

Theories of professional dominance focused on the coupling of political power and public confidence. Control over the profession's work was achieved via the efforts of political and economic elites who bolstered the profession's science-based claims for state support and organizational power. As depicted in Fig. 8.2, Freidson saw professional dominance as a two-stage process. The necessary, first condition for the establishment of the profession of medicine was to gain a legal monopoly over healing. The exclusive right to practice medicine required a political act—the passage of licensing laws. State by state in the U.S., the scientific profession of medicine drove other competitors (e.g., homeopaths, chiropractors, "granny" midwives) out of practice or drove them underground. Practicing medicine "without a license", a state conferred license, was now illegal and punishable by imprisonment. Second, even with this monopoly, the medical profession had to convince the public to use its services, not those offered by other healing traditions. Freidson saw no reason that "consulting status," as he called it, had to be conferred by government in a similar, heavy-handed manner. He argued, instead, that the public was persuaded by mass education, increasingly molded in the scientific tradition in Western societies, as well as by the visible successes of medicine which would come from scientific application and innovation.

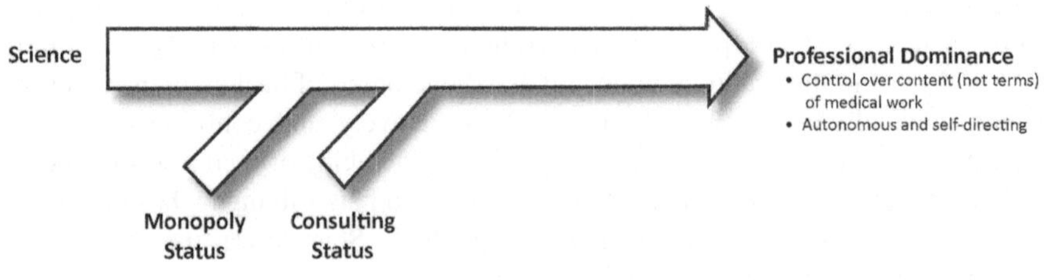

Fig. 8.2 Sociological theories of the medical profession, Phase II: Freidson's model (1970)

Phase III: Synthesis Embedded in a Cultural Twist—The Social Transformation of American Medicine

In many ways, Starr's (1982) theory represented a grand summary and synthesis of all of the work in the professional dominance tradition that preceded it (Mechanic, 1983). With no need to reject that approach, Starr argued that a key component, necessary to establish the profession of medicine, was missing in earlier theories. Specifically, only the recognition of how the larger political and cultural context had changed in the U.S. during the late nineteenth and early twentieth centuries could explain why the efforts of allopathic physicians succeeded in the early twentieth century and was accompanied by sovereignty (i.e., across-the-board acceptance, see Fig. 8.3). Starr, like Freidson, saw the public's suspension of skepticism, coupled with its willingness to defer to healing, as a matter of science. As an instrument of moral and political reform, science "was inseparable from the rise of status and power of professionals in new occupations and organizational hierarchies" (Starr, 1982: 10).

Importantly, however, he documented that early attempts to gain exclusive licensing privilege by allopathic physicians had failed. It was not enough to have physicians organize and court state legislators; rather, a larger cultural shift had to occur to allow both powerful groups and the public to grant the profession its privileged status. The Progressive Era, which he calls America's Cultural Revolution, created a growing willingness to rely on the specialized skills of strangers and replaced the commonly-held skepticism surrounding "expertise" that had characterized earlier political and cultural eras in the U.S.

Rejecting earlier views that were more idealistic, optimistic, and positivist, Starr drew from the second wave of sociological (Freidson, 1970b) and historical (Rosen, 1983) theories but combined them with newer theories of states, markets, power, and authority. He did not see the success of the profession's claims for political support as inevitable, and he dismissed earlier notions that political pre- or proscriptions would "take hold" and translate directly into popular acceptance. Rather, a cultural change, inspired by the new industrial age, allowed for the growth of cultural authority and its conversion into the control of markets, organizations, and

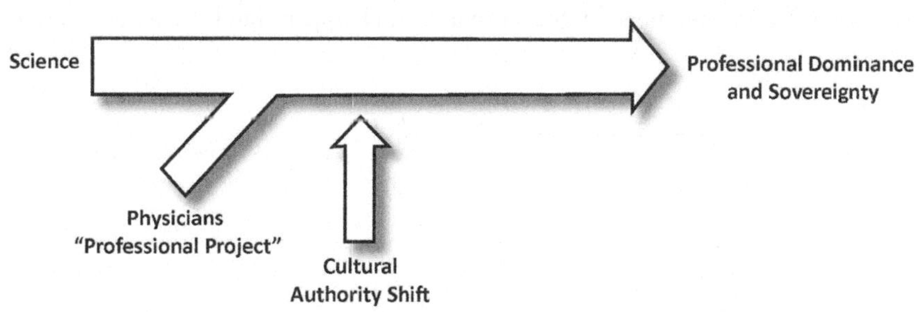

Fig. 8.3 Sociological theories of the medical profession, Phase III: Starr's model (1982)

governmental policy. Cultural authority engendered trust, compelled obedience, and fostered legitimacy, thereby increasing public acceptance of and dependence on the scientific profession of medicine. Without this larger shift, and only in this context, did the American public become willing to embrace physicians as experts and institutionalize the scientific model as preeminent.

Standing Outside Mainstream Sociological Arguments: The Marxist Alternative

While scholars in the conflict tradition were aware of the developing line of sociological theories of the profession, they focused squarely on the notion that societal structures of inequality are inevitably mirrored in the medical system. Professions and institutions, by their very nature, align with or against the dominant forms of production; and more importantly, produce disparities in life chances by social class. This theme of the illness-generating effects of capitalism goes back before the writings of Carr-Saunders and Wilson (Friedrich Engles, Rudolph Virchow) and represents a continuous and alternative stream of theory and policy (Salvador Allende, Vincente Navarro; see Howard Waitzkin, 2011). The work in this tradition placed medicine in the broader context of capitalism and imperialism, rejected the view that science and the coming of the industrial age translated inevitably into progress, and emphasized the economic interests that shaped the healthcare system. Studies documented how modern medicine was used to reward some and punish others, especially in Africa and Asia during the period of European colonialism (Lyons, 1988). However, the language of the professions was never writ large in their work. Rather, they focused on the maldistribution of medical personnel and the illness-generating effects of capitalism (see Fig. 8.4). This may account for its relative absence in standard theoretical accounts of the rise of the profession of medicine.

Nevertheless, this theoretical approach brings neglected structural understandings to theories of the rise of the profession. For example, Navarro (1978, 1983, 1993) cast the primary objective of the long educational training not as a necessity but as a way to perpetuate social roles within privileged social classes. And, in *Medicine Under Capitalism* (1976), he argued for and presented data on the pervasive control that members of the corporate and upper middle classes exert on

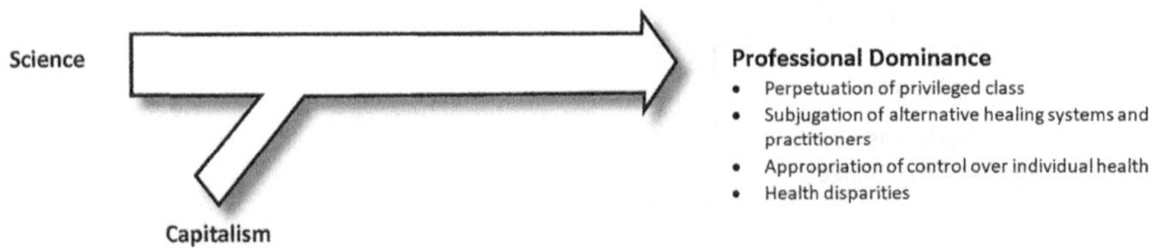

Fig. 8.4 Sociological theories of the medical profession: The Marxist alternative

policy-making bodies of U.S. health care institutions. Berliner (1983, 1985) and others went further, arguing that the great philanthropists of the early industrial era recognized the potential benefits for their own class-based interests in funding the scientific-based medical profession. Their massive donations provided not only goodwill as they amassed their wealth at great fiscal and health cost to the working classes, but also put in place an ideology of disease and a rationale for treatment that was compatible with the logic of industrial capitalism.

But it was not until the work of E.R. Brown that a political economic story of the rise of the American medical profession was articulated. Celebrated by some, ignored by most, Brown (1979) documented the role of the private philanthropy of the capitalist "robber barons" in establishing the American medical profession in *Rockefeller Medicine Men*. He argued that the Flexner Report essentially served as a medical system blueprint for the "captains" of industry and their administrative "lieutenants" who would serve their vested interests. This was accomplished through donations made by their philanthropic foundations.

The Flexner Report was commissioned, funded. and carried out by the Carnegie Foundation, whose interests surrounded education. Arguing that all proprietary medical schools were of exceedingly poor quality and should be closed, the Flexner Report prompted other philanthropies, most notably the Rockefeller Foundation, to fund the economic foundation of the modern medical care system. This included but was not limited to building university-based medical schools that embraced the same techno-scientific model that underlay industrial capitalism. Foundations provided the resources to set up the expensive laboratories and large, technologically equipped hospitals that scientific medicine required.

Philanthropists tied their donations to requirements that changed both the face of medicine and higher education. To receive funds, for example, universities were required to appoint physicians as "faculty," not an accepted or welcome practice at the time. By situating medical education in the university, the class-based profile of the modern physician was set. Practicing physicians who were female, working-class, from communities of color, or who were trained primarily through apprenticeship or attendance at proprietary medical schools were disenfranchised as they failed newly instated licensing exams based on the scientific model. Aspiring practitioners from other healing traditions or from lower social ranks, however defined, found their entry to university-based medical schools blocked by educational or financial requirements.

Comparing the U.S. and Great Britain, Hollingsworth (1986) showed how powerful class divisions played out as different nations solved the problem of financing their emerging modern systems of medicine. He looked not to scientific imperatives, but to "the social relations in which medical systems are embedded and the influence of power relationships on the structure of national medical systems" (1986: xiii). Ironically, he showed that the greater level of stratification within the early allopathic British medical profession (i.e., those affiliated with the prestigious voluntary hospitals versus general practitioners) resulted in a weaker social movement by practitioners, a stronger working class voice, and a fiscal role for the state to assure access that was clearly absent in the U.S.

In sum, those in the political economic tradition saw the newly wealthy philanthropists as purposively using their resources to reinforce and legitimate the dark side of industrial capitalism, including deflecting issues of health, disease, and treatment away from larger social issues and the damaging effects of industrialization (e.g., see Arnove, 1982; Berliner, 1983; Hollingsworth, 1986; Waitzkin, 2011). Unlike mainstream work on the rise of the profession of medicine, these accounts tend to cast physicians as either conspirators or puppets. Current work continues this discussion; for example, asking whether managed care pressures physicians to be "double agents," both protecting patients from the profit motive of for-profit health care while having to attend to its bottom line (e.g., Waitzkin, 2000).

Phase IV: Synthesis Embedded with a Network Twist—Elaborating the Internal Mechanisms of Professional Change

Curiously, Starr explicitly rejected Marxist accounts of the rise of the profession (see Pescosolido & Martin, 2004). However, professions do not "bring money to the table." As experts, they rely on their ability to persuade others of the value of their knowledge and services. By their very nature, they are dependent on economic resources that "society," whether individuals or organizations, are willing to provide. Aside from the Marxists, the sociology story of the profession of medicine minimizes the role of money, resulting in a "shock" that accompanied discussions of the health care crisis of the late 1980s. Neither the public nor the profession, itself, was prepared to shift the discourse and see issues of financial support take center stage in dealing with health, illness, and health care reform (Mechanic, 1983).

As sociological theories moved from "ideal type" to "professional project" to "cultural shift," historians, sociologists of science, and critical sociologists came forward to document that the rise of the medical profession was linked to very limited empirical proof of scientific medicine's efficacy (McKeown, 1979; McKinlay & McKinlay, 1981) and to a simultaneous, often contentious struggle of both science and medicine for legitimacy (Gieryn, 1999; Wailoo, 2004). Laboratories, autopsies, and vaccinations were not welcomed nor accepted by the public. Debates and resistance were commonplace; utilization rates were low (Warner, 1986). Physicians, as applied practitioners of little regard, were not embraced by scientists and, even within the ranks of aspiring physicians, there was skepticism about a blanket adoption of the scientific approach.

All sociological theories saw the middle class promulgating a strong belief in medical science, reforming medical education under the scientific paradigm, and working against practitioners, patients and patrons from other social classes to impose their views. But it was Brown (1979) who reminded us that homeopathy was the preferred medical sect of upper class physicians and patients. He documented how J.D. Rockefeller, himself, insisted that homeopathy as well as allopathy be supported by his donations, only to be overridden by middle class, philanthropic managers who came to control the Rockefeller Foundation.

Following on this, Jack K. Martin and I argued that unearthing the actual dynamic processes and interactions that created the conditions for the Flexner Report, modern medical education, the construction of medical infrastructure, and the public use of services was necessary (Pescosolido & Martin, 2004). Following Frenk and Duran-Arenas (1993), we saw professional dominance (monopoly) and sovereignty (consulting status) as two fundamentally different processes that did not flow in the same way as previous theories contended. A larger cultural shift, the Progressive Era, inspired the real actions of real people in the middle classes, and in turn, produced a much later and more gradual cultural shift among the broader public. The transfer of resources from the upper to the middle classes constrained the actions of individuals in all social classes.

Our premise was simple and two-fold: Social network ties among members of the middle classes created professional dominance under a fortuitous cultural context, and social network influence process shaped how individuals in the community came to culturally construct, consider, and use treatment options. However, class actions did not favor upper class preferences nor did individuals in the community rapidly embrace the new medicine with the same enthusiasm as the middle class elites (see Fig. 8.5).

Constructing Professional Dominance From the mid– to late nineteenth century an ideological shift, turning on the progress of science for the "betterment" of society, took place among the emerging middle classes. A middle class of managers grew as a result of the transition to industrial capitalism. The elite of this class formed a network of administrative leaders across formal social institutions (e.g., politics, education, law) that acted to mobilize resources (i.e., money, licensing

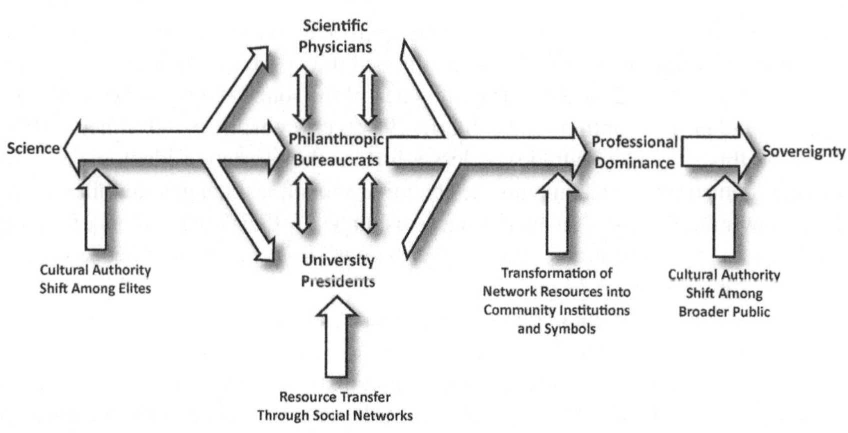

Fig. 8.5 Sociological theories of the medical profession, Phase IV: Pescosolido and Martin's model (2004)

laws, and curricular change) in support of the aspiring profession of scientific medicine.

Existing mainstream theories give more than a fair share of the credit to the concerted efforts of middle class physicians and politicians to establish the modern profession of medicine using science as the vector of differentiation. However, it took those physicians, in concert with the middle class administrators in philanthropic foundations and higher education to negotiate, cajole, coerce, and collaborate to underwrite the wholesale construction of a new medical marketplace in the U.S. Physicians engaged in a simultaneous struggle for dominance and sovereignty in line with other entrepreneurial projects of the rising middle class (e.g., the creation of the modern university; Hollingsworth, 1986; Ludmerer, 1985; Markowitz & Rosner, 1973; Stone, 1997).

Following the Marxists, we saw traditional explanations underplaying the role of the enormous transfer of resources from private philanthropy to the modern profession of medicine and the modern university (see also Stone, 1984). American industrialists of this period endowed the profession generously, but their money was directed by the visions and efforts of the middle class managers of their foundations, university presidents, and newly configured hospital boards. These middle-class elites, particularly members of other aspiring professions, all shared the ethos of scientific progress solving social problems, whether in business, medicine, education, or the larger society. Together, they re-engineered society by reshaping societal arrangements and resources to benefit this model, including establishing the dominance of scientific medicine. In the U.S., unlike the U.K., the reconstruction of the medical marketplace was accomplished almost exclusively with private monies, setting up a private system that offered no social safety net to individuals in times of sickness, as the Marxists noted.

Cultural shifts and professional organization offer far more elegant accounts of the rise of scientific medicine than the crass details of how money drove the transformation of institutions and set the terms of medical care in the U.S. All theories agree on the importance of the early foundations' economic contributions, but they part on the motivation of the capitalists, dubbed the "pseudo-aristocracy" by some (e.g., Larrabee, 1971: 228, 242). The influence of the foundations has been told as a story of either redemption (e.g., Starr, 1982) or conspiracy (Berliner, 1985). However, this story can be told with less effort, as the overlap of ideological views between industrial capitalism and the scientific model, as changes in philanthropy which saw middle class managers hijack resources to their own visions of "doing good," and as the frustration of the "robber barons" losing control of decision making in their own foundations.

The Marxists were right in seeing the deliberate and powerful influence of industrial capital; ironically, they conflated *ownership* and *control* of the means of production. With the wealth of the industrial capitalists, the managerial class held the authority to control where the charitable contributions went, changing the objective and symbolic conditions of healing. In doing so, they often subverted the wishes of the financial elites. They shaped an ideology based on their class position and activated their network ties to transfer enormous sums of money to produce the visible symbols of scientific medicine (e.g., new hospitals, ambulances, emergency rooms) which came to pervade the modern landscape of healing. They created the idea of medical schools attached to universities, against the will of most faculty; legitimated the scientific medical professor as a member of the faculty; and funded the building of the first great medical schools and hospitals in the U.S. In turn, these faculty trained the new breed of physicians and wrote the examinations that their students were well prepared to answer, but all others would fail.

In sum, this transformation resulted in what Sarfatti-Larson (1977) calls a monopoly in cognitive superiority. The middle class shared an ideological stance, believing they had the "right" answer for continued progress despite disagreement among the ranks of practicing physicians and the upper class elites (Rothstein, 1972). Presidents of universities, foundation officers, and elite members of the scientific medical profession activated their network ties to the mutual benefit of modern institutions fashioned under the scientific model. The building of large, impressive scientific medical schools and their associated complexes, as well as the transformation of hospitals from centers of last resort to "modern temples of science," embodied the cultural authority of scientific medicine. Thus, professional dominance was both reflected and reified in a huge built environment accompanied by public relations campaigns stressing the miracle of science (Stevens, 1999) that emplaced the cultural authority of scientific medicine. Local philanthropic foundations throughout the country followed the lead of the most visible foundations in funding local scientific medical schools and in building new hospital and clinic facilities where the new allopathic physicians would hold appointments (Pescosolido & Martin, 2004). This process of mimetic isomorphism (DiMaggio & Powell, 1983) differed mostly in the details across the U.S. and dramatically diverged only where market conditions were extreme (e.g., see Starr, 1982 on Kaiser-Permanente).

Understanding Public "Acceptance." The establishment of professional dominance dwarfed all competitors, eclipsing alternative sources of care. Most theories of the profession see the public as being "convinced," while Marxists see services as either denied or coerced (e.g., Waitzkin, 1970). In reality, these theories paid little attention to what transpired among the majority of individuals in the community.

That is, theories of the rise of the profession of medicine share the absence of an explicit theory of how individuals use, or do not use, medical care services. Even Freidson's (1970a) lay referral system theory, emphasizing individuals' network structures and cultural content, did not connect markets to help-seeking. Nor he did bring this theory to bear in his theory of the medical profession. In the same work (Freidson, 1970a), both sociological theories of patient and physician status and roles are explicated but remain as separate social processes. While sociologists and other social scientists contextualized how individuals respond to illness in terms of the context of their local lives, the first generation of utilization theories (i.e., how individuals use medical care) did not consider the larger market context of medical care. Similarly, theories of the professions did not weave together how the actions of individuals played into or against scientific medicine's professional project.

Implicitly, mainstream sociological theories of the medical profession appear to reflect the importance of beliefs in health care decision-making (e.g., Rosenstock's, 1966 Theory of Health Beliefs). In some way, fervor for the scientific approach was disseminated to and embraced by the public.

However, a consideration of, essentially, a second generation of theories on how individuals come to use the formal healthcare system brings a different version of the achievement of "consulting status" to light (see Pescosolido, 1991). Whatever their ideological bent, these newer sociologically-based utilization theories emphasized how geographical and financial availability shape which "services" can be accessed, and how "choices" are made (e.g., Andersen, 1968, 1995). In other words, the financial and social organization of medical systems looms large in individuals' use of services. Both what exists and what individuals perceive in terms of available services matter. Further, financial accessibility enables individuals to use some geographically available services. With the coming of third party payers (private insurance in the 1940s and public programs such as Medicare and Medicaid in the 1960s; see Quadagno, 2004), the services of modern physicians were covered while those from most other providers were not. In these theories, the sole focus is on the use of modern physicians, hospitals, and clinics in the allopathic tradition.

Bringing this understanding of utilization to theories of the rise of the profession provides a missing link in understanding sovereignty. The social re-organization of medical care, engineered to achieve professional dominance, both preceded and produced the public "choices" for modern medical services (Pescosolido & Martin, 2004). The shift in cultural authority from the working and lower classes that would give the profession its sovereignty would *follow from, but not cause,* the establishment of dominance. Freidson's "consulting status" did not have to be "earned" through demonstrated success; individuals did not have to be "convinced;" and Starr's sovereignty was not a natural outcome of the larger cultural shift in the Progressive Era. Rather, the public use of modern medicine was constructed by actively redirecting resources that changed the calculus of individual decision-making for medical care. Under conditions of illness, shifting options for medical care, and theories that conceptualize individuals seeking a solution that is only "good enough" (Pescosolido, 1992), sovereignty was subtly coerced, even if welcomed, by constraining the public's options. The role of the new institutions and practitioners overshadowed and, over time, changed public beliefs and values because they signaled the closing off, or at least limiting, of the pathways individuals could travel to "treatments."

Thus, a two-step process occurred in which physicians' monopoly was established through the efforts of middle-class elites, which in turn *guaranteed* an eventual, inevitable change among the general public. Dramatic institutional changes in the community ensured the general public's acceptance of scientific medicine in the later twentieth century. First, professional dominance dramatically altered the ideology and symbols of healing at the community level, ultimately leading to a shift in both objective and cognitive conditions. Second, these conditions shaped the public's use of the new scientific medical services under theories that conceptualized geographic and fiscal accessibility as crucial. Later developments in the U.S. (e.g., the widespread acceptance of private health insurance after World War II, the passage in 1965 of Medicaid and Medicare) reinforced the public's sole use of allopathic medicine by refusing reimbursement of practitioners of other systems. Thus, the public's use of health care represents a bargain struck between the offerings of providers of different healing systems and the preferences of individuals (Pescosolido, 1992, 2006). No other medical tradition or "paraprofessional" in modern medicine, to use Freidson's term for other occupations in modern medicine, comes close to the "functional strength" or "structural superiority" (Lee, 1982) of science-based medicine in the U.S., or for that matter, in any Western nation.

The power of individuals has been conceptualized only more recently as an active force, as social movements organize the resources and influence of specific groups (e.g., Brown, 1995). Ironically, not all of these stand in opposition to the profession; rather, they demand more voice, access, and influence in contemporary medicine. Perhaps not as surprising, those movements that draw from the middle classes are more successful in leveraging philanthropic support and disseminating its influence throughout society (e.g., Epstein, 1996 on HIV; Sulik, 2010 on breast cancer).

Phase V: The Theoretical Shift from a Concern with the Rise of Professional Power to Its Demise

By the 1980s sociologists no longer concerned themselves with theories of the profession of medicine. Indeed, by 1989, there was a concern that medical sociologists had lost interest in the healthcare system and its practitioners as a whole (Mechanic, 1989). Those who continued to focus on the profession turned their attention from understanding the rise of the profession to considerations of its "fall" from power. Specifically, sociologists targeted the three D's: Deprofessionalization, decline, and distrust (Pescosolido, 2006).

Deprofessionalization, in Marie Haug's (1976) view, represents a loss of prestige, power, and trust. It derives from rising levels of education among the citizenry and from increased reliance on technology and medical algorithms that have demystified medical care. Decline looks to external factors that erode support for the profession and to intrinsic factors related to physician supply and shrinking AMA (American Medical Association) membership (McKinlay & Marceau, 2008). Earlier, McKinlay (1982) referred to proletarianization as the inevitable fate of physicians who, like all other workers in a capitalist society, would eventually be stripped of control over their work through corporatization and bureaucratization. Lastly, distrust stems from the rapid privatization of medical care and the growth of managed care (Mechanic, 1983). Distrust undermines expectations that medical institutions and providers will act in accordance with the interests of individuals, and calls into question physician credibility, allegiance to altruistic motives, efficacy in medical encounters, and ultimately, treatment outcomes (Pescosolido & Boyer, 2001; see Wolinsky, 1993 for a review).

Much of this discussion proceeded without empirical evidence but with statements about flagging public support and confidence. The evidence, however, was equivocal. In fact, a pair of analyses using the same data came to opposite conclusions. Both documented "erosion" since the percentage of Americans who have a "great deal" of confidence in medicine had dropped since the 1970s though not in a consistent fashion. These data from the General Social Survey also revealed a statistically significant rise in the percentage of Americans who report having "hardly any" confidence in medicine. But the interpretation differed. Whether the jump from about 5% to 13% of the general public giving a "no confidence" vote is troublesome to the status of the profession of medicine, as Schlesinger (2002) argued, was not obvious to us given the absence of any viable alternative (Pescosolido et al., 2001).

Clearly, there has been a non-trivial disenchantment with medicine in the public eye. However, placed in larger cultural and organizational context, the fate of the profession appears to be not much more than a general concern with whether the glint of the modern industrial age has tarnished and the "American Century" is over (Pescosolido & Rubin, 2000). Our further analysis of public beliefs in "physician authority" between 1976 and 1996 revealed that the increase in negative responses appeared to represent a shift from the "don't know" category, not a shift from positive to negative opinion (Pescosolido et al., 2001).

Arguably, then, the profession of medicine no longer has quite the luster that McKinlay and Marceau (2002) believed it had during "the golden age." From the beginning of the concern with professional power, Freidson (1970a) made two important points that seem to be lost in the "Three D's" debates. First, in no country, even the U.S., does medicine achieve a complete monopoly (e.g., chiropractic in the U.S. was never banned in all states). Second, to return to a point made earlier, it is control over the "content" of medical work (i.e., diagnosis, prescription, authority over ancillary professions) that is key to professional dominance, not control over the "terms" of medical work (i.e., the socio-cultural arrangements). As long as the profession is relatively free of technical evaluation and control by other occupations in the medical division of labor, intrusions that change the socioeconomic terms of modem medical work do not significantly change medicine's professional character. Of course, the distinction is not pristine. Utilization review, cost controls, enormous financial settlements for medical malpractice, and formularies that allow physicians to prescribe some drugs but not others, all bespeak a demise of the extensive powers once given to physicians, particularly in the United States. And, the profession of medicine was stunned as early as 1972 when Congress passed a law allowing Medicare to cover chiropractic services (Pescosolido, 2006).

In the end, Freidson (1993) was "unimpressed" with contentions and evidence on the fall of the profession of medicine. Similarly, Mechanic (1991) suggested that even with less autonomy, contemporary societies still support the dominant medical paradigm, the centerstone of the profession's status and roles. However, in this context, both Freidson and Mechanic supported the new theoretical work of sociologists who shifted their focus from issues of rise and fall to "maintenance."

Phase VI: Re-embedding the Medical Profession in Society in the Face of Crisis—Systems Thinking Returns

In 1983, Gieryn set the stage for understanding professional dynamics following ascent to preeminence. Focusing on science, not medicine, he argued that there will always be skirmishes at the borders of professional turf. Professional boundaries are "drawn and redrawn in flexible, historically changing and sometimes ambiguous ways" (Gieryn, 1983: 781). Theories of the profession of medicine followed suit, laying out the full complement of organizations, actors, and groups that hold the potential to support, or increasingly, encroach on its boundaries. Thus, ironically like Parsons' (1951) original theory, the medical profession is embedded in the whole of society's institutions.

Abbott (1988), in *The Systems of Professions*, focuses on the dynamics of professions "growing, splitting, joining, adapting, and dying" (p.xiii; see Fig. 8.6). Because the professions make up interdependent systems, jurisdictional disputes become central, requiring the elaboration of the professional landscape. Adjacent professions (Halpern, 1992), specialties within medicine (e.g., primary care physicians, McKinlay & Marceau, 2008; Timmermans, 2008), or institutional supports (insurance companies, private philanthropies, the government, McKinlay & Marceau, 2002) require continual monitoring and defense of jurisdictional boundaries. How to maintain the "medical professionalism" of physicians (Mechanic, 2008) has replaced a concern for the status of the profession as a whole, reflected even in medical school curriculum (Castellani & Hafferty, 2006).

Similarly, the theory of countervailing powers "locates professions within a field of institutional and cultural forces and parties" (Hafferty & Light, 1995; Light, 2000; Mechanic, 1991; Timmermans & Oh, 2010). This explicit focus on institutional pillars suggests that the relative strength of the profession vis-à-vis other

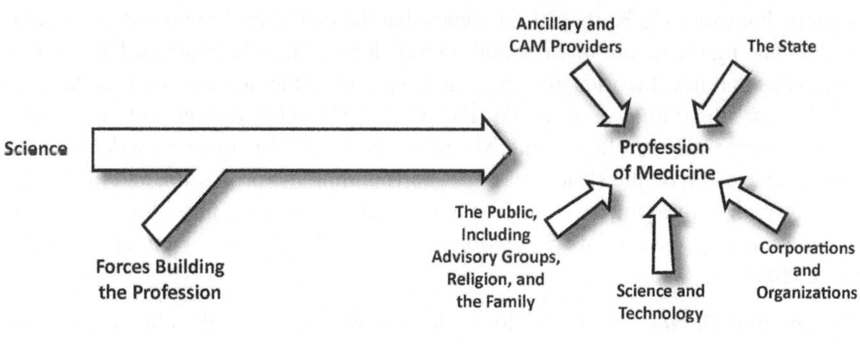

Fig. 8.6 Sociological theories of the profession, Phase IV: systems approaches

sources of fiscal and cognitive support has produced a weakened, but not less dominant, profession. On a larger scale, others theorize that the underlying, relative power in medicine has shifted from a logic of professions to a logic of institutions in controlling the terms of medical work (Quadagno, 2004; Scott et al., 2000). Some segments of the profession aspire to be free of commercial and institutional concerns, while others see direct ownership as the only protection from outside incursions. This reflects and reinforces larger cultural change. The resulting tensions, both within and at the periphery of medicine's jurisdictions, hold the potential to reformulate the terms of professional autonomy, dominance, and sovereignty. Private, unfettered, fiscal support for the profession of medicine in the U.S. has been replaced by a clear managerial perspective from private insurance to government programs that now cover the bulk of medical costs (Pescosolido, 2006).

Phase VII: The Sociological Disinterest in the Profession of Medicine, Emergent Themes, and Critical Gaps

Sociologists have not consistently monitored the fate of the medical profession over the years. Since the 1980s, and especially with the growing emphasis on the social determinants of health, medical sociologists have focused heavily on researching the social roots of illness and disease. That is, social epidemiology has dominated our analytic attention. Many editors of the *Journal of Health and Social Behavior* have noted in their editorial statements that this is not a new trend. Along with other topics—such as cross-national research, clinic or hospital-based studies, and systems of care—there has always been an imbalance in attention between social epidemiology and health services research.

At this historical juncture, a search for new research on the "profession of medicine" revealed that most work appears in compilations about medical sociology (e.g., Schupmann & Timmermans, 2023), a point that has not gone unnoticed by medical sociologists worldwide (Mühürdaroğlu, 2023). Some scholars suggest that the professional status and prestige of medicine seem to have "dissolved," raising questions about the relevance of "profession" as a social form in contemporary society. For example, Kurtz (2022) argues that the rise of professions was critical to understanding the nature of work and society during the industrial era. However, he maintains that new theories of society no longer view the profession of medicine as "the" clear illustrating case, unlike Parsons (1951), who, despite not considering himself a medical sociologist, did. Nevertheless, despite the relative neglect of sociological research on the structural issues surrounding the profession and the healthcare system, several important topics have recently emerged, providing an impetus for researching issues of professional power and practice (see also Jenkins et al., 2021).

Becoming a Doctor While we do not have new versions of the classic studies in medical school (e.g., *Boys in White, The Student Physician),* recent research addresses critical questions about the pathways to professional careers. Beginning with an examination of how first-year/freshmen students navigate their entry into the pre-medical track, Grace (2019) documents that gender and social networks are central to the retention of students in the major. Following a cohort at a large state university through their first year, he finds that women are most likely to shift away from becoming a physician, though not necessarily away from a career in health or healthcare. The women in the study report that they neither like nor excel in the initial required coursework. Additionally, Grace documents that college men's social network ties form around their career choices while women's do not. These two factors reinforce the initial gender leak in the medical pipeline.

Focusing on residents, Jenkins' (2020) detailed study on the path from medical school to residency examines how social class (in terms of organizational prestige), race, and foreign medical school degree shape the opportunities available to doctors aspiring to practice and secure a residency. The situation in the United States is fraught with irony—despite a critical shortage of residency programs, the medical system depends on foreign medical graduates to fill its lower status positions and specialties (e.g., osteopathy). This dynamic contributes to a system grappling with both a physician shortage and an underclass that perpetuates the status hierarchies in medicine.

Further, research by Mueller and colleagues (2017) reveals another gendered leak in the medical pipeline that occurs during residency. Deploying a longitudinal qualitative content analysis of narrative evaluations by attending physicians, they compare assessments collected over two years in an emergency room training program. Their findings document a shift in what attending physicians "rewarded" in their evaluations over time, as well as what kind of advice was given to those who were struggling. Initial evaluations favored women—finding them eager, responsible, and essentially "good learners." However, later evaluations found women lacking. The gender profile flipped, with men receiving more positive evaluations for qualities associated with leadership and "boldness." In addition, the feedback to residents who were struggling was also gendered. Men received "consistent" feedback from attending physicians, targeting their work performance, while women encountered "discordant" feedback, often regarding their personality traits, such as assertiveness. In sum, physician evaluators shifted from emphasizing learning potential in the early stages to prioritizing autonomy later. Ultimately, the profile of the "ideal" resident, who is more likely to become a successful physician, aligned with stereotypically masculine traits, which disadvantaged both women residents and their placement prospects.

Studies continue to show that medical specialties vary in status and prestige, which influences physicians' choices and tends to sort young doctors by gender into different fields. Surgery remains the most prestigious of all specialties and continues to be dominated by men. Perhaps more importantly, when specialties are perceived as lower in status, Olsson et al. (2019) suggest that doctors view their work not as a professional identity but more as a job.

Doctoring and Providing Care in Organizations Though still relatively rare, some recent work has begun to explore medical practice in organizational contexts. For example, recalling earlier work that contrasted physician-nurse and physician-patient relationships in medical versus surgical wards (Coser, 1958), Correia's (2017) research on physician behavior in two hospital wards found that organizations create sociocultural differences in behavior and discourse. Notably, in contrast to earlier studies, he sees these differences as challenging a standardized view of the profession of medicine. Similarly, VanHeuvelen and Grace (2020) explored how healthcare occupations shape provider responses to organizational change. Their research, which utilized survey data from nearly an entire neonatal care unit and included in-depth interviews with over 30 providers, revealed that "misgivings" about moving from an open-bay structure to individual-patient rooms were more prevalent among staff nurses compared to physicians or administrative leadership.

Medical Gaslighting and Provider-Based Stigma Medical sociologists have adapted the concept of gaslighting—traditionally focused on intimate relationships,—to a wider spectrum of relationships, including provider-patient relationships (e.g., Sebring, 2021; see Sweet, 2019 more generally). While in intimate settings gaslighting has an explicit and malevolent intent, when applied to the medical sector, it takes a more general tone of conscious or unconscious dismissal, misguided or misinterpreted understandings, and inappropriate or denied treatment. This perspective is rooted in early work by medical sociologists such as John McKinlay and Karen Lutfey, who systematically documented the inadequate care provided to women with heart disease within the medical care system (Lutfey et al., 2008; Maserejian et al., 2009; McKinlay, 1996).

Hernandez's (2013) study of how medical advances were differentially offered to pregnant women by healthcare providers provides a fascinating picture of how healthcare disparities emerge. Within multiple urban clinics, disparities arose only for one (omega-3 fatty acid supplements) but not another (Vitamin D) novel recommendation as providers expressed concern about the financial ability of disadvantaged women to afford advances that required additional resources. In this case, the disparity arose from concern rather than gaslighting. Thus, it is *not* merely the nature of the interpersonal relationship that creates healthcare disparities but rather "the result of deeply embedded and largely unchallenged ideologies underpinning health-care services" (Sebring, 2021: 1951). Similar to the earlier studies on heart disease and pregnancy, structural issues and inequalities find their way into and are carried out in interactions marked by power differentials (e.g., racial differences in opioid prescription; Kang et al., 2022).

Thought about differently, the issue of medical gaslighting which does not *require* conscious bias, raises concerns about stigma within the healthcare system. Although long understood and discussed but rarely the subject of direct research, the prejudices and discrimination that providers carry into their patient care underlie the phenomenon of gaslighting. In the highly stigmatized area of mental illness and substance use disorders, providers' views of culpability and unpredictability can lead to a lack of support for medications used for treating opioid use disorder (MOUD; Madden et al., 2021), "psychiatric boarding" (i.e., patients being held in ER hallways or other areas awaiting inpatient beds, Alakeson et al., 2010), and the persistent denial of parity in treatment (Fung et al., 2023). Stigma remains pervasive throughout the patient journey, from entry into care to aftercare, yet it has only recently been explicitly acknowledged and considered in research (Gonzales et al., 2021). Factors such as the culture of medicine, the absence of discussions around this issue in training, and a long-held, unspoken, and false assumption that healthcare providers are immune to stigma due to their career choices and training have all contributed to this research gap (Wallace, 2012).

Two Critical Topics in Need of Attention by Medical Sociologists: The Fragility of Providing Care and the Public Culture of Medicine and the Profession

Recent research has explored how feelings of powerlessness among providers contribute to burnout in patient care (e.g., Buchbinder et al., 2024; Grace & VanHeuvelen, 2019). However, there remains a dearth of sociological research that sheds light on the impending crisis in medical care. Concerns about a shortage in the medical workforce, including but not limited to physicians, point to problems arising from demographic, organizational, educational, cultural and social psychological factors (Jenkins, 2020; Kirch & Petelle, 2017; NAM, 2019).

Two issues are beginning to garner some research attention, although relatively little of it is from sociologists. The first, which flips the concerns mentioned above, is the stigma faced by healthcare providers as they deal with the stresses of their work. It may be the case that the COVID-19 pandemic heightened awareness of this issue. A 2020 survey of ER physicians conducted by their specialty organization revealed very high levels of stress and knowledge of where to seek mental health care, but also a high level of perceived stigma from colleagues and apprehension about potential structural stigma related to licensing renewal (https://www.emergencyphysicians.org/siteassets/emphysicians/all-pdfs/acep20_mental-health-poll-analysis.pdf). Despite some early research (e.g., Corrigan et al., 2014), we are only beginning to focus on the stigma that healthcare providers encounter and the stigma they themselves may hold (Hamilton et al., 2023).

The second issue relates to trust. Trust is recognized as critical for the public when seeking services and adhering to prescribed health regimes. However, not since Mechanic's sustained focus on trust (1996, 2003), have medical sociologists consistently monitored the cultural climate surrounding medicine in the US. In an era where major social institutions are strained, tested, and subjected to questions of legitimacy, understanding the public's trust—or the lack thereof—becomes increasingly important. If the Progressive Era helped to give rise to the profession of medicine, as Starr (1982) contended, then the current climate, which poses serious challenges to the core tenets of progressive ideology—including trust in science and expertise more generally—demands sociological attention. Although vaccine hesitancy and abortion issues (Hawbaker et al., 2023) have prompted a reevaluation of public trust in medicine, developing theory and conducting research on public trust remains essential (see Gille et al., 2021; Wilk & Platt, 2016 as a starting point).

Conclusion

This review of sociological theories of the profession of medicine and research directions reveals theories mirroring both the growing sophistication of sociology and the growing complexity of contemporary society. In the end, whether the medical profession, as we know it, stands or falls is inextricably tied to dominant social forms and processes, including class, economic and political structures (Waitzkin, 2011). In "The Continued Social Transformation of the Medical Profession," Timmermans and Oh (2010) returned to concerns about the role of money in professional status. Reviewing "tensions" and accepting the Phase V conceptualization of the medical profession as "one stakeholder among many stakeholders vying for market share and power in the health care field" (2010: s94), they conclude that the profession is resilient, continuing to adapt and change at the margins. But others are not so sanguine about its future (McKinlay & Stoeckle, 1988).

Our voice, as sociologists, in understanding jurisdictional boundaries and skirmishes involving the profession of medicine is critical, but not central in current debates. This is problematic for the discipline, the subfield, and for social change. Without continued sociological attention melding mainstream sociological theory and substantive expertise in medical sociology, our understanding of society, the profession of medicine, and the fate of individuals' health and health care will be impoverished. Now more than ever our theorizing must be reenergized, new data need to be collected, and those data have to be interpreted in a larger context. The debates about the future of primary care that McKinlay and Marceau (2008) and Timmermans (2008) began, the dialogue on expropriation and transformation of complementary and alternative medicine (CAM) that Wolpe (1985) initiated, and the fate of the profession in light of larger societal changes represent challenges to sociological theory.

Every society fashions its own medical social contract. Even if we experience a shift of the magnitude that parallels the one that accompanied the industrial age, for better or worse, medicine and its practitioners will be reconstituted in light of social resources, cultural context, and social cleavages. Yet, the critical ingredients will be the same, in the abstract, as we have seen here—cultural landscape, professional solidarity (or not, as AMA membership continues to slide), competing practitioners inside and outside of the scientific medical paradigm, and ownership and control of resources that will be shaped by and through networks of power. What is crucial, and what will vary, will be the specific nature of societal negotiations that construct a medical marketplace. Further, the decisions will remain the same: Will health care be a right or a privilege? Who will "own" and "control" the healthcare system? In particular, how much of a role will the State play in granting or assuring professional dominance of the full complement of healing practitioners? If the boundaries of the nation state become more porous, or less salient, as Giddens (1990) suggests, what legal or political institution will step in its place? The answers to these questions are vital in shaping the profession, the nature of medical work, and the health of populations.

Parsons' (1951) initial statement stands: All societies create institutional roles for patients and providers. For sociology to understand social institutions, the life chances of individuals in them, and the intimate connections between them, health and health care continue to present an essential window into social life. Theorizing about and empirically examining the structure, culture, and impact of these roles continues to be a central sociological task.

References

Abbott, A. D. (1988). *The system of professions: An essay on the division of expert labor*. University of Chicago Press.

Alakeson, V., Pande, N., & Ludwig, M. (2010). A plan to reduce emergency room 'boarding' of psychiatric patients. *Health Affairs, 29*(9), 1637–1642. https://doi.org/10.1377/hlthaff.2009.0336

Andersen, R. (1968). A behavioral model of families' use of health services. In *Research series* (Vol. No. 27). Center for Administration Studies, University of Chicago.

Andersen, R. (1995). Revisiting the behavioral model and access to medical care: Does it matter? *Journal of Health and Social Behavior, 36*(1), 1–10.

Arnove, R. F. (Ed.). (1982). *Philanthropy and cultural imperialism: The foundations at home and abroad*. Indiana University Press.

Astin, J. A., Marie, A., Pelletier, K. R., Hansen, E., & Haskell, W. L. (1998). A review of the incorporation of complementary and alternative medicine by mainstream physicians. *Archives of Internal Medicine, 158*, 2303–2310.

Berlant, J. (1975). *Profession and monopoly: A study of medicine in the United States and Great Britain*. University of California Press.

Berliner, H. (1983). Starr wars. *International Journal of Health Services, 13*(4), 671–675.

Berliner, H. (1985). *A system of scientific medicine: Philanthropic foundations in the Flexner era*. Tavistock.

Brown, E. R. (1979). *Rockefeller medicine men: Medicine and capitalism in America*. University of California Press.

Brown, P. (1995). Naming and framing: The social construction of diagnosis and illness. *Journal of Health and Social Behavior* Extra Issue, 34–52.

Buchbinder, M., Browne, A., Berlinger, N., Jenkins, T., & Buchbinder, L. (2024). Moral stress and moral distress: Confronting challenges in healthcare systems under pressure. *The American Journal of Bioethics, 24*(12), 8–22. https://doi.org/10.1080/15265161.2023.2224270

Carr-Saunders, A. M., & Wilson, P. A. (1933). *The professions*. Cass.

Castellani, B., & Hafferty, F. W. (2006). The complexities of professionalism: A preliminary investigation. In D. Wear & J. Aultman (Eds.), *Professionalism in medicine: Critical perspectives*. Kluwer Academic.

Correia, T. (2017). Doctors' reflexivity in hospital organisations: The nexus between institutional and behavioural dynamics in the sociology of professions. *Current Sociology, 65*(7), 1050–1069. https://doi.org/10.1177/0011392116641478

Corrigan, P. W., Mittal, D., Reaves, C. M., Haynes, T. F., Han, X., Morris, S., & Sullivan, G. (2014). Mental health stigma and primary health care decisions. *Psychiatry Research, 218*(1–2), 35–38. https://doi.org/10.1016/j.psychres.2014.04.028

Coser, R. L. (1958). Authority and decision-making in a hospital: A comparative analysis. *American Sociological Review, 23*(1), 56–63.

DiMaggio, P. J., & Powell, W. W. (1983). The iron cage revisited: Institutional isomorphism and collective rationality in organizational fields. *American Sociological Review, 48*, 147–160.

Epstein, S. (1996). *Impure science: AIDS, activism, and the politics of knowledge*. University of California Press.

Freidson, E. (1970a). *Profession of medicine: A study of the sociology of applied knowledge*. Dodd, Mead, and Co.

Freidson, E. (1970b). *Professional dominance: The social structure of medical care*. Atherton Press.

Freidson, E. (1993). How dominant are the professions? In F. W. Hafferty & J. B. McKinlay (Eds.), *The changing medical profession: An international perspective* (pp. 54–66). Oxford University Press.

Frenk, J., & Duran-Arenas, L. (1993). The medical profession and the state. In F. W. Hafferty & J. B. McKinlay (Eds.), *The changing medical profession: An international perspective* (pp. 25–42). Oxford University Press.

Fung, V., Price, M., McDowell, A., Nierenberg, A. A., Hsu, J., Newhouse, J. P., & Cook, B. L. (2023). Coverage parity and racial and ethnic disparities in mental health and substance use care among Medicare beneficiaries. *Health Affairs (Millwood), 42*(1), 83–93. https://doi.org/10.1377/hlthaff.2022.00624

Giddens, A. (1990). *The consequences of modernity*. Stanford University Press.

Gieryn, T. F. (1983). Boundary-work and the demarcation of science from non-science: Strains and interests in professional ideologies of scientists. *American Sociological Review, 48*(December), 781–795.

Gieryn, T. F. (1999). *Cultural boundaries of science*. University of Chicago Press.

Gille, F., Smith, S., & Mays, N. (2021). What is public trust in the healthcare system? A new conceptual framework developed from qualitative data in England. *Social Theory & Health, 19*(1), 1–20.

Gonzales, L., López-Aybar, L., & McCullough, B. (2021). Variation in provider attitudes and treatment recommendations for individuals with schizophrenia and additional marginalized identities: A mixed-method study. *Psychiatric Rehabilitation Journal, 44*(2), 107–117.

Grace, M. K. (2019). Parting ways: Sex-based differences in premedical attrition. *Social Science & Medicine, 230*, 222–233.

Grace, M. K., & VanHeuvelen, J. S. (2019). Occupational variation in burnout among medical staff: Evidence for the stress of higher status. *Social Science & Medicine, 232*, 199–208. https://doi.org/10.1016/j.socscimed.2019.05.007

Hafferty, F. W., & Light, D. W. (1995). Professional dynamics and the changing nature of medical work. *Journal of Health and Social Behavior, 36*, 132–153.

Haller, J. S. (1981). *American medicine in transition, 1840–1910*. University of Illinois Press.

Halpern, S. A. (1992). Dynamics of professional control: Internal coalitions and cross-professional boundaries. *American Journal of Sociology, 97*(4), 994–1021.

Hamilton, L. J., Coleman, M. E., & Krendl, A. C. (2023). Contact reduces substance use stigma through bad character attributions, especially for US health care professionals. *Psychology of Addictive Behaviors, 37*(6), 734–745.

Haug, M. R. (1976). The erosion of professional authority: A cross-cultural inquiry in the case of the physician. *Milbank Memorial Fund Quarterly, 54*, 83–106.

Hawbaker, A., Paiz, J. Y., Crawford, B. L., Turner, R. C., & Jozkowski, K. N. (2023). Medicine and abortion: Public trust in medical authority and Americans' acceptance of legal abortion. *SSM-Qualitative Research in Health, 4*, 100361.

Hernandez, E. M. (2013). Provider and patient influences on the formation of socioeconomic health behavior disparities among pregnant women. *Social Science & Medicine, 82*, 35–42. https://doi.org/10.1016/j.socscimed.2013.01.018
Hollingsworth, J. R. (1986). *A political economy of medicine: Great Britain and the United States*. Johns Hopkins University Press.
Jenkins, T. M. (2020). *Doctors' orders: The making of status hierarchies in an elite profession*. Columbia University Press.
Jenkins, T. M., Underman, K., Vinson, A. H., Olsen, L. D., & Hirshfield, L. E. (2021). The resurgence of medical education in sociology: A return to our roots and an agenda for the future. *Journal of Health and Social Behavior, 62*(3), 255–270.
Kang, H., Zhang, P., Lee, S., Shen, S., & Dunham, E. (2022). Racial disparities in opioid administration and prescribing in the emergency department for pain. *The American Journal of Emergency Medicine, 55*, 167–173.
Kirch, D. G., & Petelle, K. (2017). Addressing the physician shortage: The peril of ignoring demography. *JAMA, 317*(19), 1947–1948. https://doi.org/10.1001/jama.2017.2714
Klein, J. (2004). Open moments and surprise endings: Historical agency and the workings of narrative in "The Social Transformation of American Medicine". *Journal of Health Politics, Policy and Law, 29*(4–5), 621–642.
Kurtz, T. (2022). The end of the profession as a sociological category? Systems-theoretical remarks on the relationship between profession and society. *The American Sociologist, 53*(2), 265–282. https://doi.org/10.1007/s12108-021-09483-3
Larrabee, E. (1971). *The benevolent and necessary institution; the New York Hospital, 1771–1971*. Doubleday.
Lee, R. (1982). Comparative studies of health care systems. *Social Science & Medicine, 16*, 629–642.
Light, D. W. (2000). The medical profession and organizational change: From professional dominance to countervailing power. In C. Bird, P. Conrad, & A. M. Fremont (Eds.), *Handbook of medical sociology* (pp. 201–216). Prentice Hall.
Lindemann, M. (2010). *Medicne and society in early modern Europe*. Cambridge University Press.
Ludmerer, K. M. (1985). *Learning to heal: The development of American Medical Education*. Basic Books, Inc.
Lutfey, K. E., Campbell, S. M., Renfrew, M. R., Marceau, L., Roland, M., & McKinlay, J. B. (2008). How are patient characteristics relevant for physicians' clinical decision making in diabetes?: An analysis of qualitative results from a cross-national factorial experiment. *Social Science & Medicine, 67*(9), 1391–1399.
Lyons, M. (1988). Sleeping sickness, colonial medicine, and imperialism: Some connections in the Belgian Congo. In R. MacLeod & M. Lewis (Eds.), *Disease, medicine, and empire: perspectives on Western medicine and the experience of Western expansion* (pp. 245–256). Routledge.
Madden, E. F., Prevedel, S., Light, T., & Sulzer, S. H. (2021). Intervention stigma toward medications for opioid use disorder: A systematic review. *Substance Use & Misuse, 56*(14), 2181–2201. https://doi.org/10.1080/10826084.2021.1975749
Markowitz, G. E., & Rosner, D. K. (1973). Doctors in crisis: A study of the use of medical education reform to establish modern professional elitism in medicine. *American Quarterly, 25*, 83–107.
Maserejian, N. N., Link, C. L., Lutfey, K. L., Marceau, L. D., & McKinlay, J. B. (2009). Disparities in physicians' interpretations of heart disease symptoms by patient gender: Results of a video vignette factorial experiment. *Journal of Women's Health, 18*(10), 1661–1667. https://doi.org/10.1089/jwh.2008.1007
McKeown, T. (1979). *The role of medicine: Dream, mirage, or nemesis?* Princeton University Press.
McKinlay, J. B. (1982). Toward the proletarianization of physicians. In C. Derber (Ed.), *Professionals as workers: Mental labor in advanced capitalism* (pp. 37–62). G.K. Hall.
McKinlay, J. B. (1996). Some contributions from the social system to gender inequalities in heart disease. *Journal of Health & Social Behavior, 37*, 1–26.

McKinlay, J., & Marceau, L. (2002). The end of the golden age of doctoring. *International Journal of Health Services, 32*(2), 379–416.
McKinlay, J., & Marceau, L. (2008). When there is no doctor: Reasons for the disappearance of primary care physicians in the U.S. during the early 21st century. *Social Science & Medicine, 67*(10), 1481–1491.
McKinlay, J. B., & McKinlay, S. M. (1981). Medical measures and the decline of mortality. In P. Conrad & R. Kern (Eds.), *The sociology of health and illness: Critical perspectives* (pp. 12–30). St. Martin's Press.
McKinlay, J. B., & Stoeckle, J. D. (1988). Corporatization and the social transformation of doctoring. *International Journal of Health Services, 18*(2), 191–205. https://doi.org/10.2190/yevw-6c44-ycye-cgeu
Mechanic, D. (1983). Review of "The social transformation of American medicine". *Perspectives in Biology and Medicine, 27*(1), 163–167.
Mechanic, D. (1989). Medical sociology: Some tensions among theory, method, and substance. *Journal of Health and Social Behavior, 30*(2), 147–160.
Mechanic, D. (1991). Sources of countervailing power in medicine. *Journal of Health Politics, Policy and Law, 16*(3), 485–498.
Mechanic, D. (1996). Changing medical organization and the erosion of trust. *The Milbank Quarterly, 74*(2), 171–189. https://doi.org/10.2307/3350245
Mechanic, D. (2003). Uncertainty and changing trust relationships in medicine. In C. M. Messikomer, J. P. Swazey, & A. Glicksman (Eds.), *Society & medicine: Essays in honor of Renée C. Fox* (pp. 169–180). Routledge.
Mechanic, D. (2008). *The truth about health care: Why reform is not working in America*. Rutgers University Press.
Mueller, A. S., Jenkins, T. M., Osborne, M., Dayal, A., O'Connor, D. M., & Arora, V. M. (2017). Gender differences in attending physicians' feedback to residents: A qualitative analysis. *Journal of Graduate Medical Education, 9*(5), 577–585. https://doi.org/10.4300/jgme-d-17-00126.1
Mühürdaroğlu, A. (2023). The withering away of the physician in medical sociology: Medicalization, biomedicalization, and pharmaceuticalization. *İstanbul University Journal of Sociology, 43*(2), 421–445. https://doi.org/10.26650/SJ.2023.43.2.0034
National Academies of Sciences, Engineering, and Medicine. (2019). *Taking action against clinician burnout: A systems approach to professional well-being*. The National Academies Press. https://doi.org/10.17226/25521
Navarro, V. (1976). *Medicine Under Capitalism*. Prodist.
Navarro, V. (1978). *Class struggle, the state, and medicine: An historical and contemporary analysis of the medical sector in great*. Watson Publishers International.
Navarro, V. (1983). *Health and work under capitalism: An international perspective*. Baywood Publishing Company.
Navarro, V. (1993). Health services research: What is it? *International Journal of Health Services, 23*(1), 1–13.
Olsson, C., Kalén, S., & Ponzer, S. (2019). Sociological analysis of the medical field: Using Bourdieu to understand the processes preceding medical doctors' specialty choice and the influence of perceived status and other forms of symbolic capital on their choices. *Advances in Health Sciences Education, 24*(3), 443–457.
Ostrom, E. (2009). A general framework for analyzing sustainability of social-ecological systems. *Science, 325*, 419–422.
Parsons, T. (1951). *The social system: The major exposition of the author's conceptual scheme for the analysis of the dynamics of the social system*. Free Press.
Pernick, M. S. (1987). *A calculus of suffering: Pain, professionalism and anesthesia in nineteenth-century America*. Columbia University Press.
Pescosolido, B. A. (1991). Illness careers and network ties: A conceptual model of utilization and compliance. In G. L. Albrecht & J. A. Levy (Eds.), *Advances in medical sociology* (pp. 161–184). JAI Press.

Pescosolido, B. A. (1992). Beyond rational choice: The social dynamics of how people seek help. *American Journal of Sociology, 97*, 1096–1138.
Pescosolido, B. A. (2006). Professional dominance and the limits of erosion. *Society, 43*(6), 21–29.
Pescosolido, B. A., & Boyer, C. A. (2001). The American health care system: Entering the 21st century with high risks, major challenges and great opportunities. In W. C. Cockerham (Ed.), *The Blackwell companion to medical sociology* (pp. 180–198). Blackwell Publishers.
Pescosolido, B. A., & Martin, J. K. (2004). Cultural authority and the sovereignty of American medicine: The role of networks, class and community. *Journal of Health Politics, Policy and Law, 29*(4–5), 735–756.
Pescosolido, B. A., & Rubin, B. A. (2000). The web of group affiliations revisited: Social life, postmodernism, and sociology. *American Sociological Review, 65*(February), 52–76.
Pescosolido, B. A., Tuch, S. A., & Martin, J. K. (2001). The profession of medicine and the public: Examining Americans' changing confidence in physician authority from the beginning of the "Health Care Crisis" to the Era of Health Care Reform. *Journal of Health & Social Behavior, 42*(March), 1–16.
Porter, R. (2001). *The Cambridge illustrated history of medicine*. Cambridge University Press.
Quadagno, J. (2004). Why the United States has no national health insurance: Stakeholder mobilization against the welfare state, 1945–1996. *Journal of Health & Social Behavior, 45*(Supplement 1), 25–44. (20).
Rosen, G. (1983). *The structure of American medical practice 1875–1941*. University of Pennsylvania Press.
Rosenberg, C. E. (1987). *The care of strangers: The rise of America's hospital system*. Basic Books.
Rosenstock, I. M. (1966). Why people use health services. *Milbank Memorial Fund Quarterly, 44*(3), 94–106.
Rothstein, W. G. (1972). *American physicians in the nineteenth century: From sects to science*. Johns Hopkins University Press.
Sarfatti-Larson, M. (1977). *The rise of professionalism*. University of California Press.
Schlesinger, M. (2002). A loss of faith: The sources of reduced political legitimacy for the American medical profession. *Millbank Quarterly, 80*(2), 185–235.
Schupmann, W., & Timmermans, S. (2023). Sociology of the medical profession and para-professions. In *Handbook on the sociology of health and medicine* (pp. 199–212). Edward Elgar Publishing.
Scott, W., Richard, M. R., Mendel, P. J., & Caronna, C. A. (2000). Institutional change and health-care organization. In *Professional dominance to managed care*. University of Chicago Press.
Sebring, J. C. H. (2021). Towards a sociological understanding of medical gaslighting in western health care. *Sociology of Health & Illness, 43*(9), 1951–1964. https://doi.org/10.1111/1467-9566.13367
Starr, P. (1982). *The social transformation of American medicine: The rise of a sovereign profession and the making of a vast industry*. Basic Books, Inc.
Stevens, R. (1999). *In sickness and in wealth: American hospitals in the twentieth century*. Johns Hopkins University Press.
Stone, D. A. (1984). *The disabled state*. Temple University Press.
Stone, D. A. (1997). The doctor as businessman: The changing politics of a cultural icon. *Journal of Health Politics, Policy and Law, 22*, 533–556.
Sulik, G. A. (2010). *Pink ribbon blues: How breast cancer culture undermines women's health*. Oxford University Press.
Sweet, P. L. (2019). The sociology of gaslighting. *American Sociological Review, 84*(5), 851–875.
Timmermans, S. (2008). Oh look, there is a doctor after all: About the resilience of medical professions. *Social Science & Medicine, 67*(17), 1481–1491.
Timmermans, S., & Oh, H. (2010). The continued social transformation of the medical profession. *Journal of Health and Social Behavior, 51*(Supplement), S94–S106.
Turnbull, P. C. B., & Shadomy, S. V. (2011). From ancient times to the 19th century. In N. H. Bergman (Ed.), *Bacillus anthracis and anthrax* (pp. 1–16). Wiley-Blackwell.

VanHeuvelen, J. S., & Grace, M. K. (2020). Occupational heterogeneity in healthcare workers' misgivings about organizational change. *Work and Occupations, 47*(3), 280–313. https://doi.org/10.1177/0730888420919144

Wailoo, K. (2004). Sovereignty and science: Revisiting the role of science in the construction and erosion of medical dominance. *Journal of Health Politics, Policy and Law, 29*(4–5), 643–659.

Waitzkin, H. (1970). Expansion of medical institutions into urban residential areas. *New England Journal of Medicine, 282*, 1003–1007.

Waitzkin, H. (2000). Changing patient-physician relationships in the changing health-policy environment. In C. E. Bird, P. Conrad, & A. M. Fremont (Eds.), *Handbook of medical sociology* (pp. 271–283). Prentice Hall.

Waitzkin, H. (2011). *Medicine and public health at the end of empire*. Paradigm Publishers.

Wallace, J. E. (2012). Mental health and stigma in the medical profession. *Health (London, England), 16*(1), 3–18. https://doi.org/10.1177/1363459310371080

Walsh, J. J. (1907). *Makers of modern medicine*. Fordham University Press.

Warner, J. H. (1986). *The therapeutic perspective: Medical practice, knowledge and identity in America 1820–1885*. Harvard University Press.

Wilk, A. S., & Platt, J. E. (2016). Measuring physicians' trust: A scoping review with implications for public policy. *Social Science & Medicine, 165*, 75–81.

Wolinsky, F. D. (1993). The professional dominance, deprofessionalization, proletarianization, and corporatization perspectives: An overview and synthesis. In F. W. Hafferty & J. B. McKinlay (Eds.), *The changing medical profession: An international perspective* (pp. 11–24). Oxford University Press, 261.

Wolpe, P. R. (1985). The maintenance of professional authority: Acupuncture and the American physician. *Social Problems, 32*, 409–424.

Chapter 9
Medicalization: Changing Contours, Characteristics, and Contexts

Peter Conrad

Medicalization has become a central analytical theme in medical sociology, a topic in medical sociology courses and the subject of hundreds if not thousands of articles (Conrad, 2007; Ballard & Elston, 2005; Clarke et al., 2010). Other scholars, including historians (Nye, 2003), anthropologists (Lock, 2001; Press, 2006), medical and public health researchers (Metzl & Herzig, 2007; Maloney et al., 2011; Lantz et al., 2007), economists (Thorpe & Philwaw, 2012), bioethicists (Parens, 2011), and even literary scholars (Lane, 2007) have also examined medicalization. Medicalization has been the subject of newspaper and magazine commentaries (e.g. Welch, 2010) and discussion at President's Council on Bioethics (2003). It seems clear that medicalization has become a topic of interest beyond sociology. Within medical sociology it is a concept that has moved from the periphery of intellectual interest in the 1970s to a central area of interest in the twenty-first century.

It is difficult to pinpoint the beginning of the sociological interest in medicalization. The first sociologists to name medicalization were Pitts (1968) with his encyclopedia article on the medicalization of deviant behavior and Irving Kenneth Zola, with his now classic article on "Medicine as an Institution of Social Control" (1972). It seems clear that scholarly precursors in and out of sociology also contributed to the interest and understanding of medicalization. The work of psychiatric critic Thomas Szasz on the myth of mental illness and psychiatry as an institution of social control (1960, 1970) was widely read and cited by sociologists, as was the work of Illich (1975), whose concept "social iatrogenesis" paralleled medicalization. Foucault's brilliant and innovative history of psychiatry was also

EDITOR'S NOTE: This chapter is reprinted from the first edition in honor of the late Peter Conrad to whom this book is co-dedicated.

P. Conrad (✉)
Brandeis University, Waltham, MA, USA

W. C. Cockerham (ed.), *Medical Sociology on the Move*,
https://doi.org/10.1007/978-3-031-92456-9_9

fundamentally an examination of the medicalization of deviant behavior called madness (Foucault, 1965). Within sociology, the roots can be traced to Parsons' (1951) differentiation between sickness and crime as two forms of deviance that must be managed by society. Other important predecessors include Goffman (1961) on the moral career of the mental patient and the role of the medical model, Gusfield (1967) on the "moral passage" of social problems, and Freidson (1970) on the expanding jurisdiction of the medical profession, all of whom implicitly examined medicalization without using the term. Zola was probably the first to argue that medicalization was a process occurring beyond psychiatry (where it was recognized if not named) to the whole enterprise of medicine. In this way Zola paralleled Illich in seeing medicalization as a widespread social phenomenon of critical concern. (This is not surprising since Zola and Illich collaborated on some work in the early 1970s, e.g. Illich et al. 2000).

Most of the early sociological writings on medicalization focused on deviant behavior. By the time I began research on hyperactive children (now called attention deficit hyperactivity disorder or ADHD) and the medicalization of deviance, these building blocks, plus the dominance of "labeling theory" of deviance, were already in place. My dissertation research on hyperactivity was one of the first case studies of medicalization (Conrad, 1975, 1976). Upon completing this study I felt I knew a lot about hyperactivity as a case but not enough about medicalization as a social phenomenon. In the late 1970s Joseph Schneider and I set out to look at the historical roots of the medicalization of deviance and in 1980 published a book that examined five cases (mental illness, alcoholism, opiate addiction, homosexuality, and children's deviance) and used these to better understand the origins and consequences of medicalization (Conrad & Schneider, 1980a, 1980b). Following that research, I did not write about medicalization until 1992 (Conrad & Schneider, 1992; Conrad, 1992). Because medicalization was changing so much, beginning in the 1990s, I again became interested in medicalization and turned my research attention to the topic and how it was changing (e.g. Conrad & Leiter, 2004; Conrad, 2005; Conrad, 2007).

In this chapter, rather than reviewing the development of the sociological study of medicalization in detail, I want to clarify some issues that have emerged in the development of what some have called "medicalization theory" but I prefer to see as "medicalization studies." In some instances I will refer to the work of others and in others I will take the opportunity to speculate on points where there is little research, hoping to stimulate further work and discussion.

What Constitutes Medicalization?

While there may be numerous definitions of medicalization, in its simplest form it means "to make medical." A more formal definition sees medicalization as the process by which previously nonmedical problems become defined and treated as medical problems, usually as diseases or disorders. The emphasis in this perspective is on "process" and "definition."

In my view, medicalization is distinguished by several characteristics. (1) The *definitional* issue is central to medicalization; that is, how a problem is defined is key to what is done about it. While a medicalized condition is usually defined by physicians or medical personnel, this is not necessary. (2) Medicalization can be seen as representing a range of definitions, with some problems totally medicalized and others just barely medicalized. This suggests *degrees* of medicalization: for example, some problems are virtually completely medicalized (e.g., schizophrenia, epilepsy) where others that are mostly medicalized (e.g. ADHD) with others that hardly medicalized (e.g., internet addiction, sexual addiction), with still others contested or somewhere in between (e.g., obesity, opiate addiction). A recent paper has called this "institutional layering", where multiple institutions share control (Medina & McCraine, 2011). In short, medicalization is more of a continuum than a binary either/or distinction.

(3) Medicalized categories are *elastic* and can expand or contract. For example, ADHD was for many years seen as a disorder of children but is now seen as a lifespan disorder, including adult ADHD; and, Post-traumatic Stress Disorder (PTSD) emerged in the 1970s as a diagnostic category depicting psychic troubles of Vietnam vets and has since expanded to include survivors of violence, sexual abuse, or natural disasters. Now it can even be applied to witnesses to violence or disaster. On the other hand, hysteria, which was a common medical category in the late nineteenth century, has shrunk and almost disappeared as a diagnosis. (4) Physician involvement in medicalization is variable. With the medicalization of alcoholism, physicians were minimally involved; rather, the emergence of Alcoholics Anonymous was central to this process. Consumers can promote medicalization as well, requesting or promoting medical definitions and treatments for problems. With many other examples, however, some direct medical involvement is key. (5) Medicalization is *bi-directional*; that is, there can be medicalization as well as demedicalization. The most common example of demedicalization has been homosexuality, which, due to the 1974 of the American Psychiatric Association and subsequent changes, became "officially" demedicalized. There is no question, however, that there has been much more medicalization than demedicalization in the past four decades.

What type of conditions and problems get medicalized? One could make a long list of medicalized conditions, but Davis (2010), building on Conrad (1992), conceptualizes four different kinds of problems that have been medicalized. The first are deviant behaviors such as ADHD, alcoholism, addictions of various sorts, mental illness, eating disorders, and such. These behaviors are not inherently deviant, but are defined as deviant by society and societal norms. The second are "natural life events" such as childbirth, menstruation, menopause and andropause, aspects of aging such as baldness, and even death and dying. These conditions are "natural" in the sense they are not ipso facto medical pathology and often will occur, like menopause, in anyone who lives long enough to experience it. The third kind are "problems in everyday living," such as anxiety, normal sadness, erectile dysfunction, lack of libido, shyness, bad temper, overweight, difficulty becoming pregnant, and the like. Most of these problems were long considered common parts of life that, while sometimes problematic, were tolerated or managed. These conditions have now become medical diagnoses, often with treatments—especially of the pharmaceutical nature. Finally, there are "enhancements in healthy people", which are biomedical interventions that are meant to improve an individual's life condition or performance. These include various forms of cosmetic surgery, cognitive and performance enhancements, and potentially genetic and biogenic enhancements. This topic will be discussed more fully below. While such a conceptualization is useful for seeing the breadth and types of conditions that have been medicalized, it is not comprehensive. For example, it does not include medialized risk, a growing category, which will be discussed below.

I want to add two final comments on the range of medicalization. There is no question that some conditions have been long defined as problems and in our modern age become medical problems. For example, difficulty in becoming pregnant has been long defined as a human problem and those affected sought help of some kind. One only need know the "fertility objects" that are readily found in any anthropological museum to recognize the ubiquity of the problem. However, since the invention of in vitro fertilization (IVF) in 1978, infertility has been increasingly medicalized in western society and IVF treatments are now common practice. On the other hand, occasionally we have a condition or behavior that could fit the criteria of medicalization but has not been medicalized. Cigarette smoking has been deviantized and deemed a public health issue in the past four decades (with various restrictions and a subsequent reduction in smoking) but cigarette smoking has not become medicalized. Cigarette smoking is surely an addiction, but when we conceive of the "problem" we don't see it as an illness or disability, while other addictions like alcoholism, drug addiction and gambling addiction have, to different degrees, been medicalized. It is an interesting conundrum in a society where medicalization is so that tobacco smoking has not been medicalized.

Some Common Misunderstandings About Medicalization

In this section I will discuss a few common misunderstandings and misconceptions about medicalization.

Some researchers get side-tracked about whether medicalized problems are "really" diseases or whether they are socially invented categories. When I speak about ADHD, one of the most common questions I get is, "well, is ADHD really a disorder or not?" The same might be asked about fibromyalgia, sexual addiction, PTSD, or obesity. My answer to these kinds of questions is that it is not a social scientist's job to adjudicate whether this or that condition or behavior is a "real" disease or disorder, but rather s/he should ask how this problem became defined as a medical disorder and with what consequences? Social scientists should remain agnostic about the "real" disease question not only because it is beyond our expertise but *because* what is considered "real" can change as the definition of the condition or the social context changes.

A common misconception is that medicalization automatically means overmedicalization. This is simply not the case. While considerable research on medicalization does suggest that potential overmedicalization is an issue to be considered, medicalization studies focus on the "process" of medicalization and are not necessarily driven by concerns of overmedicalization. Sociologists study medicalization just like they study other social processes, such as industrialization, secularization, or urbanization, focusing on the origins and consequences of the phenomena. It is likely in some cases there has been an overmedicalization of some problems, while in others perhaps undermedicalization of a certain problem may be the case. Either way, it assumes there is a correct amount of medicalization on the one hand or that there is no medicalization that is correct on the other hand. Both of these are normative issues that are tangential to the main sociological focus, the process and consequences of medicalization.

Related to the overmedicalization misconception, occasionally critics will use the term medicalization as an epithet or pejorative, with the assumption that medicalization is by its nature a "bad" thing. But as I have emphasized, medicalization is a not a normative process, i.e. in itself neither bad nor good. Historically, for instance, there are many examples of beneficial medicalization, such as epilepsy and, in important ways, childbirth. It is hard to imagine that most people would prefer to return to the era when epilepsy was seen as possession or a "curse," a sign of being bewitched and a justification for institutionalization; nor would we want to revisit a childbirth era in which maternal mortality was common and infant death was a regular birth outcome. That is not to say that feminists and others have not importantly analyzed some of the consequences of what might be called the unreflective and extreme medicalization of modern childbirth. I believe that unpacking the social consequences of medicalization *is* a central issue for sociologists to pursue. This is not to say I don't see some serious social consequences to medicalization, as reviewed in the "troubles" section below.

Medicalization is still sometimes equated with "medical imperialism" (Illich, 1975) or 'more recently' pharmaceutical imperialism or disease mongering (Moynihan et al., 2002). Each of these may capture a piece of medicalization but they suffer from the fallacy of single cause. With imperialism it assumes doctors or the medical profession are the major players behind the medicalization of various conditions, with a goal of colonizing problems and increasing medical jurisdiction or social control. With "disease mongering," the focus is typically on the pharmaceutical industry as the force behind medicalization, as drug companies seek to expand the markets for their products by creating new medical categories (Moynihan & Cassels, 2005). While in specific cases there is some truth to this, such as Paxil and Social Anxiety Disorder (Lane, 2007), even in such a case, calling it disease mongering de-emphasizes the important role of consumers, physicians, the particular context, and so forth. Thus I advise spurning both of these terms and examining medicalization in its broader context. Davis (2006) argues that we should limit medicalization to only what physicians do, that this is the fundamental process of medicalizing. I see this as a too constrained and narrow view of medicalizaiton, especially as the role of physicians in the medical system is changing.

I should add, with the term "biomedicalizaiton" (Clarke et al., 2003), I believe the lens is too wide and the specifics of the process of medicalization become lost in the very large picture. I will say more about biomedicalization later.

Sometimes scholars use the term medicalization rather descriptively, to mean that medical conceptions, personnel or ideas come to dominate a certain domain. This uses the concept medicalization in a different way than I and others have used it. In my view, medicalization focuses on the definition of a problem and involves the creation, promotion, or the implementation of medical categories (usually diagnoses) to that problem. Thus, books with titles like *Medicalized Motherhood* (Litt, 2000) and *Babies for the Nation: The Medicalization of Motherhood in Quebec* (Baillargeon, 2009) do not mean that motherhood has become a disease or disorder, but rather that doctors have become the experts on mothering as a medical discourse of advice. Similarly, *The Medicalization of Cyberspace* (Miah & Rich, 2008) examines how the Internet has become a vehicle for medical communication, information and patient interaction, not that cyberspace has become a medicalized problem. A parallel use has occurred in anthropology, when medicalization is used to mean more medical involvement or concern, as in the article "The Medicalization of Anthropology: A Critical Perspective on the Critical-Clinical Debate" (Morgan, 1990). Here the author means the emergence of increasing medical concerns by anthropologists. Nancy Scheper-Hughes and Margaret Lock (1987) define medicalization as a reduction of social bodies to purely biological ones, and many anthropologists have written about the medicalization of childbirth and other human conditions (Davis-Floyd, 2004). While no one has ownership of the correct definition of the word medicalization, our concept of medicalization aligns more closely with these latter two definitions than with the more descriptive uses of the term.

Finally, as the number of studies and statements concerning medicalization has grown over the years, some writers have begun to refer to "medicalization theory" (e.g., Williams & Calnan, 1996; Clarke & Shim, 2011). While there are certainly theoretical aspects of medicalization, and there are clearly concepts and rigorous precepts (many of which are discussed in this chapter), I would hesitate to call it a theory. In the first place, it has not been consistently presented as a theory even by its purveyors; in fact, the vast majority of papers on medicalization seem to be cases studies or analyses of some aspects of the medicalization process. While many of medicalization's conceptualizations are replicable, especially when comparing cases, there has been very little direct testing of various propositions presented about medicalization. Similar to what was called "labeling theory" of deviance, medicalization is more of a conceptual framework with interconnected observations and ideas than a full-blown theory (cf., Becker, 1973). To circumvent the demands and criticisms of a "theory", I prefer the humbler claim of interconnected "medicalization studies", that together give a picture of the process of medicalization, by focusing on the origins, content, conflicts, and consequences of medical definitions and treatments of human problems. The key to increasing knowledge about medicalization is to adopt the a priori definitions of research (i.e., what constitutes medicalization) and maintain a clear focus on process and outcomes. This allows the accumulating research and conceptualizations to contribute to a growing scholarly discourse, building and strengthening our understanding of medicalization, yet eschewing the strictures of a fully articulated theory.

Relating-Zations

Along with medicalization sociologists have adopted a number of other related terms that end with—zation: Pharmaceuticaliization, Geneticization, Healthization and Biomedicalization. While there is not space here to have a thorough discussion or present a comprehensive view of various scholars usage, I think it is useful to review these terms and distinguish how they relate to medicalization.

I introduced the term healthization in a review essay (Conrad, 1992) to distinguish certain health and fitness activities from medicalization. I had been studying worksite wellness programs (Conrad, 1987) and encountered depictions of these as the medicalization of fitness. But these health and fitness activities (including exercise, diet, stress reduction, smoking cessation, etc.), while being done to improve health, proposed behavioral and lifestyle causes for ill health, I tried to distinguish these activities. Medicalization proposes biomedical causes and interventions, healthization in contrast, proposes lifestyle and behavioral causes and interventions. One turns the moral into the medical, the other turns health into the moral (1992: 223). For example, to promote meditation or yoga to reduce stress is not medicalization, but healthization. While I think the distinction between the two is real (e.g. healthization does not create new definitions of conditions as diagnoses), it seems to me a very minor tangent related to medicalization (Hislop & Arber, 2003). And, I must confess, over the years I have found it to be an unfortunately awkward term.

There is abundant evidence that the pharmaceutical industry has a more dominant and powerful impact on health affairs than it did four decades ago when the first studies of medicalization were published (Angell, 2004). Williams et al. (2008), Abraham (2010a), and others have written about the pharmaceuticalization of medicine, meaning that pharmaceutical and drug interventions are increasing in usage for a range of human problems. Abraham (2010b) argues that the drivers are medicalization, pharmaceutical industry promotion and marketing, consumerism and regulator-state policy. He notes that advances in medical science (e.g. evidence based therapeutics) play only a small part in the increased pharmaceutical usage. In my own work, I have identified both biotechnology (mainly the drug industry) and consumerism as among the shifting engines of medicalization (Conrad, 2005). While I agree that the pharmaceutical industry, in its search for expanding markets for its products, is an important driver of medicalization, I see pharmaceuticalization as a subset of medicalization and not a competing concept. Pharmaceuticalization is a strong force increasing medicalization. This is amplified by "direct to consumer advertising" on various media, which while only legal in the U.S. and New Zealand, has a much wider impact through other electronic media, especially the Internet

(Conrad & Leiter, 2008). Phamaceuticalization may be a significant factor in the globalization of medicalization.

Geneticization, defined first by Lippman (1991, p. 109) as the process by which "differences in individuals are reduced to their DNA codes, with most disorders, behaviors, and physiological variations, defined, at least in part, as genetic in origin." This also includes the application of genetic technologies "to diagnose, treat, and categorize conditions previously identified in other ways" (Lippman, 1998, pp. 84–85). As Lippman (1991) notes, geneticization is rooted in medicalization but can also serve to expand medicalization. Several scholars (Press, 2006; Nelkin & Susan Lindee, 1995; Conrad, 2000) have warned of the potential of genetics to expand medicalization.

There is no doubt that genetization of problems can impact certain conditions, perhaps especially how genetics can put individuals at risk for an illness or disorder. But as Shostak et al. (2008) point out, it is not genetic findings or conceptions per se that can lead to medicalization, but the way the genetic information is interpreted. For example, it has been 20 years since the discovery of the so-called "gay gene" (Conrad & Markens, 2001), but this had virtually no effect on the potential remedicalzation of homosexuality. It may have affected the public culture views of homosexual origin, with many believing that they were "born gay", but this has not resulted in any new medicalization. In fact, the geneticization of homosexuality could equally sustain claims that homosexuality is a normal human variation and thus would support a totally nonmedicalized definition. The point here is that genetic findings, whether they are for alcoholism, depression, or eating disorders, do not ipso facto lead to increased medicalization. It is the interpretation or meaning given to the genetic findings that make a difference, not merely the genetic claims by themselves.

Adele Clarke and her colleagues introduced the concept of "biomedicalization" in a 2003 article and followed it up with an edited book several years later (Clarke et al., 2010). Grounding their concept as much in Science and Technology Studies as in Sociology, Clarke and her associates present an ambitious analysis of what they see as a major transformation in medicine and medical care. They argue that medicalization is being transformed; they state that in about 1985 "dramatic changes in both the organization and practice of contemporary biomedicine, implemented largely through the implementation of technoscientific interventions" coalesced with an expanded phenomena which they call biomedicalization (Clarke et al., 2003, p. 161). By biomedicalization they mean "the increasingly complex, multisited, multi-directional processes of medicalization that today are being reconstituted through the emergent social forms and practices of a highly and increasingly technoscientific medicine" (Clarke et al., 2003, p. 162).

As I have noted elsewhere (Conrad, 2005, 2007), I admire the scope and ambition of the Clarke et al. conceptualization, but I find that the authors paint biomedicalization with such a broad brush that medicalization gets lost. I recognize some of the same changes they observe, only I see them as "shifting engines" of medicalization, the ascendance of certain influences (consumers, drug companies, health insurance), and the change or diminution of others (doctors, the medical profession). Clarke and colleagues suggest the medicalization era was ending around 1990 giving way to the biomedicalization era *(see also Clarke et al., 2011). Here I disagree, as I believe that medicalization is actually more intensified and widespread in the twenty-first century than it was in the 1970. In short, my claim is that there is an intensification of medicalization occurring, not a transformation.

Expanding the Medicalization Purview

As noted earlier, the early research on medicalization was rooted in the study of deviant behavior, focusing on psychiatry as an agent of social control. Zola (1972), Freidson (1970), and others pointed to the broad swath of medicalization defined and controlled largely by the medical profession. In this wider view, the medicalization lens was aimed toward childbirth, sexuality, menopause, aging, and other conditions that were beyond deviant behavior.

Feminist scholars also began to use a medicalization framework to understand how doctors and modern culture were depicting women's bodies (Ehrenreich & English, 1973; Martin, 1987) and medicalized aspects of women's lives like menstruation (Figert, 1995), menopause (Bell, 1987), and childbirth (Wertz & Wertz, 1989). Riessman 1983wrote a benchmark paper about women and medicalization, depicting medicalization as a double-edged sword. While some saw medicalization as something male doctors did to women, others (e.g. Wertz & Wertz, 1989) recognized that women often were actively implicated in their own medicalization. Riska (2003, 2011) has published several papers that examining the gender aspects of medicalization, highlighting how many more aspects of women's bodies are medicalized, yet at the same time recognizing that in recent years men's bodies seem to be increasingly medicalized (e.g., see Rosenfeld & Faircloth, 2006). Feminist oriented scholars continue to make important contributions to the medicalization literature.

In recent years, studies of medicalization have expanded from illness conditions to also include biomedical enhancements (Conrad & Potter, 2004). Enhancements include medical interventions to improve aspects of performance or the body. These interventions do not conceptualize bodily conditions as disorders or threats to health, but rather as techniques for improving a characteristic or capability. These are specifically biomedical enhancements, including much of cosmetic surgery (Sullivan, 2001), pharmaceutical body enhancements like use of human growth hormone to increase height (Conrad & Potter, 2004), and pharmaceutical performance enhancement (Wolpe, 2002) including cognitive enhancement (Greely et al., 2008). The potential of reprogenetics, especially related to genetically enhancing offspring, remains mostly potential but likely real within the next few decades (Silver, 1997). Sometimes the line between medicalized treatments and enhancements is difficult to discern; for example, there is the use of evidence drugs like Ritalin and Adderall are used by individuals who do not have ADHD as a cognitive enhancement (Outram, 2012) or the Viagra is used not only to treat Erectile Dysfunction but to improve normal sexual performance. The growth of biomedical enhancements, especially through (cosmetic) surgery, pharmaceuticals, and eventually genetics is likely to be an expanding arena of medicalization.

Several analysts have pointed to the "medicalization of risk" as an area of increased medicalization (e.g., Clarke et al., 2010). With the development of many sophisticated technologies that can screen and scan the body, such as MRI, CAT scans or genetic screenings, physicians can identify risks for future disorders at increasingly earlier stages. Often, when these risks are identified, the patient comes under medical surveillance, be it in terms of measuring cholesterol or PSA, viewing mammograms, having a colonoscopy, or genetic screening, each of these can discern more risks an individual may have in the future. Here the problem is medicalized not because an individual has a disorder, but because s/he has a higher *potential* for a medical condition sometime in the future. This may also affect the "threshold" of when a condition becomes seen as a medical problem. For instance, there is a current debate about whether to treat high blood pressure at 140 or 120 systolic. Reducing the treatment threshold to 120 would put millions more individuals under medical care. Thus, the medical management of risk increases the amount of medical surveillance (Armstrong, 1995), which is a result of medicalizing the risk. While the early detection of risk may be medically beneficial, it is also an expanding form of medicalization.

Shifting Engines: Another Engine?

Several analysts have observed that medicalization has changed since the 1980s; Clarke et al. (2003) terms it a turn to biomedicalization while I call it shifting engines of medicalization. I touched on biomedicalization earlier, and will only briefly mention the shifting engines here, since I have written about them at length elsewhere (Conrad, 2005, 2007).

In essence, I believe that the engines or social forces underlying medicalization have shifted. Rather than locating the source of medicalization, the medical profession, interprofessional or organizational conflicts, and social and professional movements, by the 1990s the most important engines were biotechnology (the pharmaceutical industry, genetics, and forms of medical technology), consumers, and managed care (including all kinds of health insurance). Physician's roles are now more subordinate in medicalization, often becoming gatekeepers for the expansion or contraction of medicalization.

We can characterize the three ascending engines as follows. Biotechnology, mainly the pharmaceutical industry and potentially genetics, has expanded enormously in the past two decades (Abraham, 2010a) along with treatments for what are often newly defined disorders. A good example of this is the promotion of Paxil for the diagnosis Social Anxiety Disorder (Lane, 2007), where the drug company (Glaxosmithkline) first promoted SAD as a common disorder and then promoted Paxil to treat it. Pharmaceutical promotion has been important in the medicalization of everyday sadness (Horwitz & Wakefield, 2007), erectile dysfunction (Loe, 2004), menopause (Bell, 1987), and baldness (Conrad, 2007), among many others.

In our modern medical world patients have increasingly become consumers, often coming to their medical provider with new demands for a specific treatment or diagnosis. Direct to consumer advertising has encouraged this with the mantra, "Ask your doctor if [name of drug] is right for you" and patients (as consumers) approaching their physicians with requests for specific diagnoses and/or medications. The Internet has also created opportunities for patients to be consumers with various kinds of electronic support groups; with contested illnesses consumers will often band together over the Internet to advocate for the legitimacy of their diagnosis, such as with fibromyalgia (Barker, 2008). Consumers are also important in the use of biomedical enhancements, since most of these (e.g. breast augmentation) are not covered by any kind of insurance. This can be seen as medicalization from below, whether it is pursued by individuals or organizations (Figert, 2011). The third engine, managed care, really is a designation of all types of health insurance. If something is covered by health insurance, such as gastric by-pass operations for obesity, it fuels the medicalization of the designated disorder. On the other hand, if insurance does not cover some conditions, e.g. infertility or transgender surgery, that may well slow the medicalization of that condition. Thus, third party payers, including both public and private insurance, can accelerate or slow the process of medicalization.

When I reexamined the three engines of medicalization for my 2007 book, I was tempted to write a chapter on a fourth engine, but I had no data to support my ideas about this fourth engine so I left it out. I briefly sketch that fourth engine here; I still do not have any empirical evidence to support its impact. In my published conception of shifting engines, I claimed that physicians were increasingly relegated to gatekeepers in the context of the other three engines. I still believe this is true. But physicians may also be an important engine in what may be another way. I believe physicians are engines toward increasing medicalization because *a major objective and mission of physicians is to reduce individual suffering.* Physicians are trained to diagnose and treat ailments, conditions, and disorders to reduce patient's discomfort, vulnerability, disability, risk, pain, and suffering.

Thus, it seems to me, physicians are incentivized to treat conditions with medical interventions because they believe their calling is to reduce suffering, especially when patients come to the doctor's office or practice. This means sometimes providing medical treatments or diagnoses for problems that may be of questionable medical origin (e.g. some of what gets diagnosed as ADHD, sadness, sleep problems, obesity, shyness, among others). It should be noted that physicians only treat certain kinds of suffering; they do not see the suffering of extended unemployment, poverty, or lack of skills as problems need medical intervention. To paraphrase Zola's (1972) observation, if problems can be connected to the body or the psyche in some way they can been seen as falling into the physicians mission to reduce individual suffering. What is not yet known is whether the boundaries of medical views of suffering contribute to medicalizing particular conditions or behaviors. The physician's definition of what kinds of suffering elicit a medical response, what that response is, and what are the consequences is a question ripe for sociological research. Where are the lines drawn between medical and nonmedical suffering?

Few Approaches to Political Economy and Disparities of Medicalization

While the roots of medicalization studies may be elsewhere, the fertile soil that has nourished it stems from a social constructionist perspective on the development of medicalized categories (Barker, 2010). I have lamented elsewhere (Conrad, 2005) that we do not have much understanding about the political economy of illness. There are two places scholars have been unearthing some specifics about economic factors. With the emergence of studies of pharmaceutical promotion of diagnoses and treatments (Loe, 2004; Lane, 2007; Horwitz & Wakefield, 2007) we can begin to examine how socioeconomic factors, especially expanding markets, can contribute to increased medicalization. This market-based approach sees medical treatments and care as a product and aligns with consumers as an engine. The other market arena is biomedical enhancements, which are typically market-based and tend to may be more or less purchased as medical commodities. This includes a significant amount of cosmetic surgery, including breast augmentations, rhinoplasties (nose jobs), face lifts, liposuction, etc., almost all of which is paid for out of pocket. As more of medicine becomes commercialized (Alper, 1987), an increasing amount of procedures and treatments will be market-based (see Conrad & Leiter, 2004).

While we don't have any exact calculations of what part of health care spending can be attributed to medicalization, a few years ago several colleagues and I made an attempt to estimate the cost of medicalization (Conrad et al., 2010). The amount of GDP spent on all health care has risen from 4% in 1950 to nearly 17% in 2011. Using 2005 data on the direct costs of 12 medicalized conditions we estimated that the total spending on these conditions was $77.1 billion or 3.9% of total domestic spending on health care. It is difficult to say if this is a lot or a little, but it is more than the total that is spent on public health. Even if these numbers are reasonably accurate estimations, we don't know how they have changed overtime and or to what extent they are the economic drivers of these costs. It would be interesting to connect these findings to the three engines of medicalization to see how much each of these contributes to health costs.

While health disparities have become a central focus of public health and health services research, scholars have been limited in their approach to the differences and disparities of medicalization. As noted above, there is a significant literature on gender and medicalization focusing on gender differences, especially how women's conditions have been more susceptible to medicalized categories. We know much less about the racial and ethnic disparities in medicalization. Are some groups' conditions more likely to be medicalized, Are some "over" medicalized, or others undermedicalized? We know very little about this. For example, with ADHD there are claims that African American children are more likely to be labeled as ADHD while much of the data we have shows fewer African American children diagnosed and treated with ADHD (Bussing & Fay, 2010). We know little about these disparities and how they are related to conceptions of disorders and access to health services, or, more generally, how they effect medicalization.

Finally, there is one socioeconomic factor that is so basic that once it is pointed out, it becomes patently obvious. In the U.S. and many other countries, the only way to get human services paid for (or reimbursed) is to define a condition or situation as a medical problem, because we only have insurance for health problems not for social problems. This creates an incentive to medicalize more problems because it is the only way to get them paid for. While this should be obvious, it is rarely mentioned and has not been well researched.

Troubles with Medicalization

Since I have written at length on what I see as some of the troubling social consequences of medicalization (Conrad, 2007, pp. 146–164), I will only touch on them here. These discontents are probably some of the most significant, but by no means the only, troubling aspects of medicalization. For example, medical treatments often have health risks, as with menopause and hormone replacement therapy (HRT) or silicone breast implants (Stults & Conrad, 2010), but these risks are not necessarily social consequences.

There are five major consequences of medicalization that I deem social ramifications, largely independent of any validity of diagnosis or efficacy of treatment. (1) *The pathologicalization of everything*. By this I mean medicalization is increasingly turning much of human difference into pathologies that need diagnosis and medical treatment. This is particularly true with behavior witness the continuing growth of the number of diagnoses in the diagnostic and statistical manual (DSM) but also true with bodily conditions. In lectures, I have rhetorically asked, does hypochondria still exist? After all, we seem to have a diagnosis for virtually every human problem, so it is difficult to become labeled as a hypochondriac for one's symptoms. (2) *The medical definition of normality*. Here is where medical norms become social norms. Often this is manifested with the pharmaceutical industry defining what is "normal". Examples of this include what is normal sadness or shyness, the quality of erections as one ages, or the correct height for children and adults. Medicine has often adopted social norms, but here medicine is increasingly in the business of creating the "proper" social norms.

(3) *The expansion of medical social control.* Medical social control has always been an element of medicalization (Zola, 1972; Conrad & Schneider, 1980b) but with developments in pharmaceuticals, surgery, genetics and neuroscience the technological reach of medical social control is expanding. Moreover, there are other elements of medical social control that are expanding as well, such as medical

surveillance be it of behavior (e.g. drinking when pregnant) or body conditions (e.g. relating to cholesterol or blood pressure) that makes medicine at least implicitly the overseer of behavior. (Remember that expanding medical surveillance is not necessarily bad, it just exists, yet this does increase medical social control.)

(4) *The individualization of social problems.* While this is obvious to sociologists, medicalization and its clinical gaze turn complex social problems into clinical entities. With problems like alcoholism, obesity, and ADHD, for example, seeing these primarily as an individual clinical problem with a medical solution ignores the social contexts and roots of the problems at hand. This makes social or environmental interventions either ignored or at best secondary and reinforces technological fixes for complex social problems. (5) *Consumerization of medicine.* As noted above, medical procedures and care are increasingly becoming consumer items, subject to market forces. Sometimes this occurs from above, e.g. with pharmaceutical or cosmetic surgery promotion, but it also comes from below, with consumers (and patients) seeking more medical diagnoses and interventions. This runs parallel to what some are calling the commercialization of medicine and the rise of medical markets (Conrad & Leiter, 2004).

These consequences are inherent inhere in medicalization and are independent of any issues of the validity or efficacy of particular cases of medicalization.

Islands of Resistance

There is some resistance to medicalization aside from scholars and social critics writing about it. It is not really organized social resistance but rather separate islands of resistance to specific issues. I will mention a few here.

Specific social movements or embodied health movements mount either organized campaigns against medicalization or seek to modify medical responses (Brown et al., 2004). The classic example historically is the success of what was then called “gay liberation” to get the APA to demedicalize homosexuality. Other movements like the disability rights movement and the body size acceptance movement are also examples of resistance to medicalization. To these one could add the long-term childbirth movement that has criticized the extremes of medicalization but is really seeking to reform childbirth care, not demedicalize it entirely. Another, perhaps more marginal group, are the Scientologists who campaign against psychoactive medication treatments for various psychological troubles. In another realm, there are some Internet sites that critique and seek to reconceptualize medicalized conditions. These include the “pro ana” websites that claim anorexia is not an illness but a lifestyle, or the neurodiversity websites that reconceptualize autism (especially Asparger’s syndrome) as just part of human diversity and not a disorder.

When certain treatments are found to increase risk for other illnesses, there may be a response that reduces medicalization. Stults has called these “risk scares”: when information about a new and usually serious risk becomes public knowledge into question a specific medical intervention and treatment is called into question

(Conrad & Stults, 2010). This occurred with silicone breast implants that were found to increase the risk of breast cancer. A broader example was when there were several "risk scares" about the effect of HRT, a common treatment for menopause, found to increase the risks of breast cancer, heart disease, and other ailments. This lead to a huge reduction of HRT use for menopause, but when a "safer" medication was developed the use increased again. Here it seems clear menopause was not demedicalized; only the use of a dangerous treatment reduced usage, which rose again when new or different "safer" medications were introduced.

Finally, insurance can impact medicalization. On the one hand it can encourage medicalization, as when Medicare and subsequently other medical insurance plans decided to consider obesity as a reimbursable illness and thus pay for gastric bypass operations for some patients. On the other hand, the fact that some insurance plans do not cover certain problems or conditions, such as infertility, probably acts as a resistance to medicalization. Some place in between is the interesting case of most insurance plans paying for medications or hospitalization but not psychotherapy for mental health problems; this could be seen as inducing greater use of psychopharmacology because it is the only treatment insurance will pay for. In short, insurance can provide an inadvertent resistance to medicalization.

As should be apparent from this section, the resistance to medicalization is dispersed and not particularly connected. There are no real organized countervailing forces (Light, 1993) restricting medicalization. Since so few cases of demedicalization (e.g. homosexuality and masturbation are examples) can be identified, it seems fair to surmise that there are islands of resistance reacting to a tidal wave of medicalization.

A Glimpse at the Future

It seems clear that medicalization will not soon abate and it may increase further in a range of areas. I will close this chapter with a brief look at some potential areas where medicalization may expand in the next couple of decades. Some of these are already visible, others are barely emergent.

Among the greatest potentials for medicalization are the further findings in genetics. While genetic findings will not automatically lead to medicalization of conditions, there are at least two ways genetics will nurture medicalization. First, genetic testing and screening will allow doctors to identify potential conditions or genetic susceptibilities that will increase the surveillance and treatment of genetic risk. These proto diseases (Rosenberg, 2000) will be medicalized even though there is no specific existing illness. The other potential contribution to increasing medicalization will be the ability to provide genetic biomedical enhancements. It may begin with genetic interventions to prevent certain medical disorders (e.g., from heart disease to alcoholism), but it will soon create a market for genetic enhancements for specific characteristics. It is my belief there will be high demand for enhancements that will create "designer babies" with medicalized enhanced traits among those who can afford it. This might ultimately lead to a new distinction between genetically enriched and non-enriched children.

Pharmaceutical medicalization will continue to and probably expand. Pharmaceutical companies, when they don't have blockbuster drugs like Viagra or Lipitor, will attempt to find new uses for their already existing drugs. A current example is the repackaging of Prozac as Serifem, the same drug under a new name now marketed for premenstrual dysphoric disorder. The development of direct to consumer advertising will facilitate the growth of new markets.

The population in the U.S., Europe and elsewhere is aging, and this will impact medicalization. There are now specialists in anti-aging medicine, a fast growing part of medicine, that are now promoting all kinds of medical treatments for various aspects of aging. (Mykytyn, 2006) They advertise that aging is a disease and not an inevitability. While some treatments related to aging already exist, this opens up an even larger frontier for the medicalization of what is essentially a normal part of the life course.

The Internet not only nurtures consumers and advertises treatments, it also is a repository of medicalized information. It is unclear how this will play out but the Internet can be a vehicle that can both be a support or critique of medical diagnoses and treatment. One thing for certain: there are few medical secrets anyone and various types of medical knowledge can be found there (e.g. professional, organizational, experiential). It would not be surprising if within a few years it will be possible to get a diagnosis via Internet websites and then order prescribed medications directly from an Internet seller, by passing face-to-face interaction with physicians.

Medicalization is going global. While medicalization used to be predominantly a North American and European phenomenon, we are seeing a globalization of medicalization. This is partly due to the Internet, the global pharmaceutical industry in search of new markets, the increased diffusion and influence of Western medicine (through professional influence and direct U.S.European training). As one anecdotal example, when I lived in Indonesia in 1990 I asked physicians (trained in the U.S., Australia, and Europe) if they diagnosed and treated ADHD and anorexia. All said they heard of it, but no it wasn't a problem here, or at least, they did not medically treat it. Recent communications with colleagues suggests this is no longer the case. The diagnoses and treatment have migrated to Indonesia (at least among those who could afford medical care).

In sum, by this point in time, medicalization has been established as a sociological analytic category that his influenced other disciplines and popular thinking about health and medicine. Reviewing the directions of medicalization studies, it seems safe to say that many conceptions about medicalization are well established yet some aspects are still unknown or under-addressed. However, there seems no doubt that medicalization continues to expand and impact society, with very few signs that this trend will be modulated or altered.

References

Abraham, J. (2010a). The sociological concomitants of the pharmaceutical industry and medications. In C. E. Bird, P. Conrad, A. M. Freemont, & S. Timmermans (Eds.), *The handbook of medical sociology* (pp. 290–308). Vanderbilt University Press.

Abraham, J. (2010b). Pharmaceuticalization of society in context: Theoretical, empirical, and health dimensions. *Sociology, 44*, 603–622.

Alper, P. R. (1987). Medical practice in a competitive market. *New England Journal of Medicine, 316*, 337–339.

Angell, M. (2004). *The truth about the drug companies*. Random House.

Armstrong, D. (1995). The rise of surveillance medicine. *Sociology of Health & Illness, 17*, 393–404.

Baillargeon, D. (2009). *Babies for the nation: The medicalization of motherhood in Quebec, 1910–1970*. Wilfred Laurier Press.

Ballard, K., & Elston, M. A. (2005). Medicalisation: A multi-dimensional concept. *Social Theory and Health, 3*, 228–241.

Barker, K. K. (2008). Electronic support groups, patient consumers, and medicalization: The case of contested illness. *Journal of Health and Social Behavior, 49*, 20–36.

Barker, K. K. (2010). The social construction of illness: Medicalization and contested illness. In C. E. Bird, P. Conrad, A. M. Freemont, & S. Timmermans (Eds.), *The handbook of medical sociology* (6th ed., pp. 147–162). Vanderbilt University Press.

Becker, H. S. (1973). *Outsiders: Studies in the sociology of deviance* (2nd ed.). Free Press.

Bell, S. (1987). Changing ideas: The medicalization of menopause. *Social Science and Medicine, 24*, 535–542.

Brown, P., Zavestoski, S., McCormick, S., Meyer, B., Morello-Frosch, R., & Altman, R. (2004). Embodied health movements: New approaches to social movements in health. *Sociology of Health & Illness, 26*, 50–80.

Bussing, R., & Fay, G. (2010). Assessing and treating attention deficit hyperactivity disorder in culturally diverse populations. In S. Evans & B. Hoza (Eds.), *Treating attention deficit disorder* (p. 20-1–20-25). Civic Research Institute.

Clarke, A. E., & Shim, J. K. (2011). Medicalization and biomedicalization revisited. In B. Pescosolido, J. Martin, A. Rogers, & D. Pilgrim (Eds.), *Handbook of the sociology of health, illness and healing* (pp. 173–199). Springer.

Clarke, A. E., Shim, J. K., Mamo, L., Fosket, J. R., & Fishman, J. R. (2003). Biomedicalization: Technoscientific transformations of health, illness, and U.S. biomedicine. *American Sociological Review, 68*, 161–194.

Clarke, A. E., Mamo, L., Fosket, J. R., Fishman, J. R., & Shim, J. K. (Eds.). (2010). *Bimedicalization: Technoscience, health and illness in the U.S.* Duke University Press.

Clarke, A. E., Shim, J. K., Mamo, L., Fosket, J. R., & Fishman, J. R. (2011). Biomedicalization: A theoretical and substantive introduction. In A. E. Clarke, L. Mamo, J. R. Fosket, J. R. Fishman, & J. K. Shim (Eds.), *Biomedicalization: Technoscience, health, and illness in the U.S* (pp. 1–47). Duke University Press.

Conrad, P. (1975). The discovery of hyperkinesis: Notes on the medicalization of deviant behavior. *Social Problems, 32*, 12–21.

Conrad, P. (1976). *Identifying hyperactive children: The medicalization of deviant behavior*. Lexington.

Conrad, P. (1987). Wellness in the workplace: Potentials and pitfalls of worksite health promotion. *Milbank Quarterly, 65*, 255–275.

Conrad, P. (1992). Medicalization and social control. *Annual Review of Sociology, 18*, 209–232.

Conrad, P. (2000). Medicalization, genetics and human problems. In C. Bird, P. Conrad, & A. Fremont (Eds.), *Handbook of medical sociology* (5th ed.). Prentice Hall.

Conrad, P. (2005). Shifting Engines of Medicalization. *Journal of Health and Social Behavior, 46*, 3–14.

Conrad, P. (2007). *The medicalization of society: On the transformation of human condition into treatable disorders*. Johns Hopkins University Press.
Conrad, P., & Leiter, V. (2004). Medicalization, markets and consumers. *Journal of Health and Social Behavior, 45*(extra issue), 158–176.
Conrad, P., & Leiter, V. (2008). From Lydia Pinkham to Queen Levitra: DTCA and medicalization. *Sociology of Health and Illness, 30*, 825–838.
Conrad, P., & Markens, S. (2001). Constructing the 'Gay Gene' in the news: Optimism and skepticism in the American and British press. *Health, 5*, 373–400.
Conrad, P., & Potter, D. (2004). Human growth hormone and the temptations of biomedical enhancement. *Sociology of Health & Illness, 26*, 184–215.
Conrad, P., & Schneider, J. W. (1980a). *Deviance and medicalization: From badness to sickness*. C.V. Mosby.
Conrad, P., & Schneider, J. W. (1980b). Looking at levels of medicalization: A comment on strong's critique of the thesis of medical imperialism. *Social Science and Medicine, 14A*, 75–79.
Conrad, P., & Schneider, J. W. (1992). *Deviance and medicalization: From badness to sickness* (Expanded ed.). Temple University Press.
Conrad, P., & Stults, C. (2010). Medicalization and risk scares: The case of menopause and HRT. In D. Light (Ed.), *The risks of prescription drugs* (pp. 120–142). Columbia University Press.
Conrad, P., Mackie, T., & Mehrotra, A. (2010). Estimating the costs of medicalization. *Social Science and Medicine, 70*, 1943–1947.
Davis, J. E. (2006). How medicalization lost its way. *Society, 43*, 51–56.
Davis, J. E. (2010). Medicalization, social control and the relief of suffering. In W. Cockerham (Ed.), *The new Blackwell companion to medical sociology* (pp. 211–241). Wiley-Blackwell.
Davis-Floyd, R. (2004). *Birth as an American right of passage* (2nd ed.). University of California Press.
Ehrenreich, B., & English, D. (1973). *Complaints and disorders: The sexual politics of sickness*. The Feminist Press.
Figert, A. E. (1995). The three faces of PMS: The professional, gendered and scientific structuring of a psychiatric disorder. *Social Problems, 42*, 56–73.
Figert, A. E. (2011). The consumer turn in medicalization: Future directions with historical foundations. In B. Pescosolido, J. Martin, A. Rogers, & D. Pilgrim (Eds.), *Handbook of the sociology of health, illness and healing* (pp. 291–307). Springer Publishing.
Foucault, M. (1965). *Madness and civilization*. Bandam Books.
Freidson, E. (1970). *Profession of medicine: A study of the sociology of applied knowledge*. University of Chicago Press.
Goffman, E. (1961). *Asylums*. Anchor Books.
Greely, H. T., Sahakian, B., Harris, J., Kessler, R., Gazzaniga, M. S., Campbell, P., & Farah, M. J. (2008). Toward responsible use of cognitive enhancing drugs by the healthy. *Nature, 456*, 702–705.
Gusfield, J. R. (1967). Moral passage: The symbolic process in the public designations of deviance. *Social Problems, 15*, 175–188.
Hislop, J., & Arber, S. (2003). Understanding women's sleep: Beyond. Medicalization-healthicization. *Sociology of Health & Illness, 25*, 815–837.
Horwitz, A. V., & Wakefield, J. (2007). *The loss of sadness: How psychiatry transformed normal sorrow into depressive disorder*. Oxford University Press.
Illich, I. (1975). *Medical nemesis: The expropriation of health*. Random House.
Illich, I., Zola, I. K., et al. (2000). *Disabling conditions*. Marion Boyers.
Lane, C. (2007). *Shyness: How normal behavior became a sickness*. Yale University Press.
Lantz, P. M., Lichtenstein, R. L., & Pollack, H. A. (2007). Health policy approaches to population health: The limits of medicalization. *Health Affairs, 26*, 1253–1257.
Light, D. W. (1993). Countervailing power. In F. W. Hafferty & J. B. Mckinlay (Eds.), *Theh changing medical profession: An international perspective* (pp. 69–79). Oxford University Press.

Lippman, A. (1991). Prenatal genetic testing and screening: Constructing needs and reinforcing tendencies. *American Journal of Law and Society, 17*, 15–50.

Lippman, A. (1998). The politics of health: Geneticization verses health promotion. In S. Sherwin (Ed.), *The politics of women's health: Exploring agency and autonomy*. Temple University Press.

Litt, J. S. (2000). *The medicalization of motherhood*. Rutgers University Press.

Lock, M. (2001). Medicalization: Cultural concerns. In N. Smelser & P. Baltes (Eds.), *International encyclopedia of the social and behavioral sciences*. Elsevier.

Loe, M. (2004). *The rise of Viagra: How the little blue pill changed sex in America*. NYU Press.

Maloney, M. E., Konrad, T. R., & Zimmer, C. R. (2011). The medicalization of sleeplessness: A public health concern. *American Journal of Public Health, 101*, 429–433.

Martin, E. (1987). The woman in the body: A cultural analysis of reproduction.

Medina, T. R., & McCraine, A. (2011). Layering control: Medicalization, psychopathy, and the increasing muti-instiutional management of social problems. In B. Pescosolido, J. Martin, A. Rogers, & D. Pilgrim (Eds.), *Handbook of the sociology of health, illness and healing* (pp. 139–157). Springer Publishing.

Metzl, J. M., & Herzig, R. M. (2007). Medicalisation in the twenty-first century: An introduction. *The Lancet, 369*, 697–698.

Miah, R., & Rich, E. (2008). *The medicalization of cyberspace*. Routledge.

Morgan, L. M. (1990). The medicalization of anthropology: A critical perspective on the clinical debate. *Social Science and Medicine, 30*, 945–950.

Moynihan, R., & Cassels, A. (2005). *Selling sickness*. Nation Books.

Moynihan, R., Heath, I., & Henry, D. (2002). Selling sickness: The pharmaceutical industry and disease mongering. *British Medical Journal, 324*, 886–891.

Mykytyn, C. E. (2006). Anti-aging medicine: A patient/practitioner movement to redefine aging. *Social Science and Medicine, 62*, 643–653.

Nelkin, D., & Susan Lindee, M. (1995). *The DNA mystique: The gene as a cultural icon*. Freeman Publishing.

Nye, R. A. (2003). The evolution of the concept of medicalization in the late twentieth century. *Journal of the History of the Behavioral Sciences, 39*, 115–129.

Outram, S. (2012). The use of methylphenidate among students: The future of enhancement? *Journal of Medical Ethics, 36*, 198–202.

Parens, E. (2011). On good and bad forms of medicalization. *Bioethics*. https://doi.org/10.1111/j.1467-8519.2011.01885.x.online

Parsons, T. (1951). *The social system*. The Free Press.

Pitts, J. R. (1968). Social control: The concept. In D. L. Sills (Ed.), *International encyclopedia of the social sciences* (Vol. 14, pp. 381–396). Macmillan and The Free Press.

President's Council on Bioethics. (2003). *Beyond therapy: Biotechnology and the pursuit of happiness*. The President's Council on Bioethics.

Press, N. (2006). Social construction and medicalization: Behavioral genetics in context. In E. Parens, A. R. Chapman, & N. Press (Eds.), *Wrestling with behavioral genetics: Science, ethics and public conversation* (pp. 131–149). Johns Hopkins University Press.

Riessman, C. K. (1983). Women and medicalization: A new perspective. *Social Policy, 14*(Summer), 3–18.

Riska, E. (2003). Gendering the medicalization thesis. *Advances in Gender Research, 7*, 59–87.

Riska, E. (2011). Gender and medicalization and biomedicalization theories. In A. E. Clarke, L. Mamo, J. R. Fosket, J. R. Fishman, & J. K. Shim (Eds.), *Biomedicalization: Technoscience, health, and illness in the U.S* (pp. 147–171). Duke University Press.

Rosenberg, C. (2000). Banishing risk: Continuity and change in moral management of disease. In A. Brandt & P. Rozin (Eds.), *Morality and health* (pp. 35–52). Routledge.

Rosenfeld, D., & Faircloth, C. (Eds.). (2006). *Medicalized masculinities*. Temple University Press.

Scheper-Hughes, N., & Lock, M. (1987). The mindful body: A prolegomenon to future work in medical anthropology. *Medical Anthropology Quarterly, 1*, 6–41.

Shostak, S., Conrad, P., & Horwitz, A. (2008). Sequencing and its consequences: Path dependence and the relationships between genetics and medicalization. *American Journal of Sociology, 114*(S1), S287–S316.

Silver, L. M. (1997). *Remaking Eden: Cloning and beyond in a brave New World.* Avon Books.

Stults, C., & Conrad, P. (2010). Medicalization and risk scares: The case of menopause and HRT. In D. Light (Ed.), *The risks of prescription drugs* (pp. 120–142). Columbia University Press.

Sullivan, D. A. (2001). *Cosmetic surgery: The cutting edge of medicine in America.* Rutgers University Press.

Szasz, T. S. (1960). The myth of mental illness. *The American Psychologist, 15*, 113–118.

Szasz, T. S. (1970). *The manufacture of madness: A comparative study of the inquisition and the mental health movement.* Harper and Row.

Thorpe, K. E., & Philwaw, M. (2012). The medicalization of chronic disease and costs. *Annual Review of Public Health, 23*, 409–423.

Welch, H. G. (2010). The medicalization of life. *Los Angeles Times, 15*, A15.

Wertz, R. W., & Wertz, D. C. (1989). *Lying-in: A history of childbirth in America* (Ex ed.). Yale University Press.

Williams, S. J., & Calnan, M. (1996). The 'Limits' of medicalization? Modern medicine and the lay populace in 'Late' modernity. *Social Science and Medicine, 42*, 1609–1620.

Williams, S. J., Seale, C., Boden, S., & Lowe, P. (2008). Waking up to sleepiness: Modafinil, the media and the pharmaceuticalisation of everyday/night life. *Sociology of Health & Illness, 30*, 839–855.

Wolpe, P. R. (2002). Treatment, enhancements and the ethics of neurotherapeutics. *Brain and Cognition, 50*, 387–395.

Zola, I. K. (1972). Medicine as an institution of social control. *The Sociological Review, 20*, 487–504.

Chapter 10
Marx, Critical Realism and Health Inequalities

Graham Scambler and Sasha Scambler

The philosophy of critical realism associated with Roy Bhaskar has been winning influence in sociological circles since his early writings in the 1970s. It remains a dynamic and evolving philosophy, taken up and developed by influential sociological theorists like Margaret Archer. It has also had a considerable impact on the sociology of health and healthcare. In this chapter we start by introducing Bhaskar's "basic" and "dialectical" critical realism and briefly comment on Margaret Archer's critical realist-informed sociology before showing why his considerable body of work is of relevance to the sociological project and to sociological practice. The bulk of the chapter is then committed to illustrating just how critical realism can serve as a useful "underlaboring philosophy" for sociologists in the health field by focusing in some detail on theories and research on health inequalities in the United Kingdom (UK).

Basic Critical Realism

Underlying Bhaskar's philosophy was an ambitious desire to construct a more satisfactory philosophical grounding for Marx's philosophy in general and for his theory of social formations, dynamics and change in particular. Basic critical realism (hereafter BCR) takes the issue of what "exists" seriously. Bhaskar coined the term "epistemic fallacy" to refer to the reduction of ontology to epistemology, or the reduction of what 'exists' to what we can or do "know" of what exists. This fallacy, he contended, has bedevilled much of western philosophy through the

G. Scambler (✉)
University College London, London, UK

S. Scambler
King's College London, London, UK

W. C. Cockerham (ed.), *Medical Sociology on the Move*,
https://doi.org/10.1007/978-3-031-92456-9_10

centuries. He also rejected the Hume's notion of causality as mere regularity and instead sought causality elsewhere. As Fleetwood (2002, p. 67), puts it, "attention turns away from the flux of events (constant or otherwise) and towards the *causal mechanisms, social structures, powers and relations* that govern them." BCR argues for a stratified ontology: the *empirical* refers to experience, the *actual* to actions and events, and the *real* to causal mechanisms, social structures, powers and relations (hereafter mechanisms). In what Bhaskar called an "open system" these strata are typically out of phase with each other. This is another way of saying that it is not possible to "map" the effects of mechanisms at the level of events and experience. This is because mechanisms act "'transfactually": once set in motion they continue to exert and influence even if other 'countervailing mechanisms' prevent this manifesting itself. For example, the mechanisms that in combination generate the tendency for the rate of profit to decline act transfactually. They are always in operation, as tendencies, even when empirically the rate of profit is rising. The reason their transfactuality is not always apparent is that the concurrent operation of other mechanisms—such as technological advance—act in a countervailing manner.

Also central to BCR and of particular relevance to the health domain is the notion of emergence. This asserts that new properties or phenomena arise at higher levels of complexity—for example, the social level—that cannot be explained by reducing them to the lower or "root" levels—for example, psychological or biological levels—from which they nevertheless *emerge*. In tennis for instance, Wimbledon is a social institution which cannot be explained by reference to the psychological attributes of its organisers or participants, let alone by reference to their biological makeups; but it is generated by, or emergent from, these "lower" or root strata. In this way Bhaskar avoided the charge of: (1) reductionism, or the view that the objects of the higher sciences are ultimately reducible to those of the lower sciences, and (2) dualism, or the view that reality is composed of different and autonomous substances that interact in an external and inessential way. Creaven (2007, p. 8) writes:

> On the one hand, reductionism is rejected because the generative mechanisms comprising a particular stratum, though generated by those of its root stratum, are nonetheless 'sui generis', a new form of complexity, with its own distinct properties and powers ... On the other hand, dualism is rejected because stratification and emergence also mean that the relations between the objects of knowledge are not inessential or contingent, but are 'necessary', with the higher order strata only 'relatively' autonomous of their root stratum.

It is a formulation that encourages interdisciplinarity. One of us (GS) has shown how mechanisms at each of biological, psychological and social strata are involved in the quality of life experienced by people with epilepsy (Scambler et al., 2010). Unlike the internal and necessary relation between objects of knowledge and their causal powers, the relation between mechanisms and their effects is external and contingent. This is because underlying phenomena in the domain of the actual are a multiplicity of biological, psychological and social mechanisms that are currently active. Thus, epilepsy-related quality of life is a complex effect of influences emanating from an array of multi-level mechanisms, where some mechanisms can either reinforce or frustrate others. Danemark and colleagues (2002, p. 56) explain:

> Taken together this – that objects have powers whether exercised or not, mechanisms exist whether triggered or not and the effects of the mechanisms are contingent – means that we can say that a certain object 'tends' to act or behave in a certain way.

Epilepsy-related quality of life cannot be understood solely in terms of social mechanisms, although sociology can make its own discrete and irreducible contribution. Biological mechanisms typically matter, and psychological mechanisms typically mediate people's handling of biologically-induced 'impairments' in socially-induced contexts. To complicate things further reference needs to be made to unannounced contingency and the play of human reflexivity and agency. There is thus a sense in which BCR exhorts, even requires, interdisciplinary investigations, whilst also factoring in the inevitable ebbs and flows in people's lives.

Moving on, the BCR ontology is transformational as well as stratified. His transformational model of social action is Bhaskar's way of going beyond conventional sociological approaches to the interaction of agents and structures. Agents do not create or produce structures out of nothing, but instead recreate, reproduce and/or transform pre-existing structures. The total assembly of structures *is* society. In Bhaskar's (1987, p. 129) words:

> … people do not create society. For it always pre-exists them and is a necessary condition for their activity. Rather society must be regarded as an ensemble of structures, practices and conventions which individuals reproduce and transform, but which would not exist unless they did so. Society does not exist independently of human activity (the error of reification). But it is not the product of it (the error of voluntarism).

BCR's stratified and transformational ontology involves a shift in focus away from the strata of the empirical and actual, and event patterns, to the stratum of the real and the mechanisms that govern events. It is the business of the social sciences, the argument runs, to "lay out the structural conditions for various conscious human actions"—for example, what economic processes must take place for Christmas shopping to be possible. Given the openness of society and the transfactuality of mechanisms, event outcomes cannot be either deduced or predicted. But mechanisms can be "inferred" from quantitative studies courtesy of "retroduction" and from qualitative studies via "abduction". These inferences tell us what mechanisms *must* exist for the results of reliable and consistent studies to be as they are. We can illustrate this from extant research on health inequalities. It is the pursuit of explanatory power via detecting and exposing mechanisms in this manner that constitutes the rationale for social science.

A preliminary comment on health inequalities research in the UK is pertinent at this point. The sociological theory of health inequalities we have ventured (because the research is largely socio-epidemiological and quantitative) has its roots particularly in retroduction. It can be expressed as a form of Kantian or transcendental argument:

> Our contention is that, given the frequently replicated statistical associations between (in critical realist parlance 'demi-regularities') linking socio-economic or occupational class status and health and longevity, there *must* exist 'real' or 'deep' structures or mechanisms of class and command (Scambler & Scambler, 2015, p. 345).

We shall have more to say of social class, which we posit as the prepotent mechanism for the distribution of health and health care in the UK below, but for clarification "command" here refers to the mechanism of the state or state relations. For now, it suffices to say that what we call the "class/command dynamic" is pivotal for a credible sociology of health inequalities in the nation state that is the UK. In other regional, community or neighbourhood contexts, the class/command dynamic can be, and is, neutralised by countervailing forces like gender, race or the politics of collective agency.

Dialectical Critical Realism

Bhaskar forged his later or dialectical philosophy in dialogue with the works of Hegel and Marx. He sought a meta-theory of the social sciences with the potential to underpin and support a truly emancipatory project. He accused Hegel of eradicating the dualisms of thought and reality and subject and object by absorbing them into a finite and self-contained form of idealism. Dialectic for Hegel was a logical process involving the unification of opposites. This is incompatible with the precepts of BCR outlined here, with its emphasis on ontological realism and open systems. There is no reason, according to Bhaskar, why all must be "conceivable" being, let alone why all being must be conceived of already. The fact that the cosmos is an "open totality" guarantees the possibility of newly emergent strata, and as far as sociology is concerned new social structures brought about by human agency. Hegel's "triumphant cognitivism", Bhaskar argued, reduces the world to a non-hierarchical flat space with fixed boundaries and dimensions, arresting the ongoing process of determinate negation in physical and social system alike.

Hegel privileged unity over difference. Bhaskar placed the emphasis instead on what he called "negative dialectics": in general terms, the absenting of absence, and more specifically, the absenting of what he called "constraining ills". Bhaskar's lively conceptual imagination must not be allowed to obscure his argument here. The negativity of absence is not simply a property of—the incompleteness of—conceptual thought, *but of the ontological status of reality itself.* He opposed what he called "ontological monovalence", or a purely positive, complementing a purely actual, notion of reality. He underlined the necessity of absence or non-being, that is, on negative dialectics, given the open-ended nature of reality. This is captured in the telling statement that "absence or non-being is an ocean – presence or being but a ripple on its surface". Articulated differently, what might have been, and might yet be, cannot and must not be lost in an obsessive focus on what presently is. Elaborating on his notion of negative dialects, Bhaskar went on to distinguish between three types of negation. The first of these, "real negation", denotes an absence from consciousness (that is, the unknown) and is the most basic and the motor of dialectic. Second, "transformative negation" refers to the transformation of some thing, property or state of affairs involving the cessation or absenting of a pre-existing thing, property of state of affairs. And third, "radical negation" represents a special case of transformative negation: it refers to the auto-subversion, transformation or overcoming of a being or condition (that is, negation as self-transformation).

Elaborating on his transformative model of social action outlined earlier, Bhaskar wrote::

> Society is both the ever-present condition (material cause) and the continually reproduced outcome of human agency … Society … provides necessary conditions for intentional human action, and intentional human action is a necessary condition for it. Society is only present in human action, but human action always expresses and utilises some or other social form (Bhaskar, 1998, pp. 34–35).

Social structures are adjudged to be "enabling", not just constraining or coercive. They are not reducible to their effects, but they only present through them.

> For Bhaskar, the transformational model of social action outperforms, sees off, the individualism of Weber, the collectivism of Durkheim and the phenomenology of Berger. The transformation model of social action goes hand in hand with a *relational* – rather than individualist, collectivist or interactionist – conception of society. So sociologists are charged with investigating social order as a "positive-practice system" (Scambler, 2018, p. 117).

It is relevant at this juncture to introduce Bhaskar's distinction between "Power 1" and "Power 2" relations. Moreover, it is a distinction with an important role to play in our discussion of health inequalities later. Power 1 relations refer straightforwardly to "the transformatory capacity intrinsic to the concept of agency as such". Power 2 relations recognise a more sociological notion of power. Recalling C Wright Mills' analyses, Power 2 relations are those that enable agents to defend their sectoral advantages by prevailing against either the covert wishes and/or the real interests of others. Creaven (2007, p. 32) elaborates:

> The significance of power 2 relations, argues Bhaskar, is not that they grant agents the capacity to exercise control over the social and natural environments, the capacity to intervene causally in the world, which is an unqualified good, but that they organise or structure an uneven distribution of the capacity of human agents to exercise transformative power over their conditions of existence, and so restrict the autonomy and free-flourishing of people subject to their governance.

Salient here too is Bhaskar's thesis that "concrete singularity", or the free-flourishing of *each*, is the relational condition of concrete universality, or the free-flourishing of *all*. He saw this as "an imminent and tendential possibility … necessitated by structural conditions … (though) held in check by global discursively moralised power 2 relations". Bhaskar was announcing here a contingent but progressive tendential movement of humanity towards what he termed "eudaimonia", or universal emancipation (see Scambler, 2018, p. 119).

Underlining this strand of Bhaskar's argument, it might be helpful to visit his definition of dialectic as the process of "absenting absence". Dialectic entails the absenting of constraints on desires, wants, needs and interests. In a summative sentence, the dialectic of freedom is powered by the interface of absence and desire, since absence is paradigmatically a condition for desire—desire presupposes lack.

> Humanity, Bhaskar maintains, is bestowed with the 'inner urge' to struggle against lack 'that flows universally from the logic of elemental … need, want'; and this is manifested 'wherever power 2 relations hold sway'. This is because power 2 relations negate the needs, ranging from those of basic survival to those defined by culture, of most humans, leading to a desire for freedom from "absenting ills" (Scambler, 2018, p. 119).

This unfolding dialectic of absenting absence on freedom, as agents struggle against successive forms of power 2 relations, combined with expanding cultural definitions of needs and wants constructed in part through this struggle, seeds and fuels a logic of more inclusive and comprehensive definitions of, and aspirations towards, freedom.

For Bhaskar, in short, to act is to absent is to presuppose universal human emancipation. To act to negate the constraining ills that threaten our own concrete singularity is to commit to recognising and acting to negate the constraining ills that threaten others who share common situations and a common human-social-being-in-nature or concrete universality. Absence is key. To press the point home:

> Absence teaches us different and difference, opens up alternate 'possible worlds': *what is need not be*. An acknowledgement of (the ocean of) absence or non-being exposes our (ripple of a) positive world as a system open for transformation (Scambler & Scambler, 2015, p. 349).

Margaret Archer's Sociology

Margaret Archer adopted a critical realist approach to sociological theory and research, albeit with a strong independent streak. One theme through her broadly critical realist or relational sociology involved the attribution of causal power to each of structure and agency (as well as to culture). She noted that causal efficacy within sociological theory had tended (1) to be granted to *either* structure *or* to agency, and (2) to be granted more often to structure than to agency (Archer, 1995). She also critiqued the idea of "conflation". She argued that the denial of autonomy to agency ("downwards conflation") had far exceeded the denial of autonomy to structure ("upwards conflation"). Archer also rejected the "central conflation" of Giddens, namely, the notion that structure and agency are "co-constitutative", that structure is reproduced through agency but is simultaneously constrained and enabled by structure. Like Bhaskar, she noted that at any given time, antecedently existing structures constrain and enable agents, whose actions produce intended and unintended consequences, which reproduce (*morphostasis*) or transform (*morphogenesis*) these structures. And she adds a timeline: structural conditioning underlying/*leading to* social interaction underlying/*leading to* structural elaboration.

> In the same vein, the initially antecedent structures were themselves the product of structural elaborations resulting from the actions of prior agents. Archer argues that this scheme—of morphogenetic sequences – permits, via the isolation of those structural and/or cultural factors that afford a context of action for agents, the investigation of how those factors mould the subsequent interactions of agents and how those interactions in turn

> reproduce or transform the initial context. Social processes are of course comprised of many such sequences. However, their temporal ordering allows for an examination of the internal causal dynamics of each sequence (Scambler, 2018, p. 92).

This thesis of Archer's allows for an analysis of health inequalities in the discrete morphogenetic cycle or sequence of post-1970s financialised or rentier capitalism.

Another aspect of Archer's theory has an obvious relevance for a credible sociology of health inequalities. No society, she contends, possesses self-awareness, but every human being does. Her distinction between structure and agency (extending also to that between objectivity and subjectivity) opens the door for her to acknowledge that people can and do reflexively examine their personal interests and concerns in light of their circumstances. They can, and do, evaluate their personal contexts in light of their projects. Personal reflexivity, Archer argued, mediates the effects of objective social forms on us. It therefore helps us grasp how structure influences agency.

> Reflexivity performs this mediatory role by virtue of the fact that we deliberate about ourselves in relation to the social situations that we confront, certainly fallibly, certainly incompletely and necessarily under our own descriptions, because that is the only way we can know anything. To consider human reflexivity play that role of mediation also means entertaining that fact that we are dealing with two ontologies: the objective pertaining to socially emergent properties and the subjective pertaining to agential emergent properties. What is entailed by the above is that subjectivity is not only (a) real, but (b) irreducible, and (c) that it possesses causal efficacy'. (Archer, 2007, p. 42).

It is via the "internal conversation" that humans make their way in the world. This inner dialogue makes us active as opposed to passive agents. And being active involves defining, refining and prioritising matters of interests and converting them into projects. When successful these projects lead to practices. But Archer stresses that these projects can be thoroughly negative as well as positive. "What people are doing in the course of their internal conversations is shaping themselves and contributing to the reshaping of the social world" (Scambler, 2018, p. 93).

Archer goes on to discern three dominant modalities' with regard to reflexivity. The dominance of any one of this trio derives from people's relationship to their natal context in conjunction with their personal concerns. They are:

(a) Communicative reflexives: people whose internal conversations require completion and confirmation by others before resulting in a course of action.
(b) Autonomous reflexives: people who sustain self-contained internal conversations, leading directly to action.
(c) Meta-reflexives: people who are critically reflexive about their own internal conversations and critical too about their effective action in society.

Analysed as generative mechanisms, these dominant modes of reflexivity have what Archer calls "internal consequences" for their practitioners as well as "external consequences" for society. Drawing on the results of a small study of social mobility involving her students, Archer suggests that autonomous reflexivity is associated with upward social mobility, communicative reflexivity with immobility, and meta-reflexivity with social volatility. She makes reference also to a fourth mode of reflexivity that gives rise to "fractured reflexives", comprising those whose internal conversations intensify their distress and disorientation rather than leading to purposeful action. When we come later to proffer a critical realist account of health inequalities, we make use of all four of Archer's modes of reflexivity.

One further aspect of Archer's work is especially relevant to this chapter. She wrote of the "morphogenetic society". What she meant by this is that there has been a shift of late: "partial morphostasis has yielded to untrammelled morphogenesis" (Scambler, 2018, p. 95). In other words, the speed of change has increased. She considered this in the context of what she termed morphogenetic sequences or cycles. This can be grasped as follows. Agents are formed against the background of structural parameters, including language-games, norms, communities, power relations and so on; but on an altogether different timescale, the structures themselves change as a result of the choices and activities of historically situated agents. The consequence is a series of cycles with varying timelines, leading Archer to venture the following "formula": *structural conditioning leads to social interaction leads to structural elaboration.*

Social morphogenesis is admittedly an umbrella term. The task of the sociologist, Archer maintained, is to identify, describe and explain which generative mechanisms are at work. She specified three orders of emergent properties in relation to such mechanisms:

> The three coincide with what are conventionally known as the micro-, meso- and macro-levels: dealing respectively with the situated action of persons or small groups, because there is no such thing as contextless action; with 'social institutions', the conventional label for organisations with a particular remit, such as government, health, education etc at the meso-level; and with the relation between structure and culture at the most macroscopic level' (Archer, 2014, p. 95).

Archer's analysis started at the macro-level, but she attached the rider that each—macro- meso- and micro-level—stratum is "activity-dependent" on that or those "beneath it" and that both "downwards" and "upwards" causation are continuous and intertwined.

Society for Archer comprises the relations between structure and culture.

> Society is the consequence of *relations between relations*, all of which are ever activity-dependent. Structures are primarily materially based, culture primarily ideational. In a nutshell, Archer contends that in what she terms 'late modernity', the interplay between economic competition and technological diffusion has fuelled intensified morphogenesis across the whole array of social institutions. At the same time, it has rapidly augmented the cultural system. Thus, the two - structural and cultural - constituents of the generative mechanism have: (a) themselves undergone morphogenesis, and (b) their synergy has extended this to the rest of the social order via knock-on effects' (Scambler, 2018, p. 96; see Archer, 2014).

Structure and culture issue in different and contrasting "situational logics of action". The for-profit sector would extend the *logic of competition* throughout the social order, including schools, universities, hospitals and so on. But the scientific and technological diffusionists are committed to a *logic of opportunity* and are in consequence hostile to bureaucratic regulation and restricted access: outcomes are not evaluated in terms of the criterion of profitability. The tension between structure and culture, and the associated discordance between the logics of competition and opportunity, has given rise to a "relationally contested order". This generative mechanism of "competition-diffusion" lends itself readily to a heightened morphogenesis.

Sociology and Health Inequalities: Orthodox Approaches

In what follows we argue that critical realism in its various forms has much to offer a rejuvenated sociology of health inequalities. Notwithstanding the growing number of studies of linkages between race and gender and health status and longevity, it is the strong relationship involving proxy measures of social class that has featured in the literature. In England and Wales an enduring program of research initially using the Registrar General's Classification of Occupations, and subsequently the National Statistics Socio-economic Classification (NS-SEC), has shown consistent linkages between these measures and life expectancy and the experience of long-term conditions. Male life expectancy at birth in 2012 to 2016 was highest among higher managerial and professional occupations (NS-SEC Class 1) at 83.6 years, 5.5 years longer than routine occupations (NS-SEC Class 7) at 78.1 years, and 9.1 years longer than males not classified to a socio-economic class (NS-SEC Unclassified) at 74.5 years. Female life-expectancy at birth over this same period was highest in NS-SEC Class 1 at 85.5 years, 4.0 years longer than NS-SEC Class 7 at 81.5 years, and 5.7 years longer than NS-SEC Unclassified at 74.5 years (ONS, 2022). Consistently with these findings, the data also show that 'lower' occupational or socio-economic groups are more likely to rate their health as 'not good' and to have long-term health conditions, and that these conditions tend to be more severe than those experienced in 'higher' occupational or socio-economic groups (Scambler, 2024, Forthcoming).

A consensus has emerged both that findings like these are statistically sound and that occupational class or socio-economic group is a key causal factor in health inequalities (Bartley, 2016). An early and influential consideration of rival explanations for these findings was offered in the Black Report (see Bartley, 2016). Its authors evaluated four possible explanations. The "artefact" explanation claimed that neither occupational class/socio-economic group nor health are easily measured and that the apparent link between the two might merely be a function of measurement decisions. The "social selection" explanation claimed that health exerts a causal effect on occupational class/socioeconomic group rather than the other way round, so poor health leads to downward social mobility. The "material/structural" explanation claimed that material deprivation and hardship and a paucity of resources leads to poor health, via low income, substandard housing and so on. Finally, the "cultural/behavioural" explanation claimed that poor or impaired health is a function of risk behaviours like smoking, bad eating habits, sedentary lifestyles and so on, which are in turn embedded in particular cultures or subcultures. Black and his colleagues did not dismiss any of this quartet, but they did rank them in line with the available evidence: first came the material/structural, followed by the cultural/behavioural, the social selection and, lastly, the artefactual.

Subsequent research has questioned hard-and fast-categories of explanation. It has been found, for example, that material/structural and cultural/behavioural factors are closely related. People who struggle with shortages of material resources are those most inclined to engage in risk behaviours for health, partly because they have less access to health-bestowing goods, options, neighbourhoods and services, and partly also because such behaviours can provide temporary respite from impoverished lifestyles and the daily grind. Over time the artefact explanation has largely been abandoned and narratives have coalesced around three headings: material factors, behavioural and cultural factors, and psychosocial factors.

The continuing salience of material factors is indisputable. These range widely over levels of wealth and income, job security, the levels of toxicity and safety of work environments, the quality of housing and so on. The era of political austerity and precarity from 2010 onwards has amplified the impacts of these factors. In fact, it has been calculated that austerity spending cuts have cost the average person in the UK nearly half a year in life expectancy between 2010 and 2019 (Berman & Hovland, 2024). Predictably, the burden of this loss in life expectancy has fallen most on those already struggling with material disadvantage. Bartley has emphasised the importance of studying the linkage between material factors and health over the whole life-course. Behavioural and cultural factors have also been extensively studied since the Black Report. Studies have covered the patterned consumption of food, drink (especially alcohol), cigarettes and vaping, but also the extent of the use of preventive medical services and immunisation, contraception and antenatal care. In her review of this literature, Bartley estimates that such behaviours account for approximately a third of the observed occupational class/socio-economic group differences in morbidity and mortality. However, to reiterate, people's individual behaviours are anchored not just in culture but in their material circumstances. As for the relevance of psychosocial factors, one significant strand of research has focused on factors like autonomy in the workplace and social support. In an important and influential contribution, Wilkinson (1996) argued that income inequality leads to social fragmentation and dislocation, and hence to a disintegration of social networks and a diminution of connection, reciprocity and trust. Expressed in alternative language, social capital is lost, which is itself known to be injurious to health and wellbeing.

Each of this trio of factors commands empirical support. There are, however two points to be made here. The first is a qualification of sorts. We have argued for thinking in terms of *flows* of health-bestowing assets (Scambler, 2018, 2024; Scambler & Scambler, 2015) and have identified seven asset flows consonant with the research literature that class is known to influence. Thus:

1. *Biological or body assets* can be affected by class. Low-income families, for example, are more likely to have low-birthweight babies, and low-birthweight babies carry an increased risk of chronic disease in childhood.

2. *Psychological assets* yield a general capacity to cope resulting in enhanced resilience. The "vulnerability factors" that Brown and Harris (1978) found reduced working-class women's capacity to cope with life events of relevance to the onset of clinical depression can be seen as class-induced interruptions to the flow of psychological assets.
3. *Social assets* or social capital refer to aspects of social integration, networks and support and figure strongly in the works of Wilkinson and others.
4. *Cultural assets* or cultural capital are frequently generated through processes of socialisation and can engender a strong sense of self-worth and belonging. They encompass formal educational opportunities and attainment and this can have important ramifications for jobs, incomes and therefore health.
5. *Spatial assets* have been shown to significant for health through numerous area-based studies. Areas with high mortality tend to be those with high rates of net out-migration; and it is often the better qualified and more affluent who exercise the prerogative to leave.
6. *Symbolic assets* stand for social status or honour and are known to impact on people's health via their sense of their social position relative to that of significant others in their reference groups.
7. *Material assets* capture the notion of relative deprivation due to impoverishment and meagre standard of living. The salience of material assets for health and longevity has long been established.

There are advantages of thinking in terms of asset flows. They are a 'good fit' with the accumulated body of socio-epidemiological research literature and the causal relevance of each flow for health status and longevity has been firmly stablished. Moreover, and crucially, each flow allows for *short as well as longer-term fluctuations* as well as *compensation between flows*. For example, while an unexpected redundancy can drastically reduce the flow of material assets, cutting income and possibly leading to the threat of no-fault eviction from rental housing, a degree of compensation might occur if there remain strong flows of psychological or social assets. Or weak flows of psychological or social flows might be mitigated by a strong flow of material assets. In fact, the literature suggests that many individuals will experience an accumulation of *either* strong flows *or* weak flows. And a clustering of weak flows in infancy or early childhood can predict impaired adult health.

A further and more telling point suggests severe sociological limitations to conventional approaches, reliance on class proxies and commitment to positivistic or multivariate research on health inequalities, and provides a take-point for our ruminations on the proper subject matter of sociology, critical realism and health inequalities. Consider Wilkinson's 'relative income hypothesis' mentioned above. Income inequality surged during Margaret Thatcher's premiership in the 1980s and has continued to rise since, notably so during the post-2010 imposition of political austerity. The UK has recently been described as the second most unequal society in Europe, following Lithuania (Brewer, 2019). But Coburn (2000) objects to Wilkinson in his relative income hypothesis taking income inequality *as the starting point in his analysis of health inequalities*. What about the causes of income inequality? Coburn notes the absence of any reference to social order and social stratification. There has been an overriding tendency in social epidemiology, which many sociologists have followed, to focus on 'the possible social-psychological mechanisms through which social factors might be tied to health rather than on examination of the basic causes of inequality and health' (Coburn, 2000, p. 137). In a later publication, Coburn (2009, p. 44) expands on this point:

> people with high SES (socio-economic status) do indeed live longer than those with less. SES, however, is a mere ranking of people according to income, educational attainment or occupational position. It reflects standard of living generally, and because these standards are related to many different types of disease, it is a good correlate of health status. But SES is itself a result of class forces. The nature of the capitalist class structure, and the outcome of class struggles, determine the extent and type of socio-economic inequalities in a given society, and the socio-economic inequalities in turn shape the patterns of health – and of health care.

Too many researchers, Coburn maintains, do not 'go far enough up the causal chain to confront the class forces and class struggles that are ultimately determinant.' Advocates of using the NS-SEC in research might reasonably baulk at the idea that it can be subsumed under the concept of SES, but his statement here provides a text for the analysis that follows in this chapter.

Sociology and Health Inequalities: Using a Critical Realist Lens

There is a broad consensus in mainstream sociology that during or around the 1970s, the postwar welfare state capitalism in the UK (and in other segments of the Global North) gave way to what has variously been called "financial" or "rentier capitalism". We will use the term rentier capitalism here. Drawing on the work of Christophers (2020), rent can be defined as payment for an economic actor, the rentier:

> who is in receipt of that rent *purely by virtue of the control exercised over something valuable*. The 'something' here is referred to as an asset. Some assets are physically constructed, in virtual if not in actual space, such as housing, telecommunications, infrastructure and digital platforms; while others are purely legal, for example, intellectual property rights and outsourcing contracts; and others simply exist spontaneously, such as land and natural resources' (Scambler, 2024, pp. 61–62).

Rent, in short, is income derived from the ownership, possession or control of scarce assets under conditions of limited or no competition. In our view post-1970s rentier capitalism, represented in this way, can properly be analysed after Archer in line with her concept of "untrammelled morphogenesis" announcing the advent of a novel morphogenetic sequence or cycle. Her formula—structural conditioning underlying/leading to social interaction underlying/leading to structural elaboration—resonates here. It is a formula that provides a frame for our applications of

BCR and DCR to the sociological understanding and explanation of health inequalities.

BCR contends that social structures can only be exposed via our experience of the patterning of events. They remain unseen or *beneath-the-surface,* but their existence and impact can be detected, affirmed and dissected *on-the-surface*, most obviously through what Lawson (1997) calls the "demi-regularities" delivered by epidemiological and quantitative sociological research. In precisely this way the consistent results of empirical studies linking proxies for class like Coburn's SES and NS-SEC and health status and longevity bear unequivocal testimony to the existence and potent causal power of structural class relations. It is a reminder of Coburn's challenge to confront and address class as ultimately determinant for health inequalities. But how to get behind proxies of class like NS-SEC to expose the social structural dimensions of contemporary class relations? In the delineation of five classes that follows we have drawn on the US-based sociology of Erik Ohlin Wright (2015, 2019) that has strong echoes in the UK of the twenty-first century:

1. *An extremely rich capitalist class and corporate managerial class,* living at extraordinarily high consumption standards, with relatively weak constraints on their exercise of economic power. The American class structure is the most polarised class structure at the top among developed capitalist countries, though with the UK in hot pursuit.
2. *An historically large and relatively stable middle class,* anchored in an expansive and flexible system of higher education and technical training connected to jobs requiring credentials of various sorts, but whose security and future prosperity is now uncertain.
3. *A working class* that was once characterised by a relatively large, unionised segment with a standard of living and security similar to that of the middle class, but which now lacks these protections.
4. *A poor and precarious segment of the working class,* characterised by low wages and relatively insecure employment, subjected to unconstrained job competition in the labour market with minimal protections by the state.
5. *A marginalised, impoverished sector of the population,* without the education and skills needed for jobs above the poverty level and living in conditions that make it extremely difficult to acquire those skills. The USA remains the most polarised at the bottom among developed capitalist countries.

We have argued that the structural genesis of health inequalities in the UK's *advanced* version of rentier capitalism can be found within Wright's class (1) (Scambler & Scambler, 2015). Specifically, an exclusive hard-core of what we call rent-oriented "capital monopolists", constituting well under 1% of the adult UK population, bear the prime causal responsibility for the UK's marked and widening health inequalities, notably exposed and amplified by COVID-19. This group comprises a largely globalised network of major shareholders and investors, financiers and CEOs, backed by what has been called a "concierge class" of managers and professionals (Byrne & Ruane, 2017). Drawing on the concept of absence from DCR, the capital monopolists are systematically "absented" from the proxies for class routinely deployed in quantitative research on health inequalities. It is *above all else* the strategic decisions taken by this group behind closed doors or digitally that have led to those policy shifts that have condemned members of Wright's classes (3) and, in particular (4) and (5), to poorer health. One of us (GS) has referred in this connection to a "class/command dynamic". This dynamic epitomises the relations between class and state in the UK. In a nutshell, class-based *capital* buys state-based *power*, involving not just governing politicians but senior civil servants, lobbyists, think tanks and sections of the mainstream media, to influence *policy* in its own interests. And, critically, *in post-1970s rentier capitalism capital gets a much better return on its investment than was the case in post-WW2 welfare state capitalism.*

The legal, tax, social and health policies of most relevance to the greater accumulation of capital on the part of the few are precisely those that compromise the flow of health-bestowing assets to the many. These include prioritising the monopolising of rentable or asset holdings; retaining tax havens; protecting tax avoidance and evasion strategies available only to the rich; keeping top rates of income tax low and privileging regressive over progressive taxation; weakening employment laws, trade unions and potentials for solidary strike action; failing to build affordable housing or to regulate private rental housing; expanding numbers and proportion of low-paid and insecure jobs, culminating in zero hours contracts; cutting public expenditure, including benefits; privatising public services, substituting for-profit for public service agendas; and criminalising political protests and demonstrations. Revealingly, the post-2023 election of a Labour government under PM Kier Starmer, following the internal "coup" against former member-elected socialist leader Jeremy Corbyn, is offering no substantive challenge to the status quo.

Our BCR/DCR-informed thesis on a credible sociology of health inequalities can be articulated by a family of theses. The first of these reiterates our view that the class/command dynamic is the prime social structure/generative mechanism for explaining health inequalities, and that its causal power has become all the more pronounced in rentier capitalism. Rentier capitalism itself can be regarded as the start of a new morphogenetic sequence or cycle characterised by a resurgence of the logic of competition. The class/command dynamic is not of course the sole mechanism accounting for health inequalities, but it is pivotal. Moreover, it *must* exist in Bhaskar's stratum of the real for the replicated empiricist findings on health inequalities to take the forms they have. In particular communities, neighbourhoods and groupings, however, there may be other countervailing mechanisms that neutralise the impact of the class/command dynamic, or even displace it; but at the national level it clearly holds causal sway. It should be added that there exists a complex "two-way" macro—meso-micro-social causal chain linking the class/command dynamic with the flows of health-bestowing assets and their sequelae.

A second thesis draws attention to the salience of a cultural shift towards a "relativization" of beliefs, values and attitudes that cannot simply be signed off as a product of the class/command dynamic, *but which is nevertheless functional for it.*

References to a postmodern culture have faded in the literature of late but the more recent focus on concepts like post-truth, fake news, cancel culture, gaslighting and so on are revealing of the ascendancy of what Lyotard (1984) called "petty" over "grand" narratives. The fixation on identity and identity-formation are natural correlations of this shift, and the emergence of identity politics as a successor to the politics of distribution is functional for those with a vested interest in a neoliberal status quo favouring for-profit dealings and the logic of competition (which in fact might reasonably be characterised as a grand narrative at the end of grand narratives). What cultural relativisation does is mitigate against the formulation and dissemination of alternate futures.

A third thesis mines Archer's writings on internal conversations to declare that the capitalist monopolists, who constitute the class constituents of the governing oligarchy or plutocracy in the UK, are socially structured—but not structurally determined—"focused autonomous reflexives" (Scambler, 2012). As such they display the following attributes:

(a) *Total commitment*—they exhibit an overriding engagement with accumulating capital and personal wealth and income and/or power. Nothing less will satisfy them. Any deficit in commitment will result in failure.
(b) *Nietzschean instinct*—deriving from a Hobbesian notion of the natural human state, or of human nature, they betray a ruthless determination to cut corners to win advantage over their rivals.
(c) *Fundamentalist ideology*—their commitment is fundamentalist in that it does not admit of compromise. It is an ideology—that is, a standpoint emerging from a coherent set of vested (class/command) interests—that cannot tolerate alternatives.
(d) *Cognitive insurance*—while cognitive dissonance is probably universal, the governing oligarchy is able, courtesy of the class/command dynamic, to take out enough insurance to draw its sting. Accusations of greed, excess and irresponsibility are rarely internalised. Such epistemological and ontological security is rare in rentier capitalism.
(e) *Tunnel vision* a concomitant of a total, Nietzschean and fundamentalist commitment is the sidelining of other matters and a reflex and frequently gendered delegation of these to assorted others.
(f) *Lifeworld detachment*—There is simply no time for the ordinary business of mundane day-to-day decision-making. In this way, the largely white, male governing oligarchy rely on and reproduce structures not only of gender but of class, race and age. Lifeworld detachment presupposes others' non-detachment.

This ideal type of focused autonomous reflexives makes an important contribution to any comprehensive sociology of health inequalities.

A fourth and related thesis again involves Archer's work on reflexivity. 'Vulnerable fractured reflexives', once more representing a non-determinant structuring of agency, may be especially susceptible to impaired health and wellbeing and at risk of premature death (Scambler, 2013; also see Rybczynska-Bunt et al., 2024). This ideal type is composed of the following attributes:

(a) *Lifeworld dependency*—they are sucked in and almost dry by the "getting by" routines of the household or private sphere.
(b) *Ships without anchor*—they lack bearings, drifting, at the beck and call and mercy of Lyotard's petty narratives. There is no core to who they are or why and what is all might amount to: it has been nibbled away by the cut and thrust of conditional circumstance.
(c) *Easily led*—they are in need of constant guidance, awaiting the arrival of the cavalry of an autonomous or meta-reflexive; but they wait without genuine hope or aspiration.
(d) *Open to ephemera*—with no set compass and disorientated, they attach themselves to fads, fashions and the discourses of the moment, but without lasting conviction; rather, they are appendages or hangers on to the convictions and commitment of others.
(e) *Lacking personal projects*—they are characterised by passivity: they are Sartrean "object-for-others", underplaying agential causal efficacy for want of personal aspiration or ambition.
(f) *Alienated*—expanding on Marx's classic exegesis, they are alienated in line with some or all of Seeman's (1959) dimensions of powerlessness, meaninglessness, normlessness, isolation and self-estrangement.
(g) *Of low self-worth and -esteem*—following on from their natal backgrounds and early life-events, impoverished sense of self, plus the self-fulfilling prophecy, they hold themselves of little account. They have feelings of imperfection and/or inadequacy.

Vulnerable fractured reflexives have been described as disconnected in an increasingly connected world. They are, in a sense, an ongoing accomplishment of the strategic behaviours on the focused autonomous reflexives. It is reasonable also to hypothesise that vulnerable fractured reflexivity is the culmination of a clustering of weak health-bestowing asset flows.

Our fifth thesis is that orthodox recommendations to alleviate health inequalities by incrementally reforming social and health policy, that is, by piecemeal social engineering, is no more likely to be effective in the future than it has been to date. An impressively researched series of official reports on "tackling health inequalities" in the UK has failed to deliver the required change (Scambler, 2018, 2024). As we have written:

> health inequalities in a nation-state like Britain can only be explained with reference to the real generative mechanism of relations of class and, as Bhaskar helps affirm, class *struggle*. In financial capitalism it is the hardened core or cabal within Britain's increasingly finance-oriented transnational capitalist executive (since named "capital monopolists") that commandeers the state's power elite to deliver its agenda., and a by-product of this agenda is a staggering boost to wealth, income and, in its wake, health inequality. It is Britain's governing oligarchy that most notably occasions, reproduces, underwrites and in today's financial capitalism intensifies its health inequalities' (phrase in brackets added) (Scambler & Scambler, 2015, p. 351).

In a nutshell, policy reforms currently under consideration invariably understate the causal power of social structures, most conspicuously those invested in the class/command dynamic. Their advocates often stress that they are being "realistic". We refer to this as realism 1, and we counter by drawing attention to and promoting what we call realism 2. Realism 1 essentially accepts a need to work with rentier capitalism's neoliberal status quo, while realism 2 draws on Bhaskar concept of "the real", rejects the status quo, and emphasises the need for what Archer calls structural elaboration.

Our sixth thesis commences with an acceptance of realism 2 and confronts what this might involve. Consider once more Bhaskar's distinction between power 1 and power 2 relations, the former capturing the human potential for exercising transformative agential power, and the latter lending itself to the defence of sectoral advantage. The class/command dynamic epitomises sectoral advantage, and neoliberal ideology—"the grand narrative at the end of grand narratives"—its rationalisation. This thesis briefly suggests how the constraining ills associated with extant power 2 relations might be absented. It is a thesis advanced with all due caution: sociologists can rarely predict future structural elaboration, let alone how it might pan out. It is explicated in more detail elsewhere (Scambler, 2024, pp. 165–180), but for present purposes its principal "ingredients" might be outlined as follows:

1. *Class action*—it will require the causal force of collective class agency to provide the momentum for structural change. Moreover, working-class leadership is critical and appeals for transformative change cannot involve a "narrative of loss" for those already most disadvantages (e.g., via blanket demands for economic 'de-growth'). For all that this kind of class engagement seems unlikely in early twenty-first century Britain, it remains a vital component of transformative agential power.
2. *Class anger, even hatred*—the causes of widespread anger are widespread and traveling "up" from Wright's class 5 to impact on classes 4 and 3. It is a form of anger/hatred that is not personal, psychological or pathological, "but a radical structural hate for what the world has become" (Mieville, 2022, p. 177). It amounts to a loathing for an uncaring and unyielding system of rule from which few are beneficiaries.
3. *A crisis of state legitimation*—the socio-political context in which things might well come to a head involve crisis of state legitimation. Capitalism is prone to intermittent crises and in late welfare state and rentier capitalism the state has come to play an increasingly risky role in assuming responsibility for economic management (witness the financial crash in 2008/9 and the COVID-19 pandemic). A "rationality crisis" can occur if people feel unrepresented, alienated and let down, and this can be accompanied by a "motivation crisis" when they disavow the capitalist "imperative to work" (Habermas, 1975).
4. *Spontaneous mass mobilisation*—class-based collective action is perhaps most likely to arise in the guise of what Abrams (2023) calls a "spontaneous mass mobilization" emergent from widespread and burgeoning anger and a legitimation crisis.
5. *Trigger events*—As Abrams founds, spontaneous mass mobilisations are typically triggered by unpredicted and unpredictable singular events, like the

introduction of an unfair or punitive piece of legislation (e.g., Thatcher's poll tax), or a race riot consequent on the police shooting of an innocent black suspect.

6. *Utopian realism*—an accessible manifesto for transformative change not constructed by professional middle-class campaigners or "outsiders", but with its roots and genesis in "insider" working-class oppositional activism. As Archer rightly insists, "ideational innovation" can exercise its own causal power (Archer, 2024, p. 96). The ideas of absence and absenting constraining ills are pertinent once more:

These six theses represent *one possible and plausible pathway* to the kind of transformative structural and cultural elaboration that we contend are a precondition for effectively reducing those material and psychosocial inequalities that impoverish and shorten so many people's lives.

Conclusion

It is only possible in the context of a single chapter to give a flavor of Bhaskar's evolving critical realism and its potential for underpinning (Bhaskar) and informing (Archer) the sociological project. We have sought briefly to introduce Bhaskar's under-laboring philosophy (from BCR to DCR), and to suggest what it has to offer the sociology of health and illness. The notion of absence (non-being) has been stressed: the present (being) need not be as it is, and the future might diverge from predictions based on current trends and unfold very differently. By way of illustrating our argument we have focused on the current widening of health inequalities in the UK and the failure of detailed socio-epidemiological and quantitative sociological research and the policy reforms deriving from them to deliver effective change. In response, we have reconceptualised and retheorised the case for transformative structural, cultural and agential change. We then closed our contribution with a sextet of theses suggesting one credible route to accomplish such change. We attach the important rider that, as ever, these are no guarantees that a mass of people spilling onto the streets out of rage, hopelessness and a desperation for a different way of organising our affairs will produce the kind of change that is required. But if people are not mobilised against constraining ills, then the neoliberal status quo will remain.

As far as sociology is concerned, we repeat our argument that Burawoy's (2005) four types of sociology—professional, policy, critical and public—be supplemented by two further types (Scambler & Scambler, 2015). The first of these is "foresight sociology", which is focused on the study and consideration of "alternate futures", or better ways of organising our social institutions and affairs. And the second is "action sociology", which extends Burawoy's advocacy of public sociology by calling for a committed strategic engagement in the public sphere to contest the ubiquitous ideology of neoliberalism and to expose those whose vested interests it serves.

References

Abrams, B. (2023). *The rise of the masses: Spontaneous mobilisation and contentious politics*. Chicago University Press.

Archer, M. (1995). *Realist social theory: The morphogenetic approach*. Cambridge University Press.

Archer, M. (2007). *Making our way in the world*. Cambridge University Press.

Archer, M. (2014). The generative mechanisms re-configuring late modernity. In M. Archer (Ed.), *Late modernity: Trajectories towards morphogenetic society*. Springer.

Archer, M. (2024). *Morphogenesis answers its critics*. Cambridge University Press.

Bartley, M. (2016). *Health inequality: An introduction to concepts, theories and methods*. Polity Press.

Berman, Y., & Hovland, T. (2024). *The impact of austerity on mortality and life expectancy*. LSE Working Paper.

Bhaskar, R. (1987). *The possibility of naturalism: A philosophical critique of the human sciences* (2nd ed.). Harvester Wheatsheaf.

Bhaskar, R. (1998). Critical realism and dialectical. In M. Archer, M. Bhaskar, R. Collier, S. Lawson, & A. Norrie (Eds.), *Critical realism: Essential readings*. Routledge.

Brewer, M. (2019). *Inequality: What do we know and what should we do?* Sage.

Brown, G., & Harris, T. (1978). *Social origins of depression*. Tavistock.

Burawoy, T. (2005). For public sociology. *American Sociological Review, 70*, 4–28.

Byrne, D., & Ruane, S. (2017). *Paying for the welfare state in the 21st century*. Policy Press.

Christophers, B. (2020). *Rentier capitalism: Who owns the economy and who pays for it?* Verso.

Coburn, D. (2000). Income inequality, social cohesion and the health status of populations: The role of neo-liberalism. *Social Science and Medicine, 58*, 41–56.

Coburn, D. (2009). Inequality and health. In L. Panitch & C. Leys (Eds.), *Morbid symptoms: Health under capitalism*. Merlin Press.

Creaven, S. (2007). *Emergentist Marxism: Dialectical philosophy and social theory*. Routledge.

Danemark, B., Ekstrom, M., Jacobsen, L., & Karlsson, J. (2002). *Explaining society: Critical realism in the social sciences*. Routledge.

Fleetwood, S. (2002). What kind of theory is Marx's labour theory of value? A critical realist essay. In A. Brown, S. Fleetwood, & J. Roberts (Eds.), *Critical realism and Marxism*. Routledge.

Habermas, J. (1975). *Legitimation crisis*. Heinemann.

Lawson, T. (1997). *Economics and reality*. Routledge.

Lyotard, J.-J. (1984). *The postmodern condition*. Manchester University Press.

Mieville, C. (2022). *A spectre haunting: On the communist manifesto*. Head of Zeus Ltd.

ONS. (2022). *Trends in life expectancy by National Statistics Socioeconomic Classification, England and Wales: 1982 to 1986 and 2012 to 2016*. Office of National Statistics.

Rybczynska-Bunt, S., Byng, R., Spitters, S., Shaw, S., Jameson, N., & Greenhalgh, T. (2024). The reflexive imperative in the digital age: Using Archer's 'fractured reflexivity' to theorise widening inequities in UK general practice. *Sociology of Health and Illness, 46*, 1772–1791.

Scambler, G. (2012). Archer, morphogenesis and the role of agency in the sociology of health inequalities. In G. Scambler (Ed.), *Contemporary theorists for medical sociology*. London; Routledge.

Scambler, G. (2013). Archer and 'vulnerable fractured reflexivity': A neglected social determinant of health. *Social Theory and Health, 11*, 302–315.

Scambler, G. (2018). *Sociology, health and the fractured society: A critical realist account*. Routledge.

Scambler, G. (2024). *Healthy societies*. Policy Press.

Scambler, G. (Forthcoming) Structure, culture, agency and health inequalities. In T. Crew & D. O'Neill (Eds.), *Handbook on class and culture*. Intellect Books.

Scambler, G., & Scambler, S. (2015). Theorising health inequalities: The untapped potential of dialectical critical realism. *Social Theory and Health, 13*, 340–354.

Scambler, G., Afentouli, P., & Selai, C. (2010). Discerning biological, psychological and social mechanisms in the impact of epilepsy on the individual: A framework and explanation. In G. Scambler & S. Scambler (Eds.), *New directions in the sociology of chronic and disabling conditions*. Palgrave Macmillan.

Seeman, M. (1959). On the meaning of alienation. *American Sociological Review, 24*, 783–791.

Wilkinson, R. (1996). *Unhealthy societies: The afflictions of inequality*. Routledge.

Wright, E. (2015). *Understanding Class*. Verso.

Wright, E. (2019). *How to be an anti-capitalist in the twenty-first century*. Verso.

Chapter 11
Reflexive Modernity and the Sociology of Health

Jason Adam Wasserman and Brian P. Hinote

The analysis and explanation of increasingly complex social phenomena represents one of the foremost challenges of sociological theory. This is particularly important in the sociology of health because definitions of health, mechanisms of disease, the nature of clinical medicine, and the structure of health care delivery are all undergoing fundamental transformations in late modernity. Undoubtedly, scholars will be better positioned to understand these developments if they also consider the broader social changes from which they emanate. Many such transformations stem in large part from the epidemiological transition, so medical sociologists should advance theory and analysis to match the complexity of contemporary health and medicine. This includes explanations that span the micro–macro divide and connect phenomena across multiple levels of analysis.

In this chapter, we draw upon the insights of Ulrich Beck (1992, 1994, 1999) to demonstrate the requisite elements of a health sociology "on the move" that can engage the multidimensional and dynamic health-related phenomena of late modernity. Beck's work on risk and incalculability is seldom utilized to understand the social forces surrounding chronic diseases [Turner, 1995 is one notable exception], a gap which becomes more pronounced when one considers the more general sociological importance of chronic diseases since the epidemiological transition. Most theories of risk and health in contemporary society, on the other hand, tend to focus on external health hazards like disasters or pandemics. We employ Beck's conceptualization of reflexive modernization to analyze critical developments in the relationship between sociological theory, medicine, and the contemporary landscape of health and illness. Connecting these various developments helps us make sense of a

J. A. Wasserman (✉)
Oakland University William Beaumont School of Medicine, Rochester, MI, USA
e-mail: wasserman@oakland.edu

B. P. Hinote
Middle Tennessee State University, Murfreesboro, TN, USA

W. C. Cockerham (ed.), *Medical Sociology on the Move*,
https://doi.org/10.1007/978-3-031-92456-9_11

contemporary health landscape that can often feel fractured and chaotic, but which is systematically curated by social forces.

Contemporary medical sociological theory can, and should, assemble the various pieces of highly complex systems by illustrating their logic when they seem fractured and chaotic. In this way, sociological theory becomes practically useful because understanding the state and direction of health and medicine broadly promotes consistent and effective strategies for moving forward. For instance, if medicine proper does not develop an episteme and institutional structure equal to the complexities of contemporary health care, it will become increasingly impotent inasmuch as complex, chronic disorders are the most significant aspect of health (Wasserman & Hinote, 2011). On the other hand, if medical sociology cannot rise to meet the same challenge, then it will fail to prove its usefulness in debates surrounding contemporary medicine, health, and illness, and will be ignored in discussions where sociological insights may be most valuable. We begin by identifying various transformations in health, clinical practice, and health care delivery, and then illustrate how Beck's ideas are particularly helpful for understanding this shifting health landscape. We then examine the challenges facing health sociology in reflexive modernity, along with how sociological frameworks can offer insights amidst the increasingly complex terrain of health and medicine.

Recent Social Transformations in Medicine

The biomedical approach to health, disease, and health care delivery has produced considerable success. But this paradigm may be reaching the upper limits of its efficacy, in part because of its limited impact on chronic illness and other health indicators (Olshansky et al., 2024). Indeed, despite general upward trends, gains in life expectancy have incrementally slowed over the last 50 years (the effects of the COVID-19 pandemic and other "mortality shocks" notwithstanding). Certainly, spending on expensive technical and pharmaceutical interventions raises questions about whether life expectancy returns are sufficient to justify the investment, particularly when we examine the trade-offs they require (e.g., decreased spending on other kinds of health programs).

In society at large, we may observe the shift from simple (or orthodox) modernity to reflexive modernity across countless social institutions. But it is also reflected in the epidemiology of disease, particularly in the shift from acute to chronic disease as dominant causes of mortality in resourced countries. Medical science's dramatic success in treating infection and injury ushered in a new paradigm of illness for which the modalities of infectious disease treatment are poorly equipped. For example, in contrast with the most common diseases of simple modernity, contemporary mortality risks are often difficult to address within the structure of the clinic. This is because the causes of these disorders, and often the interventions that prevent or manage them, are diffused across innumerable micro-decisions enacted and reproduced on a daily basis. The macro-level social factors that both enable and constrain these micro-level phenomena further complicate this picture (see Cockerham, 2013). Ultimately, the diseases most affecting health and mortality in resourced nations today are complex, multi-dimensional phenomena that have largely stymied clinical medicine, which retains a primary focus on the decontextualized individual body (Lock & Nguyen, 2010; Wasserman & Hinote, 2011).

Spawned by this epidemiological disruption, the features of reflexive modernity create challenges for professional medicine that permeate multiple institutional levels from administration to the clinic, to the overarching biomedical paradigm that constitutes the foundation of modernist medical thought. Indeed, these developments manifest a crisis in modern medicine, where novel complexities require medicine to fundamentally reinvent itself, as it did once before when germ theory and dramatic advances in bacteriology shook then-dominant notions of disease, diagnosis, and treatment (Wasserman & Hinote, 2012).

The shifting landscape of health and illness also creates new challenges for sociological theory. This also follows directly from Beck's core thesis of risk, which Mythen (2021, p. 533) characterizes as "equal parts…a critique of capitalist modernization [and] a methodological challenge to social scientists." One important task involves understanding and explaining these new, more complex transformations, not only to drive theory construction and analysis, but also to make insights relevant to clinical practice and policy developments. As social factors are increasingly recognized as important, even fundamental, dimensions of disease, social scientists can make unique contributions to contemporary debates in and around health and medicine (voices often excluded historically from pertinent practice and policy issues).

Reflexive Modernity and Epidemiological Shifts

Simple modernization spawned a new epoch of social, political, and economic developments and dramatically transformed social institutions (Beck, 1994). As a result, enlightenment rationality and technological advances in production have fed each other cyclically for the last several centuries. As science improved its capacity to produce verifiable knowledge and industry improved its capacity to produce material goods, the means-ends criterion of instrumental rationality gained an increasing share of the Western consciousness (Adorno, [1966] 1973; Horkheimer & Adorno, [1944] 2000). The result for medicine was not simply the technological *ability* to cure disease, but a scientific qua industrial *way of thinking* that established the production of cures as the ultimate goal of medical care.

But societies around the world are undergoing significant changes that undermine the logics of Enlightenment-based modernity, and writers from many disciplines have for several years struggled to conceptualize these new configurations. All agree that today and into the future, we will confront profound contradictions and perplexing paradoxes (Beck, 1999, p. 1). This is particularly evident in contemporary health and health care delivery, and the outcomes emerging from these changes seem to have one thing in common: they are unanticipated consequences of the victory of the first, simple, linear phase of modernist medicine. New forms of social, institutional, and interpersonal relations are emerging so that in various disciplines—sociology, politics, philosophy, and now medicine—we need a paradigm shift, a new way of thinking and of approaching new challenges (Beck, 1999, p. 2). The concept of reflexive modernization helps us identify and analyze these late modern problematics.

Reflexive modernization is the idea of 'creative self-destruction,' not from revolution, as Marx and Engels ([1848] 1998, 1976) predicted, but ironically from the very successes of modernism itself (Beck, 1994, p. 2). In this way, previous and ongoing techno-economic "progress" helps dissolve and transform the previous organization of institutions and social relations. These transformations help open new paths in a second modernity (Beck, 1994)—paths in the form of novel approaches to emerging problems.

Beck (1992, 1994) conceptualizes these transformations by distinguishing between "first" and "second" modernity (or "industrial society" and "risk society"). Inasmuch as modernization is defined by perpetual innovation, it is also temporal. Innovations eventually yield a new risk society (a distinct departure from first modernity), particularly because the social, political, individual, and collective risks created by innovation are increasingly unmanageable for the technologies and logics that created them. Accordingly, two developmental stages can be identified. First is a period where unforeseen hazards are systematically produced, where unintended problems arise from decisions made but where these problems are not (yet) the subject of political or public discourse. Yet there is also a second period where the hazards of industrial society can no longer be controlled, where society still makes decisions using industrial ways of thinking, and where dilemmas arising from these and previous decisions constitute a core of public, political, and private debates (Beck, 1999, pp. 72–73). In short, the institutions of industrial society produce threats that are too large and complex to manage with industrial logic.

Reflexive modernization does not refer to simple "reflection" upon the consequences of industrial modernity, but to the act of "self-confrontation." The transition from first to second modernity involves the unintended consequences of industrial society (e.g., a focus on medical-scientific progress and abstraction from its broader consequences), which dominate human thought and action and the logic of institutions. In this way, the concept is at the same time *process* (i.e., of creative self-destruction, of self-limiting development, etc.), *action* (i.e., self-confrontation of new and unmanageable hazards), and *period* (i.e., second modernity is a reflexive modernity).

Beck's theories characterize (and were inspired by) several unmanageable risks in the late twentieth century, but perhaps none as poignantly as nuclear disasters like Chernobyl. In this example, we can see how modernist science and industrial modes of thinking produced societal risks that could not be calculated or managed by the very modalities that produced them. Beck (1986, p. 156) writes about how the inability to perceive the associated risks from nuclear contamination subverts the empirical verifiability that stabilizes modernity.

> The atomic danger makes everyday life "headless." No "social organs" take the place of our senses, however. The nuclear age represents rather the end of perceptiveness and the beginning of a social construction of risk realities. The struggles and strategies over risk definitions are based upon the expropriation of the senses: information equals reality, and thus reality can be created and transformed in the shaping of information and information policy.... The construction of risk occurs in the free space of interpretations beyond countercontrol. Such constructions, however, are less and less secured through scientific authority and are still bound to the rules of credibility. Herein lies the second part of the shock: those who until now have pretended to know don't know it either. None of us—not even the experts—are experts when it comes to the atomic danger.

The inability to perceive threats gives rise to explanations that all become equally unverifiable, wherein all knowledges of risk are comparatively equal, in contrast to the industrial modernism where some were verifiably true or false. Even at the epicenter of the Chernobyl disaster, for example, some individuals died within days or weeks from radiation poisoning, while others who stood next to them are still alive today. The ramifications of unmanageable risk forced a self-confrontation that destabilized modernist institutions like the nation-state in favor of trans-national, trans-cultural, interest-based associations.

In much the same way as nuclear disaster, the epidemiological transition reflects an important shift into reflexive modernity, where the successes of modern medicine and public health unleashed chronic illness risks as primary sources of mortality. The epidemiological transition (see Omran, 1971) specifically refers to shifts in the burden of disease from infectious toward chronic ailments, when mortality and morbidity move from acute, short-term, curable sickness to more prolonged, sometimes manageable, but rarely curable, illnesses like heart disease, hypertension, and diabetes. Like the radiation that leaked across Europe from Chernobyl, many of these health risks are not perceptible to the patient themselves, at least until they become acute. Even patients with advanced heart disease and hypertension, for example, can remain entirely asymptomatic, living much of their lives "sick" while feeling perfectly well. During and after the transition, mortality risks become significantly more ambiguous and less manageable than the diseases around which modern medicine had so much previous success. The result is a health landscape of much greater complexity, perhaps most notably in the rising prominence of more complex disease processes involving health lifestyles and other social determinants of health (along with the changing nature of health risk itself).

Public perceptions of healthcare in the first half of the twentieth century fixated upon the promise of modern medicine, a phenomenon salient in the heroification of physicians such as Ehrlich in the early 1900s and Salk in the 1950s (Duffy, 1993; Witkop, 1999). But today we are likely witnessing the upper limits of traditional biomedicine's contributions to increased longevity. Gains in life expectancy from the successful treatment and prevention of infectious diseases have transformed chronic illnesses into the preeminent health risks, for which there are no "magic bullets" (Beck, 1992; Cockerham, 2005; Dubos, 1959; Turner, 1995). Ironically, modernist medical advances give rise to new illnesses that no longer conform to old clinical paradigms. Chronic disease is a constantly evolving, decades-long process that emerges from the cumulative individual, yet structurally influenced, decisions across a life course. The structure of the clinic as the singular locus of diagnosis and treatment is therefore fundamentally mismatched with the structure of illness in reflexive modernity.

The disconnect between clinical medicine and the challenges of contemporary illness is evidenced by the multiple ways that health and healthcare are now conceptualized, institutionalized, and enacted. Lifestyle is now one of the most significant predictors of health and mortality. Although medicine continues to develop and prescribe drugs aimed at illnesses like heart disease and diabetes, its success has been modest, particularly compared to past heroics where entire diseases were eradicated from entire populations. But when not distinctly providing cures, medicine proper offers only one among many treatment choices. The prominence of chronic illness means that individuals are increasingly responsible for managing their own health, and greater personal responsibility means that health has become an accomplishment, something conceptualized as earned or achieved, usually through consumption, and therefore also a symbol of status (Cockerham, 2005, 2013). Moreover, the achievement of health now invokes any number of theoretical attachments (i.e., ideas about what health is and how to achieve it) and drives consumption from any number of economic sectors (e.g., there is an entire lifestyle industry that operates outside of not only medicine but the prerequisites of modernist science).

Risk and (In)Calculability

A key facet of reflexive modernity, then, is risk incalculability. This is perhaps what signifies more than anything the need for dynamic and multilevel theories of health that incorporate this feature. This concept, perhaps more than any other, speaks generally to the fracturing of monolithic sources of knowledge and identity in contemporary Western cultures. Key to these transformations, Beck (1992, p. 171) contends, was the notion that the calculability of risks in simple modernity was beginning to become dubious. After all, the ability to predict, and therefore manage, risk is fundamental to the authority claims of experts. When scientists can reliably predict, for example, how certain kinds of bacterial exposure will lead to specific types of infections, and how various interventions will eliminate those infections, they wield significant authority.

While knowledge in modernity is still contested, its contests are contained within elite circles of experts who often share common epistemic assumptions, like positivist notions that truth exists and can be uncovered even where it is presently unknown. In other words, modernist frameworks assume that contested knowledge can and eventually will, transform into consensus. Operating from a monolithic center in first modernity, scientists search for knowledge that is universally true. Under this episteme, risks are manageable when outcomes can be predicted and their impacts lessened or anticipated. In this era, progress is the steady and unilinear improvement of scientific and technological capabilities of risk management. In turn, the authority to address social problems rests securely in the hands of experts who know, or eventually will know, what to do.

As noted, however, modernity's successes spawned situations of risk for which the experts had no answers (e.g., nuclear power, as noted above, among others). The expansive reach of potential catastrophes, combined with their incalculability, assaults large-scale social institutions like the terrain and authority of the nation-state (Beck, 1992, 1999). Under such conditions, citizens form bonds through shared risk and by organizing around risks (e.g., forming groups supporting or opposing nuclear power). Without expert answers, risk-knowledge becomes socially and politically contested by parties of ordinary people with various opinions holding relatively equal weight. When no one can claim to possess true knowledge, multiple, opposing perspectives become simultaneously legitimate.

As risks become less calculable, subcultural affiliations increasingly replace macro-level social structures and institutions as central sources of social bonds and identity. That is, individuals decreasingly identify themselves according to national citizenship, religious affiliation (e.g., Catholic, Baptist, Methodist), or political party. Rather, they derive identities from, and carried out within, subcultural enclaves, which may be religious or political, but with far less expansive qualities, concerns, or aspirations. Beck (1999) elucidates such transformations in Europe where one's identity as German or French, for example, declines in importance while organizational affiliations formed increasingly around more narrowly focused issues such as environmental causes. In the U.S., similar trends are emerging. In 2024, for example, those reporting no religious affiliation became the largest denominational group for the first time ever (DeRose, 2024). Similarly, over the last 20 years, an increasing percentage of U.S. voters identify as "independent" rather than Republican or Democrat (Gallup, 2024).

When risks shift from calculable to incalculable, *estimations* replace *calculations* that have become impossible to conduct verifiably (or at least convincingly). Beck (1992, p. 171) writes that we come to understand "calculability in the sense of *estimability*," and that "Decreasing 'calculability' is…accompanied by increasing 'estimability'," in reflexive modernity. Put another way, while consequences are more unpredictable, we must still make decisions about what to do, even when the criteria by which those decisions are justified become increasingly unstable. When risk cannot be calculated but choices still have to be made, people end up drawing on their values and preferences. On social media, there is a popular meme that reads, "Science doesn't care what you believe." But this is only functionally true when scientific methods can consistently yield conclusive answers about risk. In cases where the results are mixed or unverifiable, often because phenomena are complex and multi-causal in ways that validate multiple plausible explanations, "belief" becomes quite significant in decision-making. Moreover, when scientific methods are insufficiently authoritative, the destabilization of expertise can compromise perceptions of its authority generally, not only for those areas where it struggles to calculate risk. Science is, for example, decidedly one-sided on the issue of whether there is a human contribution to climate change, yet sociopolitical divides over the legitimacy of this knowledge proliferate. This occurs within and because of the broader destabilization of expertise, which is not issue-specific.

In situations of incalculability, people base choices on a combination of individual and cultural values supplemented by whatever evidence they individually find most believable from a field of competing possibilities, none of which can be decidedly disproven. While often utilized in ways limited to a macro-theoretical context, Beck's ideas actually traverse multiple levels of scale and speak not only to broad cultural and structural transformations, but also to individual beliefs and behaviors (see Tulloch & Lupton, 2003, who also draw down the implications of Beck's "macro" perspective to examine its implications for "everyday life"). We turn now to examine how these ideas can drive the sociology of health and illness.

Chronic Illness as Incalculable Risk

Today, chronic illnesses represent the greatest threats to mortality in resourced countries, a trend driving substantial transformations in health and medicine. Modern medicine effectively addressed most acute ailments in the form of pharmacotherapy. These were comparatively causally simple, agent-host models where interventions either targeted the microbe causing the infection (i.e., antimicrobial therapies), or made the host unsusceptible to it (i.e., vaccination). However, chronic illness is significantly more complex since many macro- and micro-sociological phenomena are seamlessly intertwined in the causal profiles of such diseases. In this section we explain the ways that chronic diseases defy modernist frameworks that rely on calculability, and how they reflect this increasingly complex and dynamic health landscape. It is to this landscape that medical sociological theory must be responsive and for which Beck's notion of reflexive modernity provides insight.

Contemporary environmental hazards like nuclear accidents clearly embody incalculable risk and hold all the ramifications for social transformation towards multi-vocaled knowledge. However, Beck's ideas are not relegated to geographically dependent threats. While this is recognized in principle—Beck notably mentions it himself—no significant body of research applies his notions of reflexive modernity and risk incalculability to chronic illness. Certainly, health demographers have identified geographically bound enclaves of chronic illness, these health risks are indeed fundamentally different from environmental toxins leeched into air or water and affecting populations within certain geographically boundaries. However, the effects of risk incalculability are more pervasive and have promoted a much more expansive fracturing of monolithic health knowledge, resulting in the legitimation of multiple perspectives on how to be healthy.

Beck (1992, p. 20) himself briefly mentions these kinds of health risks in late modernity:

> …the struggle for one's 'daily bread' has lost its urgency…For many people problems of 'overweight' take the place of hunger. This development, however, withdraws the legitimiz-

ing basis from the modernization process, the struggle against obvious scarcity, for which one was prepared to accept a few (no longer completely) unseen side effects.

In the chronic illness era, disease risk is more incalculable than ever. The estimation of consequences of this or that health behavior becomes increasingly individuated, especially in a sea of conflicting evidence about successful approaches. Lifestyle choices embody this estimation, and reflect choices about how to achieve health (or the interplay of choices and chances as we discuss later) that draw not only on data about the effectiveness of this or that diet, exercise plan, supplement regime, etc., but also on cultural frameworks, values, and identities. Indeed, amidst a sea of ostensibly conflicting data, even rationalist kinds of knowing become filtered through more individuated lenses.

Of course, these choices are not entirely individuated because they are embedded in class and other structural conditions, and because "lifestyle enclaves" (consistent with Beck's notion of subcultural affiliation) are formed around various health knowledges, which then exercise group-level influence over individual decisions (see Bellah et al., [1988] 2007). Indeed, lifestyle dispositions emerge from class structures in ways that affect the estimation process, where, for example, the poor often assume that lifestyles are relatively insignificant, particularly those that they cannot afford anyway, while more affluent and/or educated individuals deem them quite important (see Keely et al., 2009 for discussion of health fatalism as a sense-making process). Beyond class, the sheer volume of information, much of which appears contradictory, can promote a kind of retreat from the management of health risks. As Jensen et al. (2022, p. 393) describe, nearly three-quarters of U.S. adults agree that it "seems like everything causes cancer," and "there are so many recommendations about preventing cancer, it's hard to know which ones to follow." From this "information overload," the result is often a kind of health fatalism.

However, the social structural forces that set people adrift do not necessarily result in a total disregard for health lifestyles. Rather, they shape how they respond in an increasingly uncertain health landscape, where the causes of disease are multifactorial, and many of those factors are unpredictable from a particular individual's standpoint. As noted by Keely et al. (2009, p. 734), "...individuals often make fatalistic statements to express an understanding of locally or broadly limiting factors for health efficacy..." It is this indefinite fluidity that elucidates the key distinction between estimation and calculation of risk generally and for lifestyle practices in particular. This fluidity also produces social transformations in health and medicine that defy the heuristic divisions commonly utilized in many sociological theories.

Sociological thinking has for many years emphasized the importance of social factors and contexts in shaping health, but has historically struggled to work with these notions across multiple levels of scale. For example, class as a macro-level concept corresponds to mortality, while a micro-level analysis of class might examine its effects upon end-of-life experiences and decision-making. But social scientific theories and methods have been slow to produce ways of assembling these sorts of different dimensions into single conceptual or analytic frameworks (see

Cockerham & Hinote, 2009 for a discussion of related methodological issues). Certainly, theorists from Weber ([1922] 1978) to Bourdieu (1984, 1990) to Giddens (1984, 1991) provide various conceptualizations of the roles of agency and structure, while Cockerham (2005) synthesizes earlier formulations into a health lifestyles theory, explaining how specific health behavior patterns are characteristic of certain social groups. Risk incalculability plays a functional role in this multiscale framework, in that it affects the degree to which individuals can estimate risk through lifestyles (via consumption), but also facilitates the ascription of risk to particular social groups (Cockerham, 2006; Macintyre et al., 2002). In other words, class bears particular influence on chronic illness as an incalculable risk, because lifestyles represent individual attempts to estimate those risks, but where such choices are always made within structural contexts.

Working across these classical conceptual divides represents the core challenge for contemporary sociology, but medical sociological theory in particular must also engage these problematics. Epidemiological shifts increasingly render inadequate an understanding of health and illness that is confined to one level of analysis or another. That is, in the same way that practitioners cannot understand contemporary disease solely through biomedical principles, neither can sociologists understand health and illness in ways that partition those phenomena at particular levels of scale rather than across them. Beck's formulation of reflexive modernization shows us one path toward more integrated and dynamic theories of health.

The Death of the Clinic: Manifestations of Reflexive Modernity

Whereas the magic bullet hopes of the early twentieth century were extreme even then, penicillin and other antibiotics nonetheless cured an entire spectrum of infections. In the era of reflexive modernity, however, treatments increasingly emphasize long-term symptom management of incurable ailments. The result is a mismatch between old causal models and new disease profiles. The etiology of chronic illness is too complex for interventions that merely disrupt the pathways between the body and disease itself (as with vaccination, hygiene, antisepsis, and other chemotherapeutic and prophylactic treatments). For chronic diseases the lingering modernist model becomes relegated to treatments that try to disrupt the path between the disease and its symptoms. Despite being more technologically advanced than ever, medicine arguably engages in increasingly more treating and proportionally less curing because the pathogenesis of chronic illness defies the causal nature of disease that made modernist medicine successful.

In turn, contemporary health promotion defies several aspects of modern health care delivery. We have elsewhere elaborated several other manifestations of reflexive modernity, including medical education, healthcare financing, and administration (Wasserman & Hinote, 2012), but the mismatch between clinical practice and chronic illness provides perhaps the best illustration. Where the divestment of the body from social and cultural contexts gave birth to the clinic (Foucault [1963] 1994), the complex profiles of chronic illness make this approach unsustainable, thereby signaling the death of modernist forms of clinical practice. Or at least, if they remain subsidized by various forms of power and investment, those structures will be rendered increasingly ineffective.

The clinic is the traditional, sustainable, and preferable locus of treatment when dealing primarily with pre-transition infectious disorders. However, when the fundamental causes of chronic illnesses are connected to the social contexts in which patients live, the clinic's disengagement from the patient's environment poses substantive challenges that become insurmountable when medical care is quarantined exclusively in the clinic. As Greenhalgh and Papoutsi (2018, p. 1) write:

> Contemporary healthcare is experiencing several important challenges, including a mismatch between the 'patient in the guideline' and the 'patient in the bed' due to multimorbidity and interacting sociocultural influences; an inability for 'marginalised' patients to access GP services despite the super-science miracle cures ubiquitous in the media; new staff roles, organisational forms and technologies that sometimes seem to worsen the very problems they were introduced to solve; and the policy sacred cow of integrated care repeatedly proving impossible to deliver in practice.

Perhaps more importantly, while some chronic disorders are given discrete criteria, these usually are created from designated points on a scale (such as levels of cholesterol or blood sugar), not the presence or absence of some *thing* itself (as with a virus, fungus, or bacterium). All persons *have* cholesterol and blood sugar, so the question about how much is too much presents a situation of far greater ambiguity and uncertainty. Physicians' professional philosophies have little effect on the general consensus that an infection exists and should be eradicated. However, despite attempts to create consensus where various oversight bodies draw the lines between acceptable and unacceptable levels of cholesterol, blood sugar, and the like, there remains a high level of disagreement. As a result, a patient that falls in these gray areas is likely to receive different treatment from different physicians. More simply, there is no such thing as a borderline syphilitic, but borderline diabetics are common. This ambiguity is one hallmark of reflexive modernity because it engenders uncertainty that destabilizes calculation, which is then replaced with estimation.

Moreover, even when chronic disorders are discretely diagnosed, it is difficult to understand their causes or what patients are really doing day-to-day to manage them, because these ailments depend on numerous micro-events in a patient's life. Certainly, tests such as the hemoglobin A_{1C}—which gives a 3-month weighted average of glycated hemoglobin and therefore a more longitudinal picture of blood sugar than the traditional blood glucose snapshot—can in some way document the veracity of patient reports about lifestyle behaviors. However, complexity pervades and confounds even when such tests are available. For the A_{1C} test, hemoglobin glycation varies on the basis of many factors, including race and age (Ford et al., 2019). Moreover, the stable statistical correlation of glycogen to glucose within groups has limited explanatory power for any given individual. Put another way, attempts to force causally complex chronic illnesses into an infectious paradigm in clinical practice often end up falling into reductionist fallacy.

The insurgence of artificial intelligence and machine learning (AI/ML) systems into clinical decision support may portend the recovery of clinical authority (Wasserman & Wald, 2024). After all, AI/ML systems have the capacity to process data that are orders of magnitude more prolific and complex than individual clinicians or even traditional predictive algorithms that have for years supplemented clinical judgment by flagging patients' charts for risk factors. Currently utilized as clinical decision support and thus deferential to the judgment of the attending physician, the increasing accuracy of AI/ML predictive models raises questions about the future of clinical judgment. But this only brings on new questions about complexity and uncertainty, particularly where AI/ML technology is unknown or even unknowable to its users (i.e., both patients and physicians alike). This can be the result of its proprietary nature or merely because its computations employ such massive amounts of data and sophisticated modeling that it cannot be explained or understood. Thus, while the explainable AI (XAI) movement seeks to retain a notion of control and visibility that positions AI/ML as merely a tool, the technology may simply outpace any well-intended safeguards as it grows more sophisticated.

Insofar as they are multifactorial and exhibit far greater variation, treating chronic illnesses like acute disorders requires far greater aggregation, and thus only drifts further away from individual patient care in the clinical setting. Sociology came into existence struggling with this epistemic question. Comte successfully argued that we can understand society and social behaviors scientifically, but only by aggregation, by qualifying statements probabilistically. Similarly, chronic illnesses *can be* understood from a modernist scientific perspective, but only through similar processes of aggregation. Foucault (2003, p. 248) brilliantly captures this problem, writing, "Power has no control over death, but it can control mortality." Yet, while Foucault notes that death itself ultimately is outside the control of social institutions, individual patients seek individual practitioners fundamentally to avoid death. With curable infections, this typically is a sure-footed process. Chronic illness is far more complex and less predictable, and requires incorporating a broader vision where new conceptualizations of health and illness (including social and behavioral components) are central features of diagnosis, treatment, and doctor-patient communication.

As noted above, the consequences of these shifts in the epidemiology of disease and the fracturing of the epistemic authority of science in the twentieth century, may be attributed to the complexities of contemporary illness, but it is not limited to chronic illness. Rather, these shifts promote an individuation of health with wide berth. Witness the COVID-19 pandemic, an infectious disease event that nonetheless provoked variable, highly politicized responses (Jasanoff & Hilgartner, 2021). There was not only disagreement about the appropriate responses to disease risk and state authority with respect to regulating contagion. Rather, the public fractured around questions about the origins, nature, and risks of the disease itself. Moreover, the scientific community was awash in uncertainty about containment, particularly early in the pandemic (e.g., uncertainty about surface contagion, mask effectiveness, etc.). Even where the scientific community could provide clear evidence, particularly about the effectiveness of vaccination, public reaction remained fractured and mixed, something particularly pronounced in the United States (Jasanoff & Hilgartner, 2021). Even in the face of strong evidence, a significant portion of the public estimated COVID risks through their own sociopolitical lenses, for example, by taking hydroxychloroquine and ivermectin (despite no evidence of effectiveness) based on anti-government sentiments promoted (ironically) by politicians with whom they viewed themselves as ideologically aligned. Contrast this with the relative homogeneity of reaction to the rollout of the polio vaccine and one can see just how disruptive uncertainty has been to medicine at the end of the modernist era. That is, the fracturing of health epistemes in reflexive modernity is pervasive, not merely relegated to those areas of genuine uncertainty.

Medical Sociology After the End of Modern Medicine

While Beck's notion of reflexive modernity affords a good characterization of the shifting health landscape and crystallizes its challenges, another important question concerns the role of medical sociology and social theory in the future. The complexity evident in health epidemiology and related challenges for the industry of clinical medicine necessitate novel analytical approaches. In this section, we address the need to reexamine modernist notions of causality, to bridge seemingly disconnected changes in disease and medical institutions across micro-, meso-, and macro-levels of scale, and to engage previously under-explored areas of health and illness.

The medical profession grew significantly more complex, difficult to navigate, and in need of reform in the waning decades of the twentieth century. Today, we still witness calls for change in several sectors of health care delivery, including primary care and specialization, financing and reimbursement, and medical education. These social systems (among others) were, after all, fundamentally organized around practices that primarily addressed acute illness. Yet many discussions about reform seem idiosyncratic, as though the problems in a particular area can be approached in ways that are distinct from others. The lens of reflexive modernity reveals a common basis for the range of challenges in health and medicine and allows us to connect proposed reforms in its different sectors in a more comprehensive way. That is, institutional and professional crises emerge out of deeper changes that appear to signal the end of *modern* medicine and the beginning of a new era defined by unprecedented complexity and uncertainty. For its part, medical sociology must effectively articulate and theorize the changing nature of health, illness, and health care delivery, and in doing so, inform discussion and debate on various issues ranging from health policy to the economics and delivery of care.

Critiques of the biomedical model have existed as long as modern medicine. Today, however, it is the physiology and epidemiology of disease itself that underscore the limitations of traditional biomedicine (Wasserman & Hinote, 2011). As described above, this is more than just a maturing of modern medicine. Rather, the paradigmatic differences between the profiles of chronic and acute diseases suggest a seismic shift in the landscape of health, calling in turn for a corollary shift in how the institutions of medicine are arranged and function.

The nature of causality is one problematic at the core of the mismatch between the types of infection around which modern medicine was built and the new kinds of diseases that challenge it today. For infectious disease, suitable causal models have historically centered on proximate pathogenic factors. Explorations into broader contexts like environment typically were limited to where a person contracted an infectious agent (e.g., the water they drank or their associations with other infected people).

The etiology of chronic illness, however, exhibits a decidedly more complex causal structure. Notably, the cause, progression, and outcome of those diseases significantly depend on "lifestyle," which signifies the complex interplay of individual choices and social structural chances (Cockerham, 2013). In the chronic illness era, health—or disease—most often results from the dynamic interaction of hundreds of thousands of cumulative individual decisions, all of which are inextricably embedded in complex sets of social opportunities. Along with social and behavioral factors, there is an ambiguous contribution from genetics (see Conrad, 2009). Whereas professionals typically diagnose infectious diseases with universal scientific principles applicable to generalized bodies, the pathways of chronic disease are simultaneously related to individual behavior and conditioned by numerous social contexts, making them difficult to assess using the archetypical causal models of modernist medicine.

Bruce Link and Jo Phelan (1995, 2000; Link, 2008) provide ample evidence in support of social factors as critical determinants of health and disease (see also, Cockerham, 2013, for more thorough discussion of social causation). They describe how researchers achieved notable success in identifying risk factors for many major disorders, but that most research focuses upon proximal (rather than distal) causes of disease, many of which disregard social factors, resulting in hyper-individualistic notions of health and illness. Thus, while modern biomedical approaches helped conquer the epidemiological threats of one time and place (simple modernity), they also produced a situation where social contexts assume new significance in shaping health outcomes, a defining feature of reflexive modernity. That is, advances in deciphering the origins and pathways of disease manifest new and more complex ambiguities surrounding novel and increasingly complex pathogeneses.

While critics of the biomedical model have, at least discursively (which is to say, arguably, superficially) won the philosophical debate about the importance of social factors, the widespread nominal acceptance of a biopsychosocial model has not been met with widespread practices that attend to the multi-causal nature of disease that it promotes. The remaining challenges are well-described by Rocca and Anjum (2020, p. 83):

> Although the bio-psychosocial model is a step in the right direction…healthcare needs to move beyond it. The model starts with the quest for a more holistic view of health and illness that does not reduce human conditions to merely the sum of their constituent parts. Still it ends up with the fragmentation of the biological, psychological and social dimensions. Is it possible to reach a genuine integration among these three dimensions of humanity, and if so, how?

And continuing:

> This practice of isolating one causal factor from its normal complexity is a dominant epistemological norm in science when studying causality. What does this tell us? First of all, it tells us something about how we think of causality, as something that is best established by looking at the behaviour of a single factor in isolation from contextual interferences. Secondly, it reveals something about how we understand complexity. (Rocca & Anjum, 2020, 85).

Conceptualizing health and sickness in a manner that accounts for these complexities helps emphasize the ways that the contemporary epidemiology is increasingly incompatible with the reductionist approaches that embrace the proximal cause-and-effect causal models of modern medicine.

In turn, theories in health sociology have significant roles to play, including articulating new formulations of disease causality that bring into focus new causal factors, particularly social and cultural ones, that have been previously underspecified. In addition, theorizing health in reflexive modernity should consider novel conceptualizations of causality. Modernist medicine and modernist health sociology typically employ linear models of disease causation, but in a period where estimation replaces calculation, the assumption that linear patterns of causality accurately characterize social phenomena should be reexamined. Estimation is influenced more heavily by social, cultural, and psychological factors that may violate some or all of the assumptions underpinning popular forms of sociological analysis in first modernity.

Early modernist success in treating bacterial and fungal infections gave rise, epidemiologically, to viral infections and cancers with more complex pathogeneses. Moreover, success in treating viruses and bacteria produced even more complex multi-drug resistant strains (e.g., MRSA—methicillin-resistant *Staphylococcus aureus*—among others). Cancers involve complex interrelated contributions from lifestyle, genetics, and infection, but also are adaptive and dynamic (Derbal 2018) in ways that complicate (modernist) therapeutic interventions. Every point on the spectrum of acute disease has undergone its own shift toward increasing etiological complexity.

The physiological structures of simpler bacterial and fungal infections fit well with the modernist causal model because they are discrete targets of treatment; as organisms, they stand out against the human host. Alternatively, modern medicine has had less success with the more complex etiologies of viruses and cancer because these interact with bodies in ways that make them more difficult to partition and kill. While complexity on the infectious frontier necessitates fundamental shifts in the nature of medical science and practice, chronic illnesses are even more demanding in this regard. These processes open space for discussing the sociological forces that give rise to the literal existence of diseases, both chronic and infectious. That is, where these diseases result from the success of previous practices and accomplishments of health and medicine, they also reflect a variety of social values and resulting social practices. Where prevalence and even diseases themselves are the reflexive products of choices made about policy, funding, research, and development, sociology can address very literally the social creation of disease—not just as a process of unmasking theoretically latent chronic ailments, but also as producing newer, more complex infections. The choices underlying medical advances also create new health challenges and reflect social values and perspectives. Put another way, diseases, independent of socially demarcated epidemiological prevalence, are becoming increasingly sociological.

In the era of reflexive modernity, health sociology and medicine must increasingly engage the social factors fundamental to the complex etiology of chronic diseases (as it must also, though perhaps in different ways, for emerging acute ailments with increasingly complex etiologies). While there have long been calls for physicians to be more sociologically aware (McIntire, 1894), the relative causal simplicity of many infectious diseases, which gave rise to modern medicine, produced little impetus to do so. However, since the profile of chronic illnesses in reflexive modernity defies the causal logic of first modernity and fundamentally intersects social factors, it is ever more important to address these contexts within diagnosis and treatment. Most physicians recognize the social features of doctor-patient relationships, even when engagement with these is usually limited to *ad hoc* bedside strategies. Today, however, novel manifestations of chronic disease necessitate greater, deliberate inclusion of sociological influences in the diagnostic and treatment processes themselves (Wasserman & Hinote, 2012). This includes serious reconsideration of the fundamental models employed to understand the social causes of health and illness, the classical partitions of sociological phenomena in first modernity (e.g., macro, meso, and micro), and the boundaries within which sociological analysis has been previously relegated.

Conclusion

The concurrent processes of modernization and epidemiological transition set in motion an important series of transformations in health, disease, and health care delivery. As a second, reflexive modernity continues to unfold, medicine faces a number of perplexing health, lifestyle, and treatment challenges that stem in large part from the shifting structures and risk profiles of diseases now most often affecting human populations. While the significance of reflexive modernization (as process, action, and period) is underrepresented in medical sociology beyond environmental hazards, Beck's contributions to understanding the seismic shifts emanating from the epidemiological transition are important for many reasons.

First, these ideas offer a useful way to conceptualize ongoing social processes taking place at multiple levels of analysis, from fractured, individuated notions of what it means to be and stay healthy, to increasingly complex causal profiles of disease, to the paradoxes of health care delivery. Further, understanding the challenges facing health and medicine in reflexive modernity also engenders awareness of new challenges for health sociology. Accordingly, Beck's ideas raise questions about the nature of causality and its relationship to complex disease processes, health as inextricably integrated at multiple levels of scale, and social forces as insurgent factors in previously underexplored terrains of disease process.

In emphasizing these paths forward, we assert that a fractured understanding of complex, interrelated phenomena will likely lead to solutions that are minimally successful in confronting the challenges of health care delivery in the twenty-first century. Put simply, the logics of simple modernity are increasingly incapable of addressing today's most pressing epidemiological threats, at least not in a way comparable to the heroics of medicine's golden age. Undoubtedly, this age is over. The relatively simple, linear diagnosis and treatment paradigms and the industrial logics of first modernity are no longer sufficient or appropriate for the institutions of health care delivery in reflexive modernity. Rather, a fluid and changing health landscape necessitates a reflexive awareness of the complex interplay of multiple phenomena at multiple analytic levels, so that we may structure the administration and organization of healthcare accordingly. In sum, health sociology is "on the move" in the sense that it is changing alongside the health landscape itself, but also because in reflexive modernity a relevant health sociology must always be dynamic, fluid, and adaptable to match the complex and shifting nature of contemporary health and illness phenomena.

References

Adorno, T. W. ([1966] 1973). *Negative dialectics*. Routledge.

Beck, U. (1986). The anthropological shock: Chernobyl and the contours of the risk society. *Berkeley Journal of Sociology, 32*, 153–165.

Beck, U. (1992). *Risk society*. Sage.

Beck, U. (1994). The reinvention of politics: Towards a theory of reflexive modernization. In U. Beck, A. Giddens, & S. Lash (Eds.), *Reflexive modernization: Politics, tradition, and aesthetics in the modern social order* (pp. 1–55). Stanford University Press.

Beck, U. (1999). *World risk society*. Polity.

Bellah, R. N., Madsen R., Sullivan W. M., Swidler A., & Tipton S. M. ([1988] 2007). *Habits of the heart: Individualism and commitment in American life*. University of California Press.

Bodenheimer, T., Chen, E., & Bennett, H. D. (2009). Confronting the growing burden of chronic disease: Can the U.S. health care workforce do the job? *Health Affairs, 28*, 64–74.

Bourdieu, P. (1984). *Distinction: A social critique of the judgment of taste* (R. Nice, Trans.). Harvard University Press.

Bourdieu, P. (1990). *The logic of practice* (R. Richard, Trans.). Stanford University Press.

Cockerham, W. (2005). Health lifestyle theory and the convergence of agency and structure. *Journal of Health and Social Behavior, 46*, 51–67.

Cockerham, W. (2006). *Society of risk takers: Living life on the edge*. Worth Publishers.

Cockerham, W. (2013). *Social causes of health and disease* (2nd ed.). Polity Press.

Cockerham, W., & Hinote, B. P. (2009). Quantifying habitus: Future directions. In K. Robson & C. Sanders (Eds.), *Quantifying theory: Pierre Bourdieu* (pp. 199–208). Springer.

Conrad, P. (2009). A mirage of genes. In P. Conrad (Ed.), *The sociology of health and illness: Critical perspective* (pp. 438–447). Worth Publishers.

Derbal, Y. (2018). The adaptive complexity of cancer. *BioMed Research International, 2018*, Article 5837235.

DeRose, J. (2024). Religious 'Nones' are now the largest single group in the U.S. National Public Radio, January 24. www.npr.org

Dubos, R. (1959). *Mirage of health*. Harper & Row.

Duffy, J. (1993). *From humors to medical science: A history of American medicine*. University of Illinois Press.

Ford, C. N., Leet, R. W., Kipling, L. M., Rhee, M. K., Jackson, S. L., Wilson, P. W. F., Phillips, L. S., & Staimez, L. R. (2019). Racial differences in performance of HbA_{1c} for the classification of diabetes and prediabetes among US adults of non-Hispanic black and white race. *Diabetic Medicine, 36*, 1234–1242.

Foucault, M. ([1963] 1994). *The birth of the clinic: An archaeology of medical perception*. Vintage Books.

Foucault, M. (2003). *Society must be defended: Lectures at the collège de France, 1975–1976*. Picador Press.

Gallup. (2024). Party affiliation. October 9, from news.gallup.com

Giddens, A. (1984). *The constitution of society: Outline of a theory of structuration*. University of California Press.

Giddens, A. (1991). *Modernity and self-identity: Self and society in the late modern age*. Stanford University Press.

Greenhalgh, T., & Papoutsi, C. (2018). Studying complexity in health services research: Desperately seeking an overdue paradigm shift. *BMC Medicine, 16*, 95.

Horkheimer, M., & Adorno, T. W. ([1944] 2000). *Dialectic of enlightenment*. Continuum.

Jasanoff, S., & Hilgartner, S. (2021). A stress test for politics: Public reasoning, political judgment, and trust in COVID-19. *Social Studies of Science, 51*(5), 898–921.

Jensen, J. D., Shannon, J., Iachan, R., Deng, Y., Kim, S. J., Demark-Wahnefried, W., et al., for the Rural Workgroup of the Population Health Assessment in Cancer Center Catchment Areas Consortium. (2022). Examining rural–urban differences in fatalism and information overload: Data from 12 NCI-designated cancer centers. *Cancer Epidemiology Biomarkers and Prevention, 31*, 393–403.

Keely, B., Wright, L., & Condit, C. M. (2009). Functions of health fatalism: Fatalistic talk as face saving, uncertainty management, stress relief, and sense making. *Sociology of Health & Illness, 31*, 734–747.

Link, B. G. (2008). Epidemiological sociology and the social shaping of population health. *Journal of Health and Social Behavior, 49*, 367–384.

Link, B. G., & Phelan, J. (1995). Social conditions as fundamental causes of disease. *Journal of Health and Social Behavior, 35*(Extra Issue), 80–94.

Link, B. G., & Phelan, J. (2000). Evaluating the fundamental cause explanation for social disparities in health. In C. E. Bird, P. Conrad, & A. M. Fremont (Eds.), *Handbook of medical sociology* (pp. 33–46). Prentice Hall.

Lock, M., & Nguyen, V.-K. (2010). *An anthropology of biomedicine*. Wiley-Blackwell.

Macintyre, S., Ellaway, A. A., & Cummins, S. (2002). Place effects on health: How can we conceptualise, operationalise and measure them. *Social Science and Medicine, 55*, 125–139.

Marx, K., & Engels, F. ([1848] 1998). *The communist manifesto*. Verso.

Marx, K., & Engels, F. (1976). *The German ideology*. Progress Publishers.

McIntire, C. (1894). The importance of the study of medical sociology. *Bulletin of the American Academy of Medicine, 1*, 425–434.

Mythen, G. (2021). The critical theory of world risk society: A retrospective analysis. *Risk Analysis, 41*, 533–543.

Olshansky, S. J., Willcox, B. J., Demetrius, L., & Beltran-Sanchez, H. (2024). Implausibility of radical life extension in humans in the twenty-first century. *Nature Aging*. https://doi.org/10.1038/s43587-024-00702-3

Omran, A. R. (1971). The epidemiologic transition: A theory of the epidemiology of population change. *Milbank Memorial Fund Quarterly, 49*, 509–538.

Rocca, E., & Anjum, R. L. (2020). Complexity, reductionism, and the biomedical model. In R. L. Anjum, S. Copeland, & E. Rocca (Eds.), *Rethinking causality, complexity and evidence for the unique patient* (pp. 109–131). Springer.

Tulloch, J., & Lupton, D. (2003). *Risk and everyday life*. Sage Publications.

Turner, B. S. (1995). *Medical power and social knowledge*. Sage Publications.

Wasserman, J. A., & Hinote, B. P. (2011). Chronic illness as incalculable risk: Scientific uncertainty and social transformations in medicine. *Social Theory and Health, 9*, 41–58.

Wasserman, J. A., & Hinote, B. P. (2012). The end of modern medicine: The evolution of disease and transformations in medical practice. *Journal of Healthcare, Science and the Humanities, 2*, 145–156.

Wasserman, J. A., & Wald, H. S. (2024). Artificial intelligence, machine learning, and bioethics in clinical medicine. In J. Kang, T. Rattay, & B. S. Rosenstein (Eds.), *Machine learning and artificial intelligence in radiation oncology* (pp. 29–39). Academic Press.

Weber, M. ([1922] 1978). *Economy and society*. University of California Press.

Witkop, B. (1999). Paul Ehrlich and his magic bullets—Revisited. *Proceedings of the American Philosophical Society, 143*, 540–557.

Index

W. C. Cockerham (ed.), *Medical Sociology on the Move*,
https://doi.org/10.1007/978-3-031-92456-9

The manufacturer's authorised representative in the EU is Springer Nature Customer Service Centre GmbH, Europaplatz 3, 69115 Heidelberg, Germany. If you have any concerns regarding our products, please contact ProductSafety@springernature.com

Printed and bound by CPI Group (UK) Ltd, Croydon, CR0 4YY
30/09/2026
02225589-0009